"Courageous and heartwarming, *He/She/They* sheds light on the journey of gender discovery and acceptance. As a fellow advocate for transgender rights, I am inspired by Schuyler's unwavering honesty and resilience. His powerful narrative challenges societal norms, encouraging readers to embrace their authentic selves fearlessly. A must-read for anyone seeking understanding, compassion, and hope on the path to self-discovery."

—Jazz Jennings (she/her), activist, television personality, and author

"[Bailar] uses storytelling and the art of conversation to give us the essential language and context of gender, meeting everyone where they are and paving the way for understanding, acceptance, and, most importantly, connection."

—*The Next Big Idea Club*, October 2023 Must-Reads

"Tragically, it's transgender people who find themselves most targeted and scapegoated by both evangelicals and right-wingers—especially when elections roll around. Trans activist and athlete Schuyler Bailar cuts through the smears in *He/She/They*, explaining why gender-affirming medical care is lifesaving and how trans youth playing sports benefits all kids. Bailar's book isn't just for the ignorant; it also serves as a bible of trans joy."

—*The Advocate*

HE/ SHE/ THEY

How We Talk About Gender and Why It Matters

SCHUYLER BAILAR

Go
hachette
BOOKS
NEW YORK

Copyright © 2023, 2024 by Schuyler Bailar

Cover design by Terri Sirma
Cover photograph by Justin J Wee

Cover copyright © 2023 by Hachette Book Group, Inc.

Hachette Go, an imprint of Hachette Books

Hachette Book Group
1290 Avenue of the Americas
New York, NY 10104
HachetteGo.com
Facebook.com/HachetteGo
Instagram.com/HachetteGo

First Trade Paperback Edition: November 2024

Hachette Books is a division of Hachette Book Group, Inc.

The Hachette Go and Hachette Books name and logos are trademarks of Hachette Book Group, Inc.

The Hachette Speakers Bureau provides a wide range of authors for speaking events. To find out more, visit hachettespeakersbureau.com or email HachetteSpeakers@hbgusa.com.

Hachette Go books may be purchased in bulk for business, educational, or promotional use. For information, please contact your local bookseller or email Hachette Book Group Special Markets Department at: Special.Markets@hbgusa.com.

The publisher is not responsible for websites (or their content) that are not owned by the publisher.

Print book interior design by Linda Mark

Library of Congress Cataloging-in-Publication Data
Name: Bailar, Schuyler, author.
Title: He/she/they: how we talk about gender and why it matters / Schuyler Bailar.
Description: First edition. | New York, NY: Hachette Go, 2023. |
    Includes bibliographical references and index.
Identifiers: LCCN 2023018859 | ISBN 9780306831874 (hardcover) |
    ISBN 9780306831867 (trade paperback) | ISBN 9780306831881 (ebook)
Subjects: LCSH: Transgender people—Social conditions. | Transgender
    People—Civil rights. | Gender identity. | Transphobia.
Classification: LCC HQ77.9 .B34 2023 | DDC 306.76/8—dc23/eng/20230516
LC record available at https://lccn.loc.gov/2023018859

ISBNs: 9780306831867 (paperback); 9780306831874 (hardcover);
    9780306831881 (ebook)

Printed in the United States of America

LSC-C

Printing 1, 2024

CONTENTS

AUTHOR'S NOTE

IN THE CREATION OF THIS BOOK, I CONSULTED WITH COMMUnity leaders and experts; I conducted extensive interviews with community members; I integrated learnings from my near-decade's worth of interacting with thousands of trans people, from years of providing life coaching to hundreds of trans clients and their families, and from years of facilitating trans and queer support groups. I leveraged my years in academic research and ongoing work in four labs to inform the exhaustive research necessary to support my statements in this text. Finally, I engaged a handful of early readers as a sensitivity review.

Still, consensus, particularly with terminology, is elusive; many of these topics are shifting faster than I can edit. I encourage you to read this book as an invitation and guide while recognizing the dynamic nature of this work.

I am always learning, and I hope you will be, too.

꧁ ꧂ ꧁

AT FIRST MENTION, I've included pronouns for every person named. When possible, these were ascertained directly through asking individuals for their pronouns. Otherwise, pronouns were taken from bios, social media, or through research on the individual. Any mistakes are mine.

I Am Just Who I Am

WE WALK OUT ONE AT A TIME, IN ALPHABETICAL ORDER. MY last name begins with *B*, so I am first. I can feel my heart beating in my ears, the sound held inside my head by my silicone cap. A little echo chamber.

"From Washington, DC, freshman Schuyler Bailar," the announcer booms.

I know everyone is watching me. I know I've done this on a thousand occasions before. But this time is different.

Underneath my crimson warm-ups, there is no longer a one-piece swimsuit that women usually wear. Instead, I am wearing a tiny little Speedo. I am now on the men's team.

Hundreds of articles have been published about my switching from the women's to the men's team. "Transgender swimmer," they all write. Some attack me for my history, saying I'll never be a real man. Others say my history of an eating disorder just means I am a "deluded woman with body issues." Many claim there is no way I could keep up with, much less beat, other men. "From beautiful competitive woman to mediocre ugly man," one commenter wrote on a national profile about me.

As I stand by the edge of the pool waiting for the rest of my team-mates to join me, I am fifteen again, standing in my women's swimsuit behind the blocks with three girls from my relay. I remember the confidence, the feeling of knowing I could do exactly what I had set out to do. I remember the rush of the natatorium going silent as I put my hand over my heart—my pre-meet ritual—my fingers and thumb straddling my swimsuit strap on my shoulder. I had done this at the start of every single meet during the singing of the national anthem. I remember staring out at the pool as the music ended, and I took a deep breath, imagining my final stroke of my race.

I take a deep breath now, staring out at the pool as a D1 college swimmer. Everything feels so different. I've never stood alongside thirty-eight college guys before. I'm at a pool I've never raced in. And it feels like all eyes are on me. But, as always, the water resembles beautiful blue glass and I breathe a sigh of relief.

This is different, but it is also the same. The same twenty-five-yard pool. The same hundred-yard breaststroke race. The same breaststroke I have done since before I can remember. The same echoing acoustics that make hearing so difficult. The same chlorinated air that makes everyone cough. The same "Take your mark—*boop!*" before we launch off the blocks. It's all the same.

When the team is gathered along the edge of the pool, the natatorium silences. We stand in identical clothing, and the anticipation dances in my fingertips. When I am this nervous, the most nervous, I imagine my blood is rushing through my veins like white-water rapids.

When "The Star-Spangled Banner" begins to play, I instinctively begin my pre-meet ritual. But this time, my fingers seeking my shoulder strap find nothing.

In that moment, I realize that while everything is the same, it is also brand new. For the first time in my life, I am competing as just myself—without the baggage of who everybody told me to be, who everybody said I was, who I thought I was supposed to be.

Today, I am just who I am. I am Schuyler.

My eyes well with tears. More than nineteen years of stumbling to get here. Just a few months ago, I was ready to quit swimming. A year ago, I was ready to quit the world and life altogether. But today, I am standing tall, a proud Korean American queer transgender swimmer on Harvard Men's Swim and Dive—the first openly transgender athlete to compete for any D1 men's team in the NCAA.

Of course, surviving my first meet (and not getting last) did not mean that everything was easy from then on. It would take my teammates the rest of the year to consistently gender me correctly. It would take me nearly three years to feel comfortable around them. And all the years since I came out are still not enough to dispel all the hatred and bigotry about transgender people, especially in athletics.

Over the next four years, I not only became the first—and, at the time, only—transgender athlete to have competed for the team that aligns with their gender identity for all four collegiate seasons, but I also became a well-respected educator on transgender inclusion.

I never knew where this journey would take me when I began. The first speech I gave was at my own high school. The night before, I was awake until two or three in the morning, attempting to write the speech itself. Dozens of drafts in the trash, I had no idea what other people would want from me. *What should I tell them? What could they learn from me?* That speech was better received than I'd expected. Some students even said it was the best assembly they'd experienced. So, as word spread, one speech led to another. By sophomore year, speaking was the primary way I spent my free time. By graduation, 102 speeches were in the books.

Despite regular assurances that what I had to say was valuable to others, I often found myself perplexed over why people wanted to listen. I was just a college kid who wanted to swim. When news outlets would call me an "advocate" or "activist," I used to tell them no.

"You only think that I am an activist," I insisted, "because I am a transgender swimmer, and I'm talking about it."

Before every single speech, I wondered to myself, *Why are they here? Why do they care?* Only rarely, the answer was clear: I was talking to a group of swimmers or transgender folks like me; we were comrades. But most of the time, I spoke to people with whom I had little to nothing in common, or so it appeared. I tried to imagine the perspectives of the audience members—the students, coaches, administrators, teachers, mental health professionals, medical providers, or employees at a bank... *How could I connect with them?* Because, in the end, the inability to connect is what breeds hatred and bigotry. That is, connection is the essence of our humanity itself.

At a small school in northern Vermont, I gave a speech to a room filled with student-athletes. It was a standard event. I shared my story and provided training on trans literacy before opening for questions. After the event, a group of students gathered in a line, waiting to talk to me.

A young man approached and explained he was on the wrestling team. He said, "You know, before I came here today and met you..." He paused. I nodded and waited patiently.

"Before I met you," he began again, "I was nervous about people... like you. My girlfriend's best friend is bisexual and that used to make me uncomfortable. I'm not homophobic or anything, but I didn't want to hang out with her." He stared at the floor then glanced back at me as he admitted this. I didn't say anything, yet. I wasn't sure where this was going.

"But now I've met you. And you're just like me! We are both just... athletes. We're just guys." He looked directly at me now. "So now, I understand." I'd begun to smile, relieved.

At another speech at a high school in Pittsburgh, the audience was mostly students from local public schools' GSA (Gender and Sexuality Alliance) clubs, with the exception of a few athletes. At the end, two football players accompanied the GSA officers to the stage to give me a small gift. One asked if he could say something to the audience. Not knowing what he would say, I nervously agreed.

"Listen, before I came in, I was uncomfortable," he said into the mic. "You know, 'I can't do this, I can't speak, I just wanna sit over there and stay quiet.' But when I came in, it was a very inviting environment. I was like, 'Aw, I can do this! There ain't no difference!' You know, we're all the same." He then turned to me and continued, "And I want to say thank you, to you, for opening up my eyes to a brighter future." The audience's applause almost drowned out his voice as he finished, "This is reality. This is life."

I just about cried. Really, I had to try very hard not to bawl onstage. And while this is still one of the most touching moments I've experienced at a speech, such unexpected empathy has not been unique in my career. Moments like this happen over and over again—people thinking that they would find themselves uncomfortable around me, a transgender person, but then meeting me and learning I am also just someone living my life, like them. These moments serve as resounding reminders of the power of empathy and shared humanity, that there is so much more love than we might imagine—for us queer and trans folks, or for anyone, really.

Sometimes this love comes in the form of hope. After a speech in North Carolina, I spent nearly an hour with people who'd stayed after, forming a line that snaked from the stage all the way to the entrance of the large auditorium. The last person in line was a shorter, curly-haired individual with a baggy sweater and jeans. He wore a pin with "he/him" scrawled across it, presumably in his own handwriting. He burst into tears as soon as he met my eyes.

"I," he tried, before his voice caught again, and he stared at the ground.

"Take your time," I said as gently as I could. He took a deep breath.

"I drove six hours to get here," he finally managed, wiping his eyes.

"Wow," I said, genuinely surprised. "Thank you so much for coming. I'm honored that you came this far. I hope you have somewhere to stay tonight—it's late!" I smiled, trying to offer softness. He laughed and then gestured behind him. A person, who stood watching us about twenty paces away, waived as we made eye contact.

"My friend is here with me. I'm staying with her," he assured me. "You were the first trans person I found online—I'm trans, too," he shared, the words almost tumbling out of him. "For so long I didn't want to be here anymore. I didn't see trans adults...you know...living their lives. Seeing you, and reading about your story..." I felt my chest tighten as I listened. I, too, struggled back tears.

"It saved my life," he said after a few heavy breaths. "You saved my life. And I needed you to know."

Love—and sharing love in the form of hope—is incredibly powerful. Lifesaving, even. Every time someone shares experiences like these, I find myself holding back emotions that threaten to break my whole body. Sobs I'm not sure would ever end if I let them escape unrestrained. The experience is certainly optimistic and deeply meaningful—someone has chosen to stay because of me—but grief floods all the spaces in between.

This is the grief that we live in a world where trans children want to and do kill themselves. This is the grief that so many trans children do not see their own futures and their ability to thrive beyond the stereotypes of trans trauma. This is the grief that I am the first, and sometimes only, trans person so many have met and been able to find resonance with. This is the grief that I hope to turn into love through writing this book.

❖ ❖ ❖

IN 2020 AND 2021, record-breaking numbers of anti-transgender legislation were introduced in state governments around the United States. Most of these bills focused on two arenas: first, banning transgender athletes from competing in sports teams aligned with their gender identity; and second, banning children from accessing gender-affirming and lifesaving healthcare. States also introduced bills forcing teachers to out their trans students, bills banning LGBTQ+ educational content in schools, and bills banning students from using bathrooms aligned with their gender identity.

The following two years, 2022 and 2023, have only seen worse. With each editing pass of this book, the legislative bans are increasing exponentially *and* in severity. Including a comprehensive overview of every area of attack was simply impossible. At the final stage of editing, over 491 anti-trans pieces of legislation across forty states had been introduced just in 2023.[1,2] Bans on gender-affirming healthcare expanded to include trans adults in addition to minors; countless bans attempt to criminalize the presence of trans or otherwise gender-diverse people in public; bans threaten the legality of drag performances.

Anti-trans rhetoric and anti-trans violence have reached an all-time high, fueled by the media and politicians demonizing trans people and transness. Every year has been more savage than the last; 2020 and 2021 became the deadliest years on record for anti-transgender violence. Although anti-trans rhetoric has claimed anti-trans legislation to be "protecting children," or "protecting women," the transphobia has grown increasingly brazen and conspicuous, shedding this disguise of alleged protection.

In 2023, the *Daily Wire* commentator Michael Knowles (he/him) said it loud and clear: "Transgenderism [*sic*] must be eradicated from public life entirely. The whole preposterous ideology. At every level."

After I graduated from college, I went on a speaking tour. It was a busy few weeks: I gave forty-three speeches in thirty-nine days in twenty-six cities around the United States. And the majority of these events were in red cities and red states. I wanted to bring transgender awareness to places that would not otherwise have access. While I was very excited to meet new people and continue this work, I was also very nervous. I have spent most of my life living in very liberal cities—DC, New York, Seattle, and Boston. Traveling to remote and rural areas in Kansas or Illinois or Western Pennsylvania was daunting. I wasn't sure if I would be able to connect with people in such unfamiliar settings.

At one such speech, I was with a group of athletes and community members at a university in a small town in Kansas. When it came time for questions, an older lady in a purple shawl asked, "What do, um… what do people like me…" She hesitated, clearly nervous. "I don't know the right words, I—I don't want to mess up."

"That's okay," I'd encouraged her. "Let's work through it together."

"Okay." She took a breath. "What do people like me," she tried again, "do to help, uh…people, people like you?" She finally finished. I smiled.

"This is a wonderful question," I'd said. "What you're asking is how to be the best *ally*. An ally is someone who is not gay or lesbian or transgender—so, *not* LGBTQ+—but who supports us and wants to help!" The lady beamed, and before I could continue to answer her question, she interrupted.

"Thank you so much. Oh, isn't this wonderful, you've given me a new word. *Ally!* I want to be an *ally.*"

That woman in purple—and so many more like her—is exactly why I am a firm believer that most people are good people. Some just need a little help finding the right words, trans or not. Of course, finding those right words is no panacea for the horrible, often violent, discrimination trans people face, but it is most certainly a step in the right direction, the first step toward connection. So whether you're trans like me or not, I hope this book helps you find ways to connect first with yourself and then with others.

After all, connection is the essence of our humanity.

PART 1

GENDER AND ME

CHAPTER 1

Finding the Right Words: Terminology

My name is Schuyler Bailar. There are four people in my family, my brother, my mother, my father and me. My dad comes from Florida. My mom is from Korea. My mom's name is Terry. My dad's name is Gregor. Last of all my annoying little brother's name is Jinwon. I have one pet. It is a parrot. His name is Chico. I am a tomboy. I have short hair. I go to a very multi race school. It's called "Georgetown Day School." It is awesome. I have a lot of friends. Most of which are boys.

THIS IS THE FIRST PARAGRAPH OF AN ESSAY I WROTE IN FIFTH grade, titled "All About Me." During middle school, I felt it imperative that anyone I met knew I was a tomboy. It was always among the first things I shared about myself.

I needed them to know that I was not the girl that everyone expected me to be.

"My mom says we'll grow out of it," Alisha Gregg (she/her) told me. We were all standing in a line by the door, waiting for our teacher to lead us to the next classroom. "When we get to high school, we'll be more like the girls." My stomach dropped. I'm *not growing up to be like the other girls*, I thought to myself. The thought of becoming a woman terrified me. *I will* always *be myself. Like this.*

"Well, *I* won't grow out of it," I spat, upset. Alisha didn't reply because it was time to start walking, and we weren't supposed to talk in the hallway.

That moment played over and over in my head for months. *Maybe the other girls will grow out of it. But I won't.* I was then a part of a group of girls who were self-declared tomboys or labeled as such by others. Although we were often grouped together, I did not care to align myself with them. I knew something about my tomboy-ness was different from theirs. They did, too.

Years later, I'm still friends with one of those girls. After I came out as trans, she reflected on our middle school years.

"We were all tomboys, but we knew you weren't. We knew it was something else for you."

When I finally found the word *transgender*, I wished I'd had it in my early years. *This* was the word I'd been searching for. This was the permission I'd never been given as a little kid to say, "I'm actually a boy!"

Just that single word—*transgender*—has brought me so much freedom and hope. So much life and peace. Language can never define a person completely or with perfect accuracy; it is, after all, just words. But language that helps us describe our identities not only to others but also to ourselves can be lifesaving.

I've also learned that I was not alone in my ignorance regarding this word. At the end of every speech I give, I present six vocabulary words, the first of which is *transgender*. I ask for an audience member to define it and rarely are they able to. If we cannot define this word, how can we expect ourselves to have difficult conversations about complex topics regarding trans identities and our place in society?

That's right—we can't.

As I have found the words that best describe me, I have also learned that language is one of the first and most important ways we can show respect to ourselves, to one another, and to exchange stories across identities we might not share.

And so, we begin this book with language, so that you might have better words to describe yourself, as well as others.

➤ TRANSGENDER

Whenever I ask adults in an audience to define *transgender*, I often get a variation of the following incorrect answers:

> "When you were born a man or woman but you're the opposite."
> "When you change your gender."

I always thank anyone who volunteers to answer and then I provide some language suggestions.

Transgender is an adjective that describes people whose gender identity differs from the gender they were assigned at birth. I was assigned female at birth and my gender is male. Therefore, I am transgender.

You might be wondering what "gender assigned at birth" means. Usually when a baby is born, the gender is assumed (and then assigned on a birth certificate) based on the newborn's external genitalia. In the simplest terms: if the baby has a penis, or something that looks like a penis, the baby will be assigned male; if the baby has a clitoris, or something that appears to be a clitoris, the baby will be assigned female. If the baby has ambiguous genitalia (usually deemed "intersex"), the infant might be subjected to nonconsensual genital surgery to "fix" their genitals based on the doctor's assumption. I'll cover more about intersex folks later. In short, gender is most commonly assigned based on the appearance of external genitals.

The idea that one could be the "opposite gender" implies that there are only two genders. This is incorrect; gender is more complicated than just man and woman or male and female. There are trans people who do not identify as man or woman and therefore don't fit these labels.

The second answer is probably the most common misconception, and I understand why. People often describe me by saying, "Schuyler was a woman and is now a man." This does not feel accurate and most trans people I know would concur: trans people are not "changing" gender but, rather, affirming it.

For this reason, I no longer use FTM. FTM stands for *female to male,* and is a label I applied to myself in the early months of coming out. As I journeyed through my transition, I quickly realized that FTM did not feel accurate. FTM implied that I was female at some point and was then becoming male. In reality, I have never felt I am a woman. I just haven't been able always to describe my gender as what it truly is: male. This language evolved for me. Instead of FTM, I call myself a trans man. If elaboration is needed, I explain I was assigned female at birth, which is different from *being* female at birth.

Similarly, in the beginning of my journey, people told me that I was "born in the wrong body." I knew that my body didn't feel right, so I considered this to be true. But as I learned more about myself and my body, I realized this perception was flawed. I was not "born a girl," nor was my body "wrong." No, I was born myself—a boy—and was *assigned* female at birth. My body is not "wrong"; my body followed the instructions it was given quite well! And still, at one point, my body did not fit me completely. Parts of my body felt foreign and misaligned. But I did not *change* my gender when I came out. I did not wake up one day and *become* a man or *decide* to be who I am. No, I decided to tell people about it. I became more confident and found the courage to share myself with the world. But I have always been myself.

Please note that there are some (a minority of) trans people who would say they *have* "changed genders," and that is absolutely valid! Language is an *attempt* to connect and communicate ourselves, but language can only ever approximate our truths and our realities. I strongly encourage you to use the language suggested here as a baseline, but when a trans person asks you to use different language for them, you should absolutely comply.

Here's a quick rundown of some terminology suggestions:

- *Transgender* can be shortened to *trans*.
- Trans man / trans woman
  » *Trans man* or *transgender man* refers to a man assigned female at birth.
  » *Trans woman* or *transgender woman* refers to a woman assigned male at birth.

» Include a space between *trans* and *man* or *woman*, as omitting this space is often used by trans-exclusionary folks to imply that trans men are not "real" men, but rather some kind of modified version: a transman. This is akin to the derogatory term *chinaman*, which was used to refer to men of Asian descent. *Chinese man* is not derogatory; *chinaman* is.

» Some trans folks refer to themselves as "men of trans experience," or "women of trans experience." Using this implies transness is less of a central identity, or sometimes even an identity at all; it is more of an experience, and, for some, a *past* experience that might no longer feel relevant. As a result, some who use this terminology might not identify as trans, rather considering transness to be an experience of their past.

• Trans masculine / trans feminine

» *Trans masculine* is an umbrella term that can refer to someone assigned female at birth who does not identify as a girl or woman.

E.g., I use both the labels *trans man* and *trans masculine* for myself. Put simply: all trans men are trans masculine, not all trans masculine folks are trans men. Someone assigned female at birth who identifies as non-binary could use the label *trans masculine*, but not *trans man*.

» *Trans feminine* is an umbrella term that can refer to someone assigned male at birth who does not identify as a boy or man.

• *Transness* is a noun that refers to being transgender. I discourage people from using *transgenderism* because the suffix '-ism' denotes a doctrine, act, practice, belief system, or ideology—none of which apply to being transgender.

• *Transsexual* is an outdated term, most commonly used to describe a trans person who has undergone medical transition, namely surgery. For various reasons, including that many consider *transsexual* to be pejorative, I strongly advise against using *transsexual* unless someone uses it to describe themselves.

➤ NON-BINARY

Some individuals' gender does not fit society's current understandings of only "man" or "woman," and they use *non-binary* to describe their gender identity. *Non-binary* is an umbrella term that people use in different ways; I'll talk more about non-binary identity in Chapter 3.

Notes on spelling and abbreviation:

* Many folks use the term *enby* as a short term for *non-binary*. This is the phonetic spelling of the letters *N* and *B*, but typing "NB" to refer to non-binary folks is less common, as "NB" is used as an abbreviation for non-Black folks.
* Some non-binary individuals prefer to spell the word without a hyphen: *nonbinary*. Some individuals prefer to spell it with a hyphen: *non-binary*. Some folks don't seem to mind which way it is spelled, while others have brought a great deal of intention to spelling it one way or another.
* In a survey on my Instagram in 2021, I asked my non-binary followers how they preferred to write their label. The majority preferred *non-binary*, with *nonbinary* a close second, and *non binary* third. For this reason, I will use the most popular spelling with the hyphen for the rest of this text.

➤ CISGENDER

In short, if you are not transgender, you are cisgender. That is, if your gender identity matches the gender you were assigned at birth, you are cisgender.

Some cisgender folks express anger when told they are cisgender:

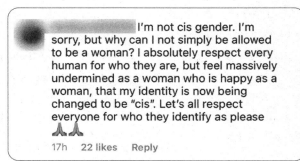

I'm not cis gender. I'm sorry, but why can I not simply be allowed to be a woman? I absolutely respect every human for who they are, but feel massively undermined as a woman who is happy as a woman, that my identity is now being changed to be "cis". Let's all respect everyone for who they identify as please 🙏🙏

17h   22 likes   Reply

While many angry comments do not give me pause, this one did—because I do want everyone to be respected in how they identify, and commenters like this believe that they are not being respected. But therein lies one of the primary centerpieces of the conflict: some cisgender people believe that being called *cisgender* is disrespectful. These are often the same folks who believe being called *white* is somehow racist. Both of these reactions reveal the same thing: when people who society generally considers the default are not treated as the default, those people get angry and feel othered.

When society talks about people who hold marginalized identities, these identities are often named, as if to clearly differentiate them from the "norm" or the default. In the eyes of the news, for example, I am not just a swimmer. I am a transgender swimmer. I am not just a man; I am a Korean American man. I am not just an athlete; I'm a queer athlete. And there is nothing wrong with naming these identities—in fact, I claim them proudly.

But then notice that naming the identities of the privileged is far less common, if ever occurring at all. No one labels Michael Phelps (he/him) as "that cisgender, straight, white athlete." He's just Michael Phelps, Olympic swimmer. No one says, "Look, a straight, cisgender football player!" Why? Because these identities are expected, assumed, and not in need of any explanation. People do not feel they need to delineate sexuality unless it isn't straight. People do not feel they need to delineate gender unless someone is not cisgender. People do not feel the need to delineate race unless the person is not white. And so on.

When we encourage folks to use the label *cisgender* and cisgender folks feel disrespected, that is because they are considering that they might not be the default, perhaps for the first time. It is crucial to remember that if you are not trans, labeling you *cis* takes nothing away from you!

Let's break down the original comment:

I'm not cis gender.
  Yes, this person is cisgender, because as she very clearly says, she identifies as what she was assigned at birth.

Why can I not simply be allowed to be a woman?

No one is trying to tell cisgender women that they cannot call themselves women. Labeling folks "cisgender" does not take away from their man- or womanhood. A cisgender woman is cisgender *and* a woman. A cisgender man is cisgender *and* a man. This is the basic function of adjectives that many folks of dominant, privileged identities often forget—the adjective just serves to add more description to the noun that follows it. I am an Asian man, an American man, a brown-haired man, and a short man. *Asian, American, brown-haired,* and *short* are adjectives that describe me, a man. They do not detract from my manhood. They simply offer more about who I am. The same applies to the adjective *cisgender* for people who are not transgender.

I absolutely respect every human for who they are, but feel massively undermined...

Using the label *cisgender* to describe cisgender folks is a way to affirm the existence of trans people. When cis women acknowledge they are *cis* women, they are also subtly, but importantly, acknowledging that cis women are not the only women out there—that trans women exist as well. When cis folks believe that using the label *cis* somehow undermines their own gender, they are erroneously making this all about themselves. The application of the word *cis* only undermines the gender of a cisgender person if they do not believe that trans people are valid in our genders.

As a woman who is happy as a woman...

Trans people are not people who are "unhappy" as what they were assigned at birth. I am not a woman who is just unhappy as a woman. No, I am a man.

My identity is now being changed to be "cis."

No one is changing cis people's identities by using the label *cis*. Cis people's identities are not changing. They are just learning a new word to appropriately and accurately describe themselves.

Let's all respect everyone for who they identify as please.
Stating, "I absolutely respect every human for who they are," and, "Let's all respect everyone for who they identify as," while deliberately rejecting a primary way of respecting trans people is manipulative and gaslighting. I assume this commenter did not intend for this, but respecting trans people includes understanding gender is not sex, that gender is not a choice, and that cisgender people have a primary role in dismantling the transphobic system created by cisgender folks in which we currently live. If you are a cis person not actively dismantling transphobia, you are perpetuating it.

Bonus: "*Cisgender* is just a made-up word!"
Yes. All words are made-up. Although *cisgender* is not all that new—it has been around since the 1960s—all words are just combinations of sounds that humans have collectively agreed have meaning. That's what language is. The words on this page—*cisgender* or otherwise—are not meaningless because they are made-up; quite the contrary is true.
Here's a quick rundown of some terminology suggestions:

* *Cisgender* can be shortened to *cis*.
* *Cis man* is a way to abbreviate *cisgender man* and refers to a man assigned male at birth.
* *Cis woman* is a way to abbreviate *cisgender woman* and refers to a woman assigned female at birth.
* *Cishet* is a compound adjective, combining abbreviated versions of *cisgender* and *heterosexual* and describes people who are neither transgender nor queer.

➤ TRANSITION

Any steps a person takes to affirm their gender identity. While many folks might think of physical or medical procedures such as surgery or hormone therapy, transitions do not always include these things and can include many others, such as different pronoun usage, wardrobe or name changes, haircuts, and more.

Many used to refer to transitioning as a "sex change." This is largely outdated now, given that sex is not simply male or female (see the section on biological sex), and most trans people do not feel that transitioning is changing their gender, but rather affirming it.

For this reason, we've even seen the introduction of the term *gender affirmation*, which some use in addition to *transition*, and others as a replacement. Although *transition* has been considered respectful and used for a few decades already, *gender affirmation* resonates for many. *Transition* implies a beginning and an end and not everyone feels that gender affirmation entails this; additionally, *transition* used to be, and often still is, short for *gender transition*, implying changing gender itself, which, again, many folks, including myself, do not feel is accurate.

Gender affirmation is an umbrella term that is more likely to be accurate and inclusive, in that it encompasses exactly what it is: a vague and therefore individualized process of affirming one's gender—an identity that existed before any affirmation processes began. Still, *transition* remains accurate for many, especially when dropping its original prefix of *gender*. You'll see a combination of *affirmation* and *transition* throughout this book as a result.

➤ GENDER IDENTITY

The internal sense of one's own gender. *Gender identity* is often shortened to just *gender*, although this can sometimes result in confusion because many folks mistakenly believe that gender is the same as sex. This is false!

➤ BIOLOGICAL SEX

Often shortened to just *sex*, this technically refers to one's reproductive and sexual anatomy, physiology, and biology, usually categorized into a binary of either "male" or "female," but is most often used to refer to a person's gender assigned at birth. Biological sex is far more complex than we are often taught. I'll discuss more about why biological sex is not binary or simple in Chapter 2.

➤ SEXUALITY

The classification of one's romantic, sexual, or emotional attraction toward others (e.g., gay, straight, bisexual, pansexual, queer, asexual, etc.).

When I came out as transgender, several of my friends asked, "Wait, but aren't you just . . . gay?" Some people ventured further and demanded, "Why aren't you just a butch lesbian?"

Sexuality is not the same as gender expression. Yes, transness and gayness are included in the same "LGBTQ+" acronym, but that doesn't mean we all have the same experiences. Trans people come in all sexualities, just like cis people do! A trans person can be gay, straight, pan, and so on.

Gender identity is an arrow pointing inward: it is who I am. Sexuality is an arrow pointing outward: to whom I am attracted. If I change something about who I am, that doesn't necessarily change the direction of the arrow pointing outward, though the label assigned to that arrow might shift. For example, I have always been attracted to women. Before I transitioned and while I called myself a woman, the label assigned to the sexuality arrow was *gay* or *lesbian*. Once I realized I'm not actually a woman and am instead a man, the label assigned to that arrow became *straight*, though I rarely use *straight* to describe myself these days. You'll read more about why later.

For a majority of trans people, coming out as trans and affirming our genders does not "cause" sexuality to change. Many trans folks, however, do experience shifts in their sexuality through their affirmation journeys. Affirmation might enable the discovery of expanding sexual expression because the individual feels more aligned with who they are. Additionally, the more gender itself can be deconstructed, the less it is necessary to label a sexuality as gay or straight—and the more fluid it can become.

➤ QUEER

While I am a man and have only dated women, I use the label *queer*. *Queer* is an umbrella term that can encompass a variety of sexual and gender identities. For some, queerness is sexuality, for others, queerness is gender, and for still others, queerness is everything. For me, queerness encompasses my history of being perceived as a woman, as a lesbian, as all the presentations of myself that I have embodied.

Queer comes from 1500s Scottish or Low German, meaning "strange, peculiar, odd, eccentric." In 1922, *queer* took on its first pejorative alignment with sexuality, denoting deviance. As a result, *queer* can carry with it deep pain, especially for some older generations.

In 2017, I spoke at a conference in South Florida to an audience mostly composed of trans women in their forties and older. Following my talk, several women shared with me that hearing the word *queer* was jarring. Some even reported that it was disrespectful and they wished that the younger generation would cease to use it in a positive or even neutral manner.

In 2023, *queer* has entered mainstream vernacular as overwhelmingly positive, and it seems that we have (mostly) successfully reclaimed the word. Still, if you are not queer and someone tells you they dislike the use of that word, respect this and reflect back the language they prefer.

➤ GENDER EXPRESSION

This refers to how folks present their gender, including how we talk, how we act, how we look. Gender expression is bound to gender roles by social construction and can change based on time period, culture, geographic location, and other socially influenced factors. You'll read more about gender expression in Chapter 5.

LANGUAGE IS AN EVOLVING TOOL

Trans non-binary actor, singer, and content creator Elle Deran (they/she) says, "*I* am not non-binary. *Non-binary* is a word I use to describe myself. But *I* am not that word."[1] Here, Elle speaks to the limiting nature of language. Language is a tool, at best, an approximation of reality—a forever inaccurate and imprecise attempt at communicating ourselves to others.

"Language inherently isn't limiting," Elle elaborated. "It's when we fully identify with the language that it limits ourselves."

This approach concentrates power in a person's knowing of themselves—in Elle's or my own feeling of knowing who we are, instead of in potentially arbitrary sounds and words. This empowerment is key when considering how language is often used to create narrow categories with which to divide communities and relegate people into small boxes.

For now, we can recognize that these terminologies, while important, are also a starting point. Language evolves as people do—which means language is also constantly changing. The language I've provided here is widely used and accepted as common and respectful, *but* if someone you meet uses different language to describe themselves, I always suggest reflecting that language.

Listen to the trans people around you.

CHAPTER 2

Biological Sex: More Complicated than Grade School Science!

IT WAS THE SECOND OR THIRD DAY OF A WEEKLONG SUMMER camp. I was probably ten years old, wearing my favorite basketball shorts and a soft T-shirt. My hair was short and shaggy—I'd selected a haircut from the men's section of the magazine at the barber and was pleased with the result. Most people thought I was just a little boy. I often didn't correct them.

We were outside the tennis courts, waiting for instructions from the counselors. I stood with Justin (he/him) and Daniel (he/him), two boys I'd befriended the day before. They wore the same kind of shorts as I did and we chattered about what we might do that day.

Eventually, the camp counselor gathered us in a huddle and said, "Okay, today we're going to play a little tournament!" Everyone cheered happily, including me. *Fun!* I loved competition. "We're going to play in two groups," he continued. "Boys come with me and girls go with Julia!" My heart sank.

"Let's go!" Justin elbowed me as I lagged behind. The other boys had already run off to the other court with the boys' camp counselor.

I didn't move. I looked off toward Julia and the girls, dreading joining them.

"What are you doing, we're going to miss the first game!" Daniel had run back to me, and Justin and was tugging on my arm.

"I can't—" I tried.

Like most people did by default at the time, they had been calling me by he/him pronouns and, as usual, I hadn't corrected them. I knew it was possible that the camp counselors knew my legal gender marker since the application paperwork requested that information, but sometimes the counselors didn't check. Or they might have assumed a mistake: I looked like a boy to them.

"I don't . . . I'm not—" I started again. "I'm not a boy," I said finally.

"What?" Justin laughed. "Yeah, right, okay. Come on!" he said.

"No, really, I—"

"You're funny," Daniel added. Neither believed me.

"I'm a girl," I said, the words twisting in my mouth. They always tasted funny, but they were the only options I had.

"You're lying. Come on!" Justin said again. His laughter had turned into annoyance. "You're a boy, like us. Let's go."

"I'm not a boy, I'm a girl!" I said more loudly this time. I was frustrated and deeply uncomfortable. A few of the girls were looking our way in disgust.

"Yeah? Okay, prove it," Daniel said. "Pull down your pants!"

"Okay!" I said angrily. Not actually intending to do so, I reached for my waistband. Justin and Daniel's eyes widened.

"No, no, no—never mind! Jeez!" Justin said, his hands up, blocking his own view of me. They ran off to join the other boys.

⁂

I HAVE BEEN asked to prove my gender for most of my life. Whether disclosing the parts I was born with or my gender identity as a man, I have rarely been granted the space to simply know my own gender.

In my childhood and ignorance, I tried to identify my gender the way I was taught: by my genitals and resulting gender assigned at birth. Unfortunately, neither of these were accurate, but it would take time, healing, and significant unlearning to arrive at a place where my gender was something I could fully accept, and my assigned gender a label I could finally discard.

At an after-school speech for parents of students, one audience member asked, "Why do you say 'assigned' gender? Why is it not just 'gender at birth'? 'Assigned' sounds so forced and inaccurate!"

The answer to this common question? Complex and simple. First, as I mentioned briefly in the previous chapter, the reason I and many others say "assigned" is because "assignment" most accurately describes the act. Babies are rarely karyotyped and their internal reproductive organs are rarely imaged at birth. Instead, when a baby is born in a hospital, a doctor or nurse examines the external genitals of the newborn. If the primary external genitalia appear to be long enough to be a penis, the doctor writes "M" on the birth certificate—*assigning* the baby "male" for their gender. Similarly, if the genitalia appear small enough to be a clitoris, the doctor writes "F," assigning the baby "female."

So yes, gender is literally "assigned"—by either a doctor or another person who assumes the baby's gender based on the appearance of the newborn's external genitalia. This is contrary to what many of us were taught. You might assume that XX denotes woman and XY man—or perhaps that penis means man and vagina means woman, but biological sex is in fact more complicated than what we were taught in grade school! (Most things are!)

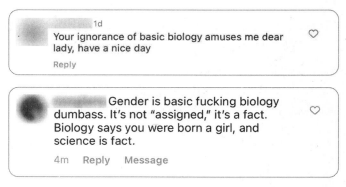

> 1d
> Your ignorance of basic biology amuses me dear lady, have a nice day
> Reply

> Gender is basic fucking biology dumbass. It's not "assigned," it's a fact. Biology says you were born a girl, and science is fact.
> 4m   Reply   Message

Second, biological sex is not binary and cannot be reduced to one single factor. There are five main components of biological sex!

WHAT MAKES UP BIOLOGICAL SEX?

Chromosomes

These refer to the sex chromosomes, specifically. Most people know of two variations of sex chromosomes: XX and XY, but several other variations also exist: XXY, XXX, XYY, and X. In 2019, former president Donald Trump (he/him) proposed that we should genetically test people for their gender—using chromosomes. This endeavor is based on not only the erroneous belief that biology alone dictates gender identity, but also the factually incorrect assumption that biology is as simple as "XY = male" and "XX = female." Biology is far more complex than this binary.

Hormones

You've likely heard of testosterone and estrogen. You've also likely been taught that testosterone is the "male" hormone and estrogen is the "female" hormone. But most people actually have *both*, just in differing concentrations. Hormone variations exist between cis women and cis men, but also within each of these groups as well. Testosterone and estrogen are also *not* the only sex hormones—there are many types! Androgens include testosterone, androstenedione, and dehydroepiandrosterone, and estrogens include estrone, estradiol, estriol, and estetrol. These, along with a few other hormones, can all impact development of sexual characteristics. These hormones also have numerous other functions outside of sexual differentiation.

Hormonal Expression

This refers to the effects of hormones, sometimes called secondary *sex characteristics*, such as voice deepening or increased body hair with testosterone exposure. As with all factors of biological sex, variance exists: some people have thicker beards, some have no facial hair at all, breast sizes vary, some Adam's apples are more pronounced than others, and so on.

You might wonder why hormonal expression is a separate category from hormones. The presence of a hormone alone will not result in effects. Hormone receptors that not only function but also match the corresponding hormone are necessary for expression.

A SLIGHTLY DEEPER DIVE

A relatively common diversity in receptors is called *androgen insensitivity*, wherein folks with XY chromosomes partially or completely do not respond to androgens, including testosterone, and therefore do not exhibit many or all of testosterone's typical effects. Those with complete androgen insensitivity have internal testes, a vulva, a clitoris, no uterus, litte to no body hair, no body odor, and no oily skin that would produce acne. People with complete androgen insensitivity are often described as hyperfeminized and, in most cases, identify as women.[1,2]

Internal Genitalia

This includes the internal reproductive organs such as undescended testes, vasa deferentia, fallopian tubes, uteri, and ovaries.

External Genitalia

Society seems to focus most on this category when discussing the concept of biological sex. External genitalia refer to reproductive organs and related structures on the outside of the body: e.g., the penis, scrotum, and the vulva (the clitoris, labia, and vaginal opening).

Distinguishing between internal and external genitalia is crucial because these do not always develop in tandem; they do not always "match." Some people born with testes also have a vagina and clitoris.

While most bodies develop in neat categories labeled "male" and "female," not all bodies do! The folks whose bodies do not fit these categories are called *intersex*, which literally means "between sex."

I appreciate your effort but I just don't think it's relevant. We teach that people have 2 hands and five fingers on each and that provides the most utility for the application of medicine and research. Yes people born with no hands, amputees, and persons born with an excess and not enough fingers exist, but I don't think that's a basis to say that genetic code doesn't predispose humans for 5 fingers. Mutations aren't the objective, there an anomaly.

27w   19 likes   Reply

pinkmantaray ✓ I hear you! You're welcome to your own opinions. However, I'd encourage you to consider that many characteristics of human biology are rare but considered "normal." But then when sex is involved, suddenly this diversity in biology is considered an "anomaly" or an "aberration." Consider the fact that red-headed-ness occurs at the SAME frequency as intersex folks do. Red-headed-ness is not excluded from discussions of biology and human phenotypic expressions because it's a natural expression of human biological diversity. This should be the same with intersex characteristics. The fact that "we do not teach" people about intersex folks does not reflect issues with the concepts or materials themselves but rather the faulty system of education that excludes facts seen as threatening to existing power structures. I hope this makes sense! Email me more if not schuyler@pinkmantaray.com 🙏 🖤

27w   228 likes   Reply

"STOP ERASING BIOLOGY. THERE ARE ONLY TWO SEXES."

When I discuss biological sex as a spectrum, naysayers will reply with a statement along the lines of, "Intersex is just abnormality. Stop erasing biology. There are only two sexes." Though intersex folks do not make up the population majority, the assertion that there are only two sexes is simply false. Recognizing the complexity of biological sex does not negate or erase biology. Quite the opposite is true: defining sex by absolute categories of "male" and "female" erases biology.

Despite the common accusation, I am not arguing that biological sex itself is made-up. Biological sex is very real—it just isn't as simple or binary as people make it out to be.

Instead of a false binary, biological sex can be described by a bimodal distribution, with most bodies resembling two prototypes commonly labeled *male* and *female*. But these labels and prototypes are neither comprehensive nor absolute: diversity exists within and beyond them. Denying so is denying biology.

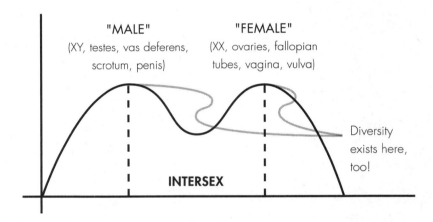

Scientists estimate that about 2 percent of the population is intersex. Many intersex advocates assert that this is a significant underestimation because so many individuals do not know that they are intersex; advocates suggest the number is closer to 5 percent of the population. But even if we consider only the lower estimate, 2 percent of the world population is still roughly 160 million people (in the 2020s), which is larger than the population of Russia. Just because Russians make up only 2 percent of the population does not mean they don't exist. In similar statistical comparisons: about 2 percent of the world population has red hair, about 2 percent has green eyes. No one is claiming red hair or green eyes don't exist. Similarly, just because intersex folks make up 2 percent of the population doesn't mean they don't exist. Intersex bodies exist and we should be learning about them, too.

Using biological sex to deny or invalidate the identities of transgender folks is not only disrespectful but also unscientific. Like most everything in our world, biological sex is not binary nor does a singular factor decide its makeup.

TERMINOLOGY SUGGESTIONS

INSTEAD OF	TRY THIS	BECAUSE
"Biological sex" "Biologically female" "Biological woman" "Biologically male" "Biological man"	Say what you really mean. If you're talking about people who have experienced testosterone-driven puberty, say that. If you're talking about people who have penises, say that. If you're talking about people who can get pregnant, say that. If you're talking about people assigned male at birth, say that.	As presented in this section, biological sex is not binary. Classifying someone as "biologically" male or female is imprecise, often transphobic, and potentially inaccurate.
"Birth sex" "What they were born as"	"Gender assigned at birth" "Assigned gender at birth" or "AGAB"	This avoids unnecessarily (or even inaccurately) referencing someone's genitals and discussing someone's private biology that is (a) likely irrelevant and (b) might not be something they want to discuss.

For me, first learning about biological sex and the complex processes of sexual differentiation was fascinating—and a bit world-shattering. I was raised, as I expect most of you were as well, to believe that biological sex was fixed, binary, and simple. Learning that it wasn't took a while to truly digest. I continue to learn about the vast diversity that human biology encompasses. This chapter was not intended to be a comprehensive discussion of the nuances of biological sex—instead, it is a place to begin.

CHAPTER 3

What Is Gender?

A TALL PERSON WITH DARK CURLY HAIR APPROACHED ME first. I'd just finished a parents' night training at a school in DC and, as always, I had offered the audience the opportunity to come up and ask me questions. This person had a particularly serious look on their face—one that I've grown very familiar with and, in all honesty, weary of.

"Okay, so, listen. I'm a man, and—and—I get that you're a man," he began, his expression somewhere between confused and frustrated. "But you say that you don't define your manhood by your...your parts. And you say your manhood isn't defined by how you act or what you wear." I nodded. I had indeed said this. "So...how *do* you define manhood?"

I smiled and nodded again. *Ah, the infamous question. If you don't have a penis, how do you* know *you're a man?*

"Thank you for coming to ask me this question," I replied. "It's a good question—and a common one. Could I ask you a few questions first?"

"Sure," he said, very unsurely.

"Great! Do you identify as a man?"

"Yes," he said quickly. "Yes."

"Okay, great, and because you've asked me this question, I'm assuming you're not transgender, yes?"

"I'm not, I'm just a man," he replied.

"Okay! I'm also 'just a man,' I'm just also transgender," I noted. He stared at me. "So, you're a man. You must know how to define your manhood. How do *you* do it?" I asked with sincerity.

"Uh, well, I was born a man," he said.

"Okay! This usually means that you were assigned male at birth, which only really means the doctors looked at your genitals when you were born, saw a penis (or something that resembled a penis), and said, 'This is a boy!' So, being 'born a man' really means being born with a penis, yes?"

"...I guess so?" he answered, uncomfortable now. "But I mean..." He trailed off.

"Let's go with this for a moment. You define your manhood by having a penis. Would you stop being a man if you were to get into an accident and lose your penis?"

"Well, n-n-no..." he stuttered.

"Okay! Then your manhood isn't defined by your penis. How else do you define it?" I spoke with a practiced kindness.

"Well, I *look* like a man and I *act* like a man and—"

"Okay! If we dressed you in stereotypical women's clothes, maybe a long flowing dress and some makeup and told you to 'act like a woman,' would you suddenly become a woman?"

"No! I mean—" He was frustrated now, his tone shifting and volume increasing.

"All right, that's okay. So, your manhood *isn't* defined by your penis, your clothing, or how you act. I'm a little confused," I said gently. And then with curiosity: "So, how *is* it defined?"

"I don't know! I just know I'm a man!!" he burst out. His fists were balled up and a few of the people behind him waiting in line looked startled. He took a few deep breaths, now aware of his outburst. I grinned.

"Bingo. *You just know.* Same as I do, same as other trans folks. We don't all have long explanations to give you about gender theory and the bio-psycho-social roots of gender identity or biological sex. But we *do* know who we are, just like cisgender people do."

The man seemed to be calming himself. I continued.

"I do need to get to the next person, but I encourage you to remember that cisgender people—like you—never have to defend their knowing of their gender. But transgender people must always explain ourselves. The frustration you felt as I pushed, asking you all those questions, is the frustration many transgender people feel every day when we are demanded to explain and defend our identities constantly. I hope you think more about this as you move forward."

"I will, thank you." He said and left.

Over the years, I've come to the conclusion that asking a transgender person how they *know* they are their gender is a microaggression.* This question implies that a transgender person cannot simply know their own gender the way a cisgender person does. It does not grant transgender people the basic respect of assuming we know ourselves best. Consider that practically no one asks cisgender people, "So, how do you *really know* that you're a man? How do you *really know* that you're a woman?" No one expects cisgender people to have long explanations about the validity of their gender supported by peer-reviewed academic articles. But they sure expect it from trans folks!

As a result, I strongly discourage people from asking trans people how we know we are the gender we are unless that conversation is explicitly invited by the trans person. These conversations can be taxing and exhausting. Understand that it is *a privilege* not to have to walk the world constantly explaining your identity.

This can be a lot to unpack, so first, let's start with some key historical context—because trans and non-binary identities are far from new.

---

* According to the *Merriam-Webster* dictionary, a *microaggression* is "a comment or action that subtly and often unconsciously or unintentionally expresses a prejudiced attitude toward a member of a marginalized group (such as a racial minority)." In the words of my best friend Kevin (he/him), if you are talking about a marginalized group and you say something you don't think is offensive but it still offends someone from that group, it's a microaggression.

GENDER AND COLONIZATION
The Gender Binary

When I was in kindergarten, each of my classmates and I were paired with what the school called a "buddy." Your buddy was someone who was a few years older, and about once a month, our buddies would come and hang out with us. They were a combination of a peer-mentor and friend. Your buddy was also supposed to be the same gender as you. So because I was not out as transgender at the time, my buddy was a girl. I was fairly disappointed when I learned this—there was nothing wrong with my buddy, but I didn't understand why I had to be paired with someone based on gender. But it quickly became apparent to me that gender was one of the most important categories in life—at least to those around me.

From infancy, books, toys, clothing were segregated by assumed gender. Our kindergarten alphabet learning cards perpetuated gendered examples: "*T* is for *Truck*. Tommy plays with his toy trucks," or "*J* is for *Jewelry*. Jessica wears her jewelry." In many ways, gender is one of the first things most children are taught, and they begin to categorize accordingly—but if we think critically about the categories created, most of the rules are quite arbitrary and have shifted over time. In the end, anyone can play with toy trucks or wear jewelry—so where do these rigid classifications originate?

EURO-COLONIAL SOCIETY—THAT is, so-called "Western society," developed and created by white European colonizers in the fifteenth and sixteenth centuries and onward—exhibits a very narrow and strict definition of gender. In this framework, only two genders exist: male and female, dictated by a reductive view of biological sex that relies solely on an individual's external genitalia at birth. This framework is most often referred to as the *gender binary*.

According to Dr. Shay-Akil McLean (they/he), a Black non-binary trans masculine evolutionary biologist, geneticist, biological anthropologist, and sociologist, the gender binary we know today was "created, enforced, and then *re*inforced across institutions for the convenience of domination."[1] That is, this concept of "gender" was largely constructed by European colonization with the original intent of gaining power and control.

Dr. McLean's statements align with my own experience as well as anthropological evidence—countless societies included and affirmed the existence of genders outside of the Euro-colonial binary. What would now be called *non-binary* and *transgender* identities were welcomed and thrived in many cultures around the world. But because this diversity threatened colonial power structures, colonizers often responded with violence, killing trans and queer individuals first.[2]

When I was a kid, I realized that gender was used as a method of categorizing people, and often a reason for bullying them. I was socialized as a girl, which, in more frank terms, meant that I was socialized to quiet myself around boys and men—to feel small and less significant. I was socialized to believe that I could not achieve what boys and men could, nor could I be included in their endeavors because they were boys and I "was a girl." In some ways, my disconnection from the identity of "girlhood" assigned to me helped me take a step back. For most of my childhood, I saw how gender was used for power.

Gender Is a Social Construct—So Is It Made-Up?

One day, my brother and I had been playing in the backyard of our childhood home when my mom came out to get us. It was time for us to get our haircuts. As I followed her back inside, she said, "What do you think of getting a short haircut? Would you like that?"

"Yes!" I said without any hesitation.

Sitting in the waiting room, I flipped excitedly through the old-school barbershop Rolodex of haircuts. I pointed to number forty-three—a little rectangle in the men's section showed the messy hair falling into his eyes, shaggy around his head. I loved it. I remember running around the house, exuberant. When I dried my hair, I shook it like I'd seen other boys do and felt a new kind of freedom.

But the next morning, I was suddenly terrified. What would everyone else think of me, a girl, with such short hair? *This haircut was for boys!* An embarrassed shame began to take root and instead of proudly wearing my new haircut, I went to school that day in a pink hat—the most feminine thing I could find.

The courage to remove my hat took time.

"I cut my hair short," I whispered to Dane on the third day.

"Oh cool," he replied. "Let me see!" I glanced around the classroom. Everyone was working in groups, and no one was watching me in particular. I pulled my hat off slowly.

"Nice," he said, rather ambivalently. I hadn't wanted a big response— even a positive one. Satisfied with his answer, I left the hat off. In the days that followed, the first and likely most impactful gender moment occurred: I was gendered as male. Presumably because of my short haircut, many who did not previously know me assumed I was a boy and would refer to me as such. And over the next several months, I'd quickly discover that my hair was not the only thing that was crucial to how people decided to gender me. What shirts I wore, what pants I wore, the shoes I had on, the overall tightness of my clothing, how I sat, the people around me, what I talked about...all these things seemed to have an effect on how other people perceived my gender, despite the fact that *I* was always the *same exact person*. What did this mean about gender?

❧   ❧   ❧

UNDERSTANDING GENDER'S HISTORY is key to contextualizing this question, which is not all that dissimilar from the one the dark curly-haired man asked me at my speech in DC. *What does it truly mean to be a man?*

Well, it depends on who, where, and when you're asking.

According to Dr. McLean, gender is "an array of mental and behavioral characteristics that relate to and differentiate from and go beyond understandings of masculinity, femininity, and neutrality."[3] This definition, created with the historian Blair Imani (she/her), is grounded in the larger history of world societies rather than the narrow scope of Euro-colonialism.

Gender, Dr. McLean and many others assert, is socially constructed. This statement causes much tension across, as well as within, communities—and, admittedly, has even been an internal struggle for me. Fourth-grade Schuyler would have agreed without hesitation that gender was made up by people to categorize us more easily, but by the time I was attempting to accept my trans identity and considering transition, I wasn't so sure. *If gender is just a* construct, *why would I transition at all?* I felt deeply conflicted, worried that this meant my identity was invalid.

But the reality is that most people do not know what a social construct truly is.

According to the *Merriam-Webster* dictionary, a social construct is "an idea that has been created and accepted by the people in a society."[4] A social construct exists because humans agree that it does.[5] Social constructs depend on people engaging with each other, and, without this interaction, they would be meaningless. However, because humans *do* interact with each other, social constructs are not, in fact, meaningless.

Those who use the framework of gender as social construct with the aim of *dismissing* the importance or validity of gender identity altogether fail to recognize that many important (life-dependent, life-altering) systems and concepts are completely socially constructed.

Money, currency, land borders, nationality, citizenship, beauty, fashion, jobs, religion, marriage, and government are all social constructs that most people would consider highly important, incredibly real, and have daily impact on our lives. These are not inherent entities created by nature without humans. But the fact that money would not exist without human interaction does not mean that someone wouldn't starve to death if they didn't have enough of it. Because of the socially constructed importance money holds, most humans cannot exist without it. Simultaneously, if we collectively agreed one day that our rectangular green paper and circles of shiny metal alloy no longer carried any value, the dollar would become meaningless.

Gender, like other social constructs, is not meaningless; quite the contrary is true: social agreements between humans are some of the strongest and most powerful forces we know.

Still, many cling to the assertion that gender is *not* a social construct—that something biological must undergird it. For trans folks, this insistence is often a result of internalized transphobia, begging us to answer: *If gender is just a construct, why transition at all?*

The evoked self-doubt is insidious and painful. In this context, trans people are only afforded validity if we can *prove* our gender through biology. I spent a long time trying to do this when I was in college; for a few years, I even considered studying the biological underpinnings of gender identity. But to the extent that this endeavor provided me with identity affirmation, it was all but fruitless.

I eventually realized I needed to trust myself and my understanding of my gender rather than trying to rely on (misinformed, transphobic, largely-by-white-cisgender-men) "scientific" research to prove my own identity—something I'd known forever. Affirmation and validation came when I finally granted myself that permission to *just know*.

Why Do We Transition If It's All Just a Construct?

"If I had not been incorrectly gendered at birth, I would not have needed to transition," Dr. McLean told me. I was quite taken aback by their answer. "What?" I wanted to interrupt, incredulous.

When I was first beginning to digest my own trans identity, I had asked myself a central question: *If I were alone on an island with no people, no society, no outside expectations or input, who would I be? What body would make me feel most comfortable?* And my answer was always the same: I would be a man. *What did Dr. McLean mean that they wouldn't transition if they'd been gendered correctly?* I jumped to the only conclusion I could fathom in the moment: that they transitioned to appease society.

Of course, I was wrong.

If we did not gender babies based on their external genitalia at birth and instead allowed them to express themselves however they feel best, "the whole framework for what it would mean to transition would be completely different."[6] Without strict boxes created from a reductive understanding of biological sex, gender-affirming surgeries and hormone treatments would not be considered parts of a *gender transition*, but rather, simply another part of one's journey in self-expression and exploration.

The term *transition* itself depends on the existence of a start and a destination: one begins at the gender assigned and transitions into expressing true gender identity. But if we were not conscripted into our genders without consent, as Dr. McLean mentioned, there would be no need to transition from or to. Dr. McLean was emphatic that they would have undergone top surgery and testosterone therapy regardless—but in a world without forced gendering at birth, these steps wouldn't be a "transition to male." They would simply be self-expression.

Why Do We Still Talk About Biology All the Time Then?

While considerable anthropological evidence exists to support the social construction of gender categories throughout history, little to no scientific evidence exists supporting a biophysiological or biochemical underpinning of gender identity.[7] (Note: unlike in the previous chapter, we are *not* talking about biological sex here, but rather gender identity. These entities are not the same thing. The science of biological sex is well researched; biological underpinnings of gender identity are not.) Still, trans and cis folks alike often attempt to rely on biology to discuss the validity (or lack thereof) of trans identity.

Why? Because it is a powerful tool, Dr. McLean reminds. At one point, it was a tool I used (albeit incorrectly) to invalidate myself, too.

"But there's no biological reason that I'm like this," I said to my therapist, exasperated. I was sitting in her office and my therapy session was almost done. It'd been a few months since I'd first used the word *transgender* to maybe—just maybe—describe myself and I was panicking.

"Maybe, maybe not," Jo (she/her) replied. "I'm not a biologist, Schuyler, but I do know one thing. You are allowed to pursue something that makes you happy even if you don't have a biological reason to do so. You need to give yourself permission to be happy."

"Ugh," I said more harshly than I meant to. She laughed.

"I get it. It's all a huge mindfuck," she said to me. Despite how upset I was, I chuckled. I always appreciated that she didn't censor herself with me. "How does anybody *really* know? They don't. They get *mostly* sure. So maybe there's a reason you're transgender. Maybe there's not. But at the end of the day, it doesn't really matter—you're going to have to find a way to validate yourself regardless."

Even though I knew she was right, I still racked my brain. *What made me this way? Did something happen in my brain's biochemistry that made me this way? Are my chromosomes different? Is there a transgender gene?* Finding nothing to support a biological reason for my transness, I had attempted to discard it. *I'm not trans; I can't be!* This line of thinking combined with the anti-trans rhetoric that trans people have "just made it all up" made me feel hopeless. It took a great deal of self-trust to move beyond biology as a tool of validation and instead learn to rely on myself—my own knowing of myself. This process demanded that I prioritize my own happiness and alignment over what I understood of biology—something I'd internalized as the ultimate truth.

"What if I *were* just making it all up," I sometimes think to myself. "I'm not, but *if* I were, what would that matter? I'm happier this way. And I'm hurting no one."

While I don't truly believe I'm making up my gender experience, I love considering what the world would be like if I were, if anyone were, and if that would just be...okay. Good. Fine. Normal. Who cares if someone is more comfortable presenting themselves in this particular way or in that one? Who cares if they are making it up or if that is "real"? What impact does it have on another person unless you demonize trans identity and queerness?

GENDER HISTORY AND NON-BINARY IDENTITIES
Trans People Existed Before the Gender Binary

"I support trans men and women, but non-binary is just a new made-up trend!"

I receive variations of this comment on a fairly regular basis—still, I'm surprised every time, not necessarily due to the obvious transphobia, but rather the lack of historical context. The earliest records of non-binary identities date back to ancient Mesopotamia in the twenty-third century BC.[8]

Some societies around the world have recognized a third gender for centuries, and, in these societies, gender is not categorized by sex but rather by gender identity, and even through spirituality. As a result,

those who identified with a third gender were not acting or identifying as something other than what they were assigned—because nothing was truly assigned. As such, society did not categorize third-gender
individuals into another category of "transgender," but rather just as
themselves.

This was a fairly radical idea even for me to digest when I first
learned it—we are so conditioned to believe that gender is determined
from birth and that the way we dress, act, and sound inherently indicates gender. But imagine a world in which gender is more expansive
from the beginning—where your gender is simply an expression of who
you are, not a conformity to or defiance of what society dictates. In that
world, I would not be transgender for defying gender roles and my gender
assigned at birth. I would just be me.

A History of Non-binary Identities Through Language and Indigenous Cultures

Two Spirit or 2S

Prior to 1990, the European American term *berdache*, which is often
considered offensive, was used to refer to Native individuals whose traditional gender or sexuality did not conform to Western gender binary and
heteronormativity.

Two spirit was later adopted by Indigenous people at the Third
Annual Inter-tribal Native American, First Nations, Gay and Lesbian
American Conference in 1990.[9] This term, restricted to Indigenous
individuals because the identity only makes sense when "contextualized
within a Native American frame," attempted to provide a pan-Indigenous
unifying word instead of the individual words from individual tribes.[10,11]

The term *two spirit* has also received criticism as it still reflects the
Euro-colonial gender binary of two genders, male and female, imposed
by colonizers upon the Indigenous peoples. This is inconsistent with
many Indigenous cultures' conception of gender. Additionally, *two spirit*
collapses a host of diverse and distinct Indigenous identities into one
English label. Some argue this further reduces the identity and ignores
important differences and cultural significance that varies from people
to people.

Maorocati

A Taino name for a deity that is believed to be third gender or even trans is Maorocati. Indya Moore (she/they), an afro-Taino genderqueer woman, identifies as two spirit but notes that many Indigenous descriptors of gender-variant people have largely been lost or erased.

"I really appreciated learning [this word]," Indya told me, finding solace in the fact that trans people were once regarded by society in a more positive light.[12]

Quariwarmi

In Peru, the pre-colonial Inca civilization had yachaq, or shamans, called Quariwarmi—also spelled Qhariwarmi or Qariwarmi. Meaning "men-women," Quariwarmi took on a mixed-gender role in society. Co-founder of Queer Nature, Pınar Ateş Sinopoulos-Lloyd (they/them) is a non-binary person who is both Quechua and Turkish. Though often referred to as "two-spirit" by Native folks from North America, Pınar prefers terms of their own Native language and most often uses Quariwarmi. Pınar's use of Quariwarmi is a reminder that Quariwarmi not only exist historically but continue to exist in our present and future.

Winkte

The Winkte people of the Lakota are those who would be categorized as male by the Euro-colonial binary but assume traditional women's roles such as cooking and caring for the children.[13] Winkte also assumed special roles in society such as naming children, resolving conflict, and praying for the sick.[14]

Nádleehí

Non-binary trans femme scholar, writer, and Diné content creator Charlie Amáyá Scott (they/she) shares that the Diné people affirm the existence of Nádleehí—similar to the Winkte. Diné, like many other Indigenous cultures, embrace genders beyond the Eurocolonial gender binary.[*][15]

---

[*] Indigenous peoples might not have used the language of gender and sexuality to describe their relationships to each other the way we do today.

Muxes

The Indigenous Zapotecs of modern-day Oaxaca, Mexico, have long accepted and even celebrated the Muxes, those who are "born male" (as they would be categorized by the Euro-colonial binary) but like the Winkte assume roles traditionally associated with women.[16] The acceptance of the Muxes—pronounced MOO-shays—and their identities could stem from the fact that Muxes have been seen as a "part of the culture and its traditions, not separate from it," according to an article from Los Angeles County's National History Museum.[17]

Several Indigenous societies across the Americas include genders that do not exist within the Euro-colonial binary, including the Lakota, Crow, Apache, Chickasaw and Choctaw, Cree, Dakota, Flathead, Hopi, Illinois, Inuit, Diné, and many more groups.[18] Indigenous acceptance and celebration of non-binary identities extends globally: the **Mahu** of Hawai'i, **Metis** of Nepal, **Hijra** of South Asia, **Ashtime** of Ethiopia, **Mino** of Benin, **Bangala** of the Democratic Republic of Congo, **Ankole** of Uganda, **Sekrata** of Madagascar, **Acault** of Myanmar, **Bakla** of the Philippines, **Whakawahine** of Aotearoa (also known as New Zealand), **Skoptsy** of Russia, **Burrnesha** of Albania, **Femminiello** of Italy, **Köçek** of the Ottoman Empire, and the **Mamluk** of Egypt.[19] These lists are far from comprehensive, and books could (and should!) be written about each.

I often wonder what kind of cultural landscape we'd have today if our trans ancestors had not been so discriminated against and, worse, exterminated. How many more words might we have to describe more accurately our gendered experiences, and how much more room might there be for expression.

"Meaning God"

Today, trans people are often portrayed as not family friendly—as unsafe for children, a threat to family life. In contrast, many Indigenous societies revered gender-variant people as healers or another part of a higher power. They were at the center of "what it meant to keep people alive as opposed to being a definition for destruction and death and impending doom the way that we are described today."[20]

This deified view of transness was found all around the world. Dr. shawndeez (they/them), an Iranian American independent scholar who completed their PhD in gender studies at UCLA, told me that in various indigenous societies around the world "our transness was a fixture of our spiritual height."[21] Trans people were seen as "really useful vessels between this world and the spiritual—our transness gave us this extra access to this divine wisdom." shawndeez believes transness demands that we cultivate "a consciousness that is so open, so spacious, [it] invites higher dimensional thought that we're not really seeing in the everyday mundane very earthly realm." The invitation is about understanding that gender—and our existences—do not have to be limited by whom we are told we must be, whom society decides we are on the basis of our genitalia or appearance, and what box the Euro-colonial gender binary has attempted to lock us into.

Non-binary People Today

One in six members of Generation Z identify as LGBT[22] and 76 percent of non-binary adults are between eighteen and twenty-nine years old.[23] Many critics have argued that being non-binary must then be a trend or a fad. Is it? If not, why is everybody suddenly non-binary? What does it mean to be non-binary? Aren't there only two sexes? Gen Z can't just "make up" genders . . . right?

In short, wrong.

The *Merriam-Webster* dictionary defines *non-binary* as "relating to or being a person who identifies with or expresses a gender identity that is neither entirely male nor entirely female."[24] Today, *non-binary* is largely regarded as an umbrella term. For some folks being non-binary means identifying somewhere between the binary "ends" (male and female) of gender, for some it means identifying as a combination of genders, and for others it means feeling a complete lack of gender altogether. For many folks, being non-binary entails liberation from the stereotypes and gender roles attached to the gender they were assigned at birth.

The term *non-binary* denotes a gender we don't have a name for right now. "There was a name for it"—there were actually many, many names for it!—"but a lot of that information was lost," Dr. McLean told me sadly. And still, non-binary people continue to exist and thrive beyond any limitations language might present. Here are some folks sharing what being non-binary means to them:

> *"I define non-binary as freedom."*
>
> —B. HAWK SNIPES (they/she),
> entertainer, style icon, and actor[25]

> *"The English language does not provide a great deal of vocabulary for explaining non-binary identity. I always put a distinction: 'English' pronouns or 'English' identities. [...] In Diné, we have very long and lengthy introductions, and one of the most comforting things is the ending, where you tell people who you are and your role and responsibility [in society]. Ákót'éego diné Nádleehí nishłį. Roughly translated, this means, 'one who transforms or one who is constantly changing.'"*
>
> —CHARLIE AMÁYÁ SCOTT (they/she), an Indigenous
> [Diné] trans femme, non-binary scholar,
> writer, and content creator[26]

> *"My own personal definition [of non-binary] fluctuates between 'I have all the genders' and 'I have no gender' at the same time."*
>
> —DYLAN KAPIT (they/them), queer, trans non-binary,
> Jewish autistic educator and researcher

> *"Being non-binary means I don't identify with being exclusively man or woman. Those labels [of man/woman] exist within me and I exist beyond them. Language inherently isn't limiting; it's when we fully identify with the language that it limits ourselves. Human beings are so much more than words. [...] I am not non-binary; non-binary is a word I use to describe myself."*
>
> —ELLE DERAN (they/she), trans non-binary actor,
> singer, content creator committed to producing
> educational, entertaining, queer-affirming content[27]

"I'm not a fan of rule-out or knockout definitions, but this is not one of the situations where we're avoiding defining a thing because non-binary itself needs no further definition. To close the definition closes the possibility. And there are so many different ways to be non-binary."

—Dr. McLean (they/he), a Black non-binary trans masculine evolutionary biologist, geneticist, biological anthropologist, and sociologist[28]

"Transgender isn't *my gender identity—that would be* non-binary. *To me,* transgender *describes my journey of transcending the gender label I was assigned at birth and coming home to my gender—of coming home to me."*

—Addison Rose Vincent (they/them), a trans feminine non-binary LGBTQ+ inclusion educator and consultant

"Transness or non-binary-ness is transcending whatever you are 'supposed to be' according to society."

—Devin-Norelle (ze/zim/zis), trans masculine Black and mixed-race writer, model, and trans advocate

"We're taught we need to act like other people in order to be accepted. People don't allow themselves to truly ask themselves: 'What does it mean to be me?' Being non-binary means being my most authentic self—and exploring what that means with celebration, instead of forcing myself into this cookie-cutter shape where I'm no longer me. Being non-binary is my 'me-gender.'"

—Meg Lee (they/them), Asian American trans non-binary artist and activist

Are Non-binary Folks Trans?

In addition to the substantial invalidation cisgender folks direct at non-binary identity, many well-known trans folks (who do not identify as non-binary) have attacked non-binary folks for aligning themselves beneath the trans umbrella. It is not worth naming these individuals, though they are easy to find with a quick Google or YouTube search.

These statements usually begin by arguing that someone must have gender dysphoria in order to be trans. Because some non-binary folks do not experience gender dysphoria, some trans people will exclude them, saying they are not trans.

The second, and perhaps more self-defeating argument, is that there are only two genders: male and female. As you learned earlier in this chapter and in Chapter 2, this is false and not easily defensible as even sex is not binary.

I have met a significant number of non-binary individuals who are afraid to call themselves trans due to backlash they might experience from other trans folks who have decided to transition. Dylan agreed. "I think [non-binary] people are more likely to not say 'trans' until they start medically transitioning," they told me.

Every non-binary person I interviewed for this book felt that non-binary does, indeed, fall beneath the trans umbrella. Their reasoning was all quite similar. Given that *transgender* describes an individual who does not identify as the gender they were assigned at birth and that no one is assigned non-binary as their gender at birth, non-binary folks do not identify with the gender they were assigned at birth and thus would be considered trans. (Of course, if a non-binary person you meet does not call themselves trans, that is also valid!)

"I like to use *trans* as more of the umbrella term," Charlie told me. "*Trans* describes someone who is beyond gender...someone whose gender identity was dictated by someone else other than them." This includes non-binary individuals, Charlie affirmed.[29] B. Hawk said, "If the opposite of cisgender is transgender, and non-binary folks are not cisgender, [then] we are special unique individuals under this amazing world of transness."[30]

Is Non-binary a Descriptor of Identity or Expression?

In addition to the word *non-binary*, you may have also come across *gender nonconforming*. Like *non-binary*, *gender nonconforming* is also an umbrella term with a wide diversity in how individuals use it. In general, *gender nonconforming* includes people whose gender identity and/or gender expression does not align with societal standards or norms for gender—essentially anyone who steps outside of the gender binary in some way. Some people use *gender nonconforming* as an identity itself, and others use it exclusively to describe gender expression and how someone presents or communicates their gender to others.

Similarly, the term *non-binary* is most frequently used to describe gender identity, but some also use it as an umbrella term to talk about their gender expression. Dr. McLean says, "I put gender expression and identity in the same category—whatever your gender is, you're expressing it."

Others such as Dylan are not quite as enthusiastic about eliminating a distinction between the terms. "I worry that using *non-binary* as a gender expression is feeding into the 'I look non-binary' discourse."[31] Here, Dylan is referencing the common misconception that being non-binary necessitates some kind of non-binary "look"—usually one that appears androgynous. But androgyny is subjective and culturally dependent; identifying people by their ability to present their gender in a specific manner does not leave much room for self-identification. Still, Dr. McLean's point is well-taken: in an ideal situation, our gender expression would just be our gender, expressed. Expression can include wearing dresses, flannels, makeup, tank tops, high heels, "rugged clothing," or none of the above. Society has gendered these things, but what if they were just clothing? Just makeup? Just ways of presenting and expressing ourselves.

Each of the non-binary folks I interviewed used both labels, *trans* and *non-binary*. Using both enhanced their ability to describe themselves, and, for several who are often received in a much more binary manner, using *non-binary* in conjunction with *trans* allowed them to distinguish between being a trans man or trans woman and being non-binary.

"Honestly the biggest misconception I get is that I'm a trans man. Happens all the time," Dylan said. "Part of why I use non-binary so strongly is because I know what I look like, and I think people make a lot of assumptions about me based on the fact that I have a beard and I wear 'men's' clothes."[32]

B. Hawk shared similar sentiments: "A lot of people like to throw me into this trans womanhood story but that's not who I am in totality." They shared with pride, "There are times when people want to box me as a trans woman, and I have to remind them I'm not. I'm B. Hawk until further notice."[33]

Non-binary Misconceptions

The diversity of opinions over how to write the label *non-binary* reflects the diversity of the identity itself. A few misconceptions and corrections about non-binary folks:

Not All Non-binary Folks Are Thin, White, and AFAB*

When B. Hawk first met someone who used they/them pronouns, B. Hawk remembers feeling skeptical. "I thought it was just something white trans people were making up." It wasn't until a year or so later when they saw Black trans and non-binary advocate, personality, and fashion influencer Milan Garçon (they/them) that B. Hawk was able to start to see themself.[34,35] "[Milan Garçon] said, 'I'm Black and non-binary,' and I was like, 'Oh! Black people can be non-binary, too!'" B. Hawk laughed. "That's why I think representation is so important."

B. Hawk hits on an issue that persists beyond gender: most representation, even for marginalized identities, focuses on other dominant identities. For trans and non-binary folks, this means that representation in media and society is largely white, cisnormative, heteronormative, conventionally attractive, thin or straight-sized,† and more. Lack of seeing others like themselves can result in thinking that we cannot access these identities, or, if we were to, that we would not be taken seriously.

---

* AFAB is an acronym for "assigned female at birth."
† Refers to people who are not fat and do not experience fatphobia or sizeism.

The reality is people of all gender assignments and biological config-urations, of all races, of all sizes, and all abilities can be non-binary.

Not All Non-binary Folks Are Androgynous

While many assume that being non-binary demands that a person looks androgynous, not all non-binary folks do and not all people who look androgynous are non-binary.

It's crucial to remember that androgyny is a socially constructed cat-egory of gender presentation or gender expression. What "looks androgy-nous" in one culture or time period could look differently in another.

Non-binary folks do not owe others or themselves androgyny. Any-one can present their gender however they'd like. A non-binary person is no less non-binary if they are not read as androgynous.

Not All Non-binary Folks Use They/Them Pronouns

As you might assume, many non-binary folks use they/them pronouns exclusively. Dylan, for example, uses only they/them pronouns. Other non-binary folks, like model, trans advocate, and writer Devin-Norelle, use neopronouns (see pages 68–69). Some non-binary folks might be comfortable using gendered pronouns either solely or in combination with gender-neutral ones. Charlie, B. Hawk, and Dr. McLean each use a combination of they/them pronouns with a gendered pronoun.

Not All Non-binary Folks Are "Genderless"

Being non-binary does not necessarily mean experiencing a complete absence of gender. Some non-binary folks do identify as *agender*, which is usually described as an absence of gender, but many non-binary folks identify their gender itself as non-binary; others experience their gender as feminine, masculine, a combination of the two, perhaps at different times or in different intensities.

Non-binary Folks Can Also Identify as Other LGBTQ+ Identities

Many non-binary folks also identify as trans masculine or trans femi-nine, as lesbian or gay, queer, pansexual, asexual, bisexual, etc.

Some Non-binary Folks Transition and Some Don't!

Some non-binary folks shift their presentation as a part of a gender-affirming process. Some get surgeries or take hormones, and some don't. Non-binary folks are valid regardless of what they do or don't do with their bodies. No one has the authority to tell someone else how they identify based on our own assumptions or conclusions about that individual.

Non-binary Identities Are Not a Trend

As discussed earlier, non-binary identities have been recognized and documented for millennia in cultures across the world. The fact that more people are now defining themselves as non-binary shows only a manifestation of available language, not of newfound or newly created identities.

And even if they were new—what would this mean? Consider that all labeled identities are made up and socially constructed at some point. Take, for example, the label *Korean*. I am a Korean man and this label is very meaningful to me. It describes the culture from which I come, the location, and suggests something about my ancestors. But *Korean* is a word that only surfaced in English in the 1600s,[36] and the Korea we know today is different from the Korea of even my North Korean grandmother's time. What it means to be Korean is a socially constructed identity. It has been made up by humans. And yet it is deeply valuable and important.

Many other labels are invented by humans to describe experience. Man and woman are also made-up categories. Non-binary people are not and have never been expressing their identities for attention or to be cool. Non-binary identities deserve respect like any other gender identity. Just like my manhood is not for you or anyone else, non-binary people's identities are not for you or anyone else: they are for them—their own self and their own peace.

WHILE SOME ARE committed to false realities such as "there are only two genders!" and "non-binary is made-up," or even the false history that "bring back manly men" implies, in reality, gender has never truly been binary, simple, or defined by the gendered stereotypes that govern life today. Gender expansiveness, diversity, and variance have always existed, whether we acknowledge that today or not. Though some of this chapter might come as a surprise, as it did to me when I was first learning, I do not want to live my life dismissing history. I want to live my life constantly integrating new information and updating my thoughts, beliefs, and opinions. I hope you will join me.

CHAPTER 4

Surgery? Hormones? Haircuts?

I N 2012, AFTER A SUMMER OF TAKING AP BIOLOGY ONLINE (before online class was something the world knew how to do), I was ready to get out and do something else. And that something else was downhill mountain biking with my brother, Jinwon (he/him). He had all the right gear, competed regularly, and would even go on to do so semi-professionally, albeit briefly. My bike was off-the-rack from a local sporting goods store.

If you're thinking this was a bad idea, you're right. Downhill mountain biking is one of those extreme sports. Not just down a hill—down a mountain at insane speeds, twisting around banked turns, blindly hurtling over jumps, you get the picture.

On our second run down the mountain, I was doing fairly well, still staying upright—until we hit a pretty big banked turn. Jinwon shouted, "Watch out!" I careened around the corner, going way too fast to maintain control of my bike. I rumbled over logs and into the brush. I thought I'd recovered but then I was airborne. I tucked, bracing myself against the impact I knew was coming.

I can still remember exactly what it smelled like as I went face-first into the flora: sagebrush and pine, with a touch of dusty mountain earth. Somehow, I saved my head from hitting the ground, and, instead,

I landed, lower back first, hard. Really hard. I don't remember much pain. The only thing I could focus on was the feeling of the wind being knocked out of me.

"She crashed!" the guy behind me had stopped and shouted out to my brother. (Though I always encourage people to refer to trans folks by the pronouns we currently use, I've left the way he referred to me unadjusted to reflect how I was perceived at the time.)

"Schuyler?" Jinwon called out for me. I was still catching my breath. "*Schuyler!* Are you okay?! *Schuyler!*" he tried again. Hearing the panic in his voice, I tried to respond.

"Noooooo," I said as loud as I could. It came out more as a moan. I was just trying to make sure he heard me. Then I returned to just trying to get my breath back, but for some reason, it wasn't coming.

It took what felt like a very long time for the medics to come. A guy with a buzz cut and facial hair began asking me typical medical emergency questions.

He examined my helmet for any evidence of a possible head injury and then poked around on my back to find where it hurt. He asked me why I was crying and shaking—was it because of the pain level or because I was scared? I said a little of both.

Truth be told, I was crying because I was sorry about everything—sorry I'd screwed up Jinwon's bike day, sorry I'd held his friends up (who seemed annoyed with the prospect of bringing along a girl), sorry I was wasting the medics' time. I was crying because I was afraid Mom and Dad would be mad at me; I was crying because I was mad at myself for being careless enough to go faster than I knew I could handle.

It felt like forever for them to get me on the backboard. Eight people lifted me from the ground and carefully carried me up to the trail and over to the access road where a truck waited for me.

My parents met me at the base of the trail. I could see how worried they were—Jinwon had, after all, told them I couldn't move. Which wasn't exactly false: I knew that moving would have been a bad idea. But it wasn't true in the ways they feared, either.

"You're going to be okay," they cooed at me in singsong voices. "It's all right, it's okay." *I know!* I wanted to shout back at them. *I'M FINE! I'm not going to die from a stupid fall!* I knew they were trying to help but I was trying hard not to fall apart.

After a very precarious ride down the mountain in the gondola with my feet sticking out because the backboard was too long, an ambulance took me to the nearest hospital where I was wheeled into a room. There, they removed my pants and cut off my T-shirt.

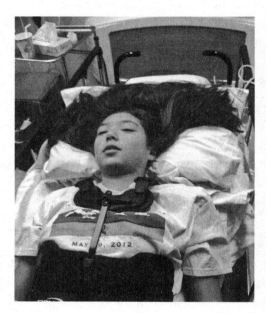

August 24, 2012, in the hospital bed, fitted with my back brace

Through the myriad of tests—CT scan with iodine contrast, X-rays, and the good old "Does this hurt?" poke test—all I could think was that my swim coach was going to be very upset. I'd had a shit season, ending by missing the qualifying times for Summer Nationals. I'd struggled to make it through even the lower-level Sectionals meet, not posting a single best time or winning a single race.

"You were on your period," my coach had said to me. "It's fine." But his tone hadn't agreed with his words. He'd been disappointed—having expected me to be one of his star swimmers that summer.

On top of this, I'd only recently joined that group, one that was widely regarded as the best in the area—and our national championship titles three years in a row would name us the best in the country, as well.

My poor performance that summer not only disappointed my coach, it also embarrassed me. I'd finally begun to feel like I belonged on my new team. But it was a cutthroat group and I was terrified of what would happen if my performance continued to stagnate.

Back in the hospital room, I awaited the doctor's results. *A few days? A week? I've got to get back in shape so I can qualify for Winter Nationals.* I tried unsuccessfully to distract myself by watching TV but the neck brace they insisted I keep wearing was very uncomfortable.

"You've broken your back." The doctor entered and, without any introduction, had spilled the beans.

I was stunned. *I broke my back?*

"How long until I can swim again?" were the first words out of my mouth.

"You're lucky, it's a stable fracture—so not that long. About four to six, maybe eight—" I breathed a sigh of relief. Four days didn't sound so bad!

"Weeks," he finished. *TWO MONTHS?* He left me in my shock to go verify the results with the radiologist. And that was when I started really crying.

"Coach's going to kill me . . ." I sobbed to my father who sat with me. I was so angry with myself.

My dad comforted me before the nurses brought me a back brace that I was instructed to wear until my next appointment. Dejected and somehow still convinced I'd return to practice sooner than two months, we went home.

In many ways, breaking my back broke everything else, too. That fall, as I began my junior year in high school, I spiraled deep into depression, self-harm, and a vicious eating disorder. Not swimming ripped a hole in my life. No longer was I eating for swimming, sleeping for swimming, and completing my studies efficiently so that I could have time for swimming. I felt empty and purposeless.

For the remainder of my high school years, I went in and out of therapy, never quite understanding what was wrong with me and why I was so relentlessly miserable. Still, I continued to succeed academically, and when I was able to swim that winter—a short three months or so after the accident—I swam faster than I'd ever swum before. These successes provided momentary glimpses of happiness that quickly faded as I fell back into my discomfort. Nothing felt right.

While I was fortunate to have access to mental healthcare, improvement was elusive. By my senior spring, I had gone to the hospital more than once for mental health issues. Clearly, I wasn't getting better.

After one hour-long intake session with yet another therapist, I was told, "You need residential treatment. You've got *way* too much going on, hon. I can't help you here. You need to go figure this all out at a place where nothing else can distract you."

I knew she was right. I'd been taking AP classes, applying to college, and swimming at least twenty hours a week for my nationally ranked team. But residential treatment meant deferring a year from Harvard, where I'd been offered a spot on the women's swim team.

"If you don't prioritize your mental health," this therapist told me, "you're going to go to Harvard and either swim slowly or do badly in school, all while being miserable."

On Monday, June 9, 2014, the day after graduation, my family flew with me to Miami, Florida, where I checked into Oliver-Pyatt Centers, a residential treatment center for eating disorders. I had decided to take the therapist's advice and deferred from Harvard to take a gap year for my mental health.

It was during my time in treatment that I would first discover my transness, and finally learn what it meant to affirm this in my body and self as I walked the world.

Following this discovery, I would often find myself browsing Instagram late at night, looking for people like me. One night, I stumbled upon a trans guy's account. His name was Kieran. In most of his photos, he was shirtless and, at least to my eye, had no evidence of ever having had breasts. I was absolutely stunned. And deeply jealous. I had no idea that people like me—people assigned female at birth—could undergo procedures that would allow us to truly see ourselves. I'd wanted my breasts gone before they had even begun to bud. Surgery to remove my breasts that were now larger than DDD-cups was a dream.

I had spent my preadolescence and adolescence ashamedly wishing I might get breast cancer one day so that I wouldn't have to keep my breasts. I was that desperate for a reason to remove them. Later, I'd find out I wasn't so alone in this wish. Lots of trans masculine folks I'd meet would share this deeply held secret with me. Though none of us ever intended to dismiss the tragic reality of cancer, the wish to have been sick instead of having to keep our breasts might help explain the pain we were in at the time. The surgery that Instagrammer Kieran received and that many other trans masculine folks receive is a double mastectomy that is commonly referred to as *top surgery*. Upon learning about the existence of this surgery, I was certain I wanted it.

❖   ❖   ❖

As DISCUSSED EARLIER, a transition or gender-affirmation process includes steps a trans or non-binary person takes to affirm their gender identity. For many people, gender affirmation is lifesaving. Even just learning that transition was possible as I consumed more content like Kieran's brought me freedom. *I could have that. I could feel like myself, too,* I thought.

Of course, transgender people are not a monolith, so it follows that our gender-affirmation processes will not be identical. There is no one way to transition and not every trans person transitions. Gender affirmation can include a myriad of things: haircuts and wardrobe changes, hormones and surgery, or nothing physical at all.

Generally, transitions can be grouped into two main categories: (1) social and (2) medical or physical.

A month or so after I began to truly accept and welcome my trans identity, I went shopping with a few friends. Laura (she/her) and Adrienne (she/her), who had remained updated with my gender journey at the time, accompanied me to the men's section of my favorite store and excitedly encouraged me to buy the jeans I so clearly wanted. I did and was thrilled. Over the next several months, I braved buying more clothes that felt more aligned with my gender and how I wanted to present myself.

In October of 2014, I booked myself an appointment at a local salon and cut my long hair short once again. Instead of the old-school barbershop Rolodex, I selected one from the internet. I'm embarrassed to admit I showed the stylist a photo of Zac Efron (he/him). *High School Musical* influence aside, I remember feeling so much gender euphoria looking into the mirror. Soon after, I began sharing my trans identity with close friends and asking that small group to call me he/him pronouns. This began my social transition.

Social transitioning usually includes shifts that result in changing how one presents and is received socially. As it did for me, social transitioning often includes coming out as transgender, asking for different pronouns, new haircuts or hairstyles, and wardrobe updates. Social transition can also involve sharing a different name, or grouping oneself into a different gendered category; for example, using a different restroom, playing on a different sports team, involving oneself in a different gendered extracurricular activity, and so on. Social transitions can also not include any of these, and as with any transitional step, it is up to the person transitioning to decide what is best for them.

In March 2015, I received top surgery in Davie, Florida, from Dr. Charles Garramone (he/him). This was the first step of my medical transition. Medically (also known as physically) transitioning entails undergoing medical procedures to alter one's body, usually including hormones and/or surgeries. Due to ignorance and misinformation, many people see medical transition as the only valid method of transition. Some will go so far as to claim that those who do not or do not want to medically transition are not actually transgender. This is inaccurate, transphobic, and cisnormative—assuming that everyone must be cisgender and/or conform to cisgender expectations of body. Transness is an identity, not an action.

I was transgender before I got top surgery, and I am still transgender now. Medical transition is not more valid than social transition, and the transness of those who do not or cannot medically transition is no less valid and should be no less respected. The expectation that every trans person will transition medically is harmful and inaccurate.

As with social transitioning, medical transitions do not all look the same. The agency of the trans person should always be considered first and foremost. As a result of harmful cisnormative standards, trans people have been restricted to specific paths of medical transition for decades. These do not work for everyone.

When I first began seeking access to top surgery, I was told I had to have been "presenting as my affirmed gender" for at least one year prior to getting top surgery. Much of the literature at the time also mandated that I undergo hormone therapy for at least one year prior to surgery. At the time, I was not sure if I wanted to take testosterone—then or ever—and this policy made it very difficult for me to attain top surgery because several therapists refused to write the required letter of support since I was not taking testosterone.

While some trans folks do not engage with hormones, many do and many find it lifesaving.

GENDER-AFFIRMING HORMONES

On June 3, 2015, I drove with a close friend to my old pediatrician's office with a rust-colored tile roof on Maple Avenue to see the doctor that I'd gone to ever since early childhood. This time, though, I was no longer a little kid. I'd just turned nineteen and had my testosterone prescription in hand.

I sat on the examiner's table with my pants around my ankles. The sanitary wax paper stuck to my bare legs as the nurse showed me what she was doing.

"Testosterone is a thick serum," she explained as she punctured the top of the tiny bottle. "Kind of like honey!" It looked like one of those miniature liquor bottles, but even smaller. "It takes a little while to draw up into the syringe. Just be patient."

"Okay," I said. My palms were sweaty now, also sticking to the paper I sat on.

"When you've got your dose, pull it out like this," she showed me the measuring line and then removed the needle from the little bottle. "You can get rid of air bubbles like this." She used her fingers to flick the body of the syringe. "The air bubbles will float to the top." I nodded.

"And then, it's time to inject! Are you ready?"

"Yes," I said, glancing at my friend who squeezed my hand and grinned. "Let's do it!"

The nurse cleaned a portion of my thigh with an alcohol swab and then swiftly injected the testosterone. It didn't hurt much—though I wasn't expecting it to. Just a small pinch like they always say. I selected a Minions Band-Aid and the nurse sent me on my way. My journey with testosterone had begun.

Hormone replacement therapy, often abbreviated as HRT, or sometimes as GAHT (Gender-Affirming Hormone Therapy), entails administering a cross hormone—one that is not produced at high concentrations during an individual's puberty. For folks assigned female at birth like me, this means testosterone (commonly abbreviated as T), and for folks assigned male at birth, an estrogen such as estradiol, progesterone, or another estrogen (commonly abbreviated as E). Taking a cross hormone causes an individual to go through either testosterone-driven puberty or estrogen-driven puberty.*

Hormones can be administered in a number of different ways:

Topical comes in either gels or creams that you spread on your body, typically daily. Many individuals who use this method experience

---

* You might notice that "testosterone-driven" and "estrogen-driven" puberty are used instead of what you might have expected: "male" or "boy's" puberty or "female" or "girl's" puberty. This is for two reasons. First, "male puberty" implies that those who undergo this process are men or male, which is not always the case. Trans women might undergo this type of puberty, and they are not men or male—trans women are women. Second, *male puberty* is not a very specific term. What does this mean? Does this mean a man going through puberty? Does this mean enlargement of genitalia associated with men? Does this mean the deepening of one's voice? Usually, it means testosterone-driven, and so that is the most accurate term to use.

slower effects of the hormone, which can be beneficial for those who want to ease into the process more gradually.

Injection is the method I use. This is probably the most common form of testosterone delivery and is usually the most affordable as well. Injections can also be a method of administering estrogen. Injections can be done at a variety of frequencies but are most commonly weekly or every other week in the United States. Injections are administered either subcutaneously (into subcutaneous fat, usually around the midsection/belly) or intramuscularly (into muscle, usually the thigh or buttocks).

Pellets of crystallized hormones (either testosterone or estradiol) the size of a grain of rice are surgically inserted beneath the skin by a doctor—usually several months apart, depending on the desired dosage and metabolism of the patient. The pellets slowly dissolve in the body, releasing the hormones over time. Individuals usually begin with another form such as injections or topicals and then graduate to pellets when their levels are consistent and stable.[1,2]

Oral pills are probably the most common form of estrogen administration. These pills function similarly to birth control pills; in fact, before HRT was more accessible to trans feminine folks, many would use birth control that was designed for cis women. This is not advisable, as individuals should always consult a doctor before beginning any kind of hormone therapy, but it is an important piece of trans history. A form of testosterone permitted for oral administration was approved in March 2019, but is significantly less commonly used among trans masculine individuals.[3–5]

BUT DON'T HORMONES CAUSE CANCER?

"Dude, I haven't gotten a pap smear yet." One of my close friends and I were driving from his home to a small town where I'd be giving a speech later that evening. He admitted this, chuckling to himself nervously.

"You're probably fine. But why not?" I replied.

"I don't want anyone up in my business down . . . down there. It freaks me out." I nodded. I have heard this from numerous trans friends, trans clients, and trans support group attendees. "I know I should, I want to take care of my body, I just...I can't do it," he said.

"That makes sense," I validated.

"What about you?" he asked me.

"I am due for my next one soon. I've gotten one once, as well."

"Where did you get it?"

"The same doctor that first prescribed me T. He works at—"

"He's a man? Is he a cis man?" Teddy asked, incredulous.

"Yeah, actually, come to think of it, every doctor who's had to do anything with my genitals recently has been a cis man."

"Wow," Teddy said, impressed. "I just couldn't imagine that. I'd be afraid of...assault. Or something else. I don't know." I nodded again, understanding. Trans people are twice as likely to experience sexual assault, so Teddy's fears weren't unfounded. I have read too many stories of inappropriate comments and unwarranted touching (sexual abuse) suffered by transgender patients at the hands of their doctors. Fear of doctors and their reactions to us, the potential for their abuse of us, and general medical transphobia has kept many of my friends away from seeking regular medical care.

"I have considered that risk, too. And sometimes it means I don't go. But at the end of the day, that means they win. And I hate that. If I want to get the care I need, I have to brave the transphobia. And so I treat the doctors the way they treat me: as a transaction. I'm not there to have them see my vagina and think I'm still me. I'm not there to prove to them I'm man enough. I'm just there so they can check to make sure I don't have cervical cancer."

Cancer, unfortunately, is a tragedy that can strike anyone anytime. But the common myth that taking exogenous hormones can "give you cancer" is exactly that, a myth. Little to no research supports this claim; however, it *is* common for trans individuals to avoid staying up-to-date with routine checkups that involve body parts not traditionally associated with their gender. I know a significant number of trans men who refuse to see a gynecologist for a routine pap smear or other checkups because either they are (validly) fearful of the doctor's reaction to their transness and body, or they do not want to confront their body parts themselves, or both. While research supporting the "testosterone causes cancer" argument is insignificant, there *is* robust research that supports increased health risks when care is difficult to access.[6,7,8]

> Transgender individuals experience discrimination and mistreatment in healthcare, including verbal harassment, denied services, violence, and more.[9]
>
> Trans folks who must educate their providers on what it means to be trans are four times less likely to seek care.[10]
>
> About 30 percent of trans folks delay care they need because of discrimination or fear of discrimination.[11]
>
> Trans women are more likely to experience being unhoused or being unemployed, reducing access to healthcare.[12]

GENDER-AFFIRMING SURGERY

The most well-known option in transition is likely surgery. In fact, many people will reduce all transness to surgery, which is inaccurate. When I first came out to my community over Facebook, a family friend texted me, "So are you going to get the surgery??"

Well…, I thought. *There are at least fourteen gender-affirming surgeries!* But of course, we know what she meant: she wanted to know if I was going to get surgery to change my genitals. A parent of a close friend put it even more directly: "Are you going to get a stick-on one??"

While genital surgery can be extremely affirming to some trans folks, it is by no means the only available or even most common surgery we undergo. (Regardless, knowledge of a person's transness is never an invitation to ask them about their genitals or other private medical information. But more on this later.)

Surgeries fall into categories roughly aligned with areas of the body, sometimes referred to as top, middle, and bottom surgeries.

Top Surgery

Top surgery is used by both trans masculine and trans feminine individuals to describe chest reconstruction surgery, though the term is less
common in the trans feminine community where *breast augmentation*
or simply *BA* is used more often. For trans masculine folks, surgery in
this area is a double mastectomy; for trans feminine individuals, it is the
aforementioned breast augmentation.

The most common top surgery for trans masculine individuals is a
double-incision mastectomy, most often with nipple grafts. As the name
implies, two incisions are made to excise the breast tissue, and the areo-
lae and nipples are resized and reattached. This is the surgery I received,
but there are several other methods that depend primarily on the size of
one's chest prior to surgery.

Top surgery for trans feminine folks is breast augmentation. A number of different techniques for breast augmentation exist, but the primary
distinguishing factor rests on the type of implant: silicone or saline. Scar-
ring for breast augmentation is often quite minimal and mostly unde-
tectable as the surgeon usually makes a small incision around the areola,
beneath the armpit, or in the breast crease, and uses this opening to
insert the implant beneath skin and muscle to create the breast shape.[13]

Middle Surgery

Though not a widely used label, middle surgery refers to the removal
of one's internal reproductive organs—and is a term that, to my knowledge, is only used in trans masculine spaces. This is because individuals
assigned male at birth do not usually have internal reproductive organs
that require a separate procedure for removal. Middle surgery for trans
masculine folks can include hysterectomy (removal of uterus), oophorec-
tomy (removal of ovaries), and salpingectomy (removal of fallopian tubes).
Many people undergo middle surgery as a release (spiritual or otherwise)
of one's assigned gender. Removal of these organs can also chemically aid
in medical transition due to the estrogen-producing function of ovaries
that can compete with prescribed exogenous testosterone. Some people
experience better results from the testosterone once their ovaries are
removed.

I have not chosen to undergo any of these, mostly because I have no active desire to. And I have not had any problems with my testosterone treatment or internal reproductive organs thus far.

During my first nationally televised interview in 2016, Lesley Stahl (she/her) asked me if I wanted to have kids. I laughed. "I'm nineteen," I'd answered. "I have no idea."

Nearly eight years later, I'm still not entirely sure. So I have not discarded the prospect of having children with my own body and would need these organs in order to do so. Though many trans men might feel a disconnect with their internal reproductive organs, I feel the opposite. My uterus and surrounding parts are symbolic of where I come from, and I cherish this. But this is just my own perspective and, like all demographics of people, transgender men are not a monolith.

Bottom Surgery

Bottom surgery is surgery to reconstruct genitalia. This is sometimes called *gender/sex reassignment surgery* or *genital reassignment surgery* but these are antiquated and/or inaccurate terms. Reconstruction of genitalia does not "reassign" gender identity; surgery is an affirmation of gender identity. I am a man whether or not I get bottom surgery. If I do ever choose to undergo that procedure, that will be an act of affirmation, not an act of reassignment.

For trans masculine folks, bottom surgery usually includes a vaginectomy (removal and sealing of the vaginal cavity) and testicular implants, in addition to some type of phallus construction.

The two primary types of bottom surgery for trans masculine folks are metoidioplasty (often abbreviated "meta") and phalloplasty (abbreviated "phallo"). In both, the urethra is usually lengthened (urethroplasty) so that the individual can urinate from the end of the phallus and standing up, and most commonly, the labia majora are fused to create scrotum with testicular implants (scrotoplasty).

The distinguishing factor between the two types of bottom surgery is the construction of the phallus. In a metoidioplasty, the phallus is constructed from the hormone-enlarged clitoris and will be approximately four to six centimeters in its final form, while in a phalloplasty, the phallus is constructed using a large skin graft from the patient's forearm, thigh, abdomen, or back, and will be approximately the size of an average phallus.

If trans feminine folks decide to undergo bottom surgery, they most likely will undergo a vaginoplasty, which also usually includes an orchiectomy—removal of the testicles. Though this surgery has many iterations, the most commonly performed is a penile inversion vaginoplasty where the penile shaft is inverted and used to create the vaginal cavity. (I first learned of this technique while attending a talk by Marci Bowers [she/her], the first trans woman to perform this surgery on other trans people. It was amazing—what a genius concept to simply invert what is already there to create what someone needs! And another testament to how truly incredible, adaptive, and flexible our bodies are.)

Facial Surgery

Facial surgeries are most commonly accessed by trans feminine folks, although there are some versions that trans masculine folks undergo. These surgeries are usually grouped together and referred to as facial feminization surgery (FFS) or facial masculinization surgery (FMS). FFS can include forehead contouring (usually a reduction), cheek augmentation, rhinoplasty (changing the shape of the nose), lip augmentation, jaw contouring, chin surgery, chondrolaryngoplasty (a "tracheal shave"), and more. FMS often includes a similar set of surgeries with alterations to create a more classically "masculine" look.

HOW DO I TALK TO TRANS PEOPLE ABOUT THEIR SURGERIES?

I cannot count the times I've been asked, "Schuyler, what if I'm curious about a trans person's surgical journey? When is it appropriate for me to ask, and how?"

While I'm grateful for the foresight to ask me this question instead of just asking every trans person about their surgical journeys, it is also a frustrating question to receive. I usually take a deep breath before I offer the following response:

"May I ask you a question?" The individual is almost always a bit surprised but nods.

"Great. Thank you!" I'll say, "I'm curious if you ask random strangers for their medical histories or what their genitals look like?" The individual's initial surprise grows far larger.

"What?" they'll answer, incredulously.

"Well, I'm just curious—you asked me when you are allowed to ask trans people about our genitals and so I'm asking you if you ask other people about their genitals—"

"No, I said surgery—" If they're thoughtful, that's usually when they'll pause and realize. "Oh..."

"Exactly." I'll smile and say gently: "When you ask trans people about our surgeries, we all know what you really mean. You're effectively asking us the same question. It's very invasive, inappropriate, and none of your business. Yes, you're welcome to be curious, but you must also remember that your curiosity doesn't mean you deserve an answer."

They usually nod aggressively in embarrassed agreement.

Asking trans people about their surgeries is inappropriate and rude, unless the conversation was invited by the trans person. Curiosity does not necessitate an answer. If you are curious, great! Be curious! Then go do some research or read a book like this instead of burdening the trans people in your life.

CHAPTER 5

Pronouns—and Why They Are So Important!

I N 2021, FORMER FOX NEWS PERSONALITY TUCKER CARLSON (he/him) declared that "the pronoun thing" would appeal to people who "still believe in destroying nature's gender roles."[1] He has also claimed that he would "be forced to participate [in using gender-neutral pronouns] at gunpoint."

Not surprisingly, no cases have been documented involving trans people holding cis people at gunpoint in order to respect us appropriately, much less gender us correctly. There are, however, countless reports of cis people holding trans people at gunpoint because they are resistant to us, and *then firing said gun*, murdering us.

Carlson also said that pronoun choice was "a war on nature," but let's not forget that none of the gender roles we employ or adhere to commonly are made by or even *in* "nature." You might know that Tucker Carlson wore a suit and tie every time he appeared on television. He sported a short haircut. Most people could consider these "men's clothing" and a "men's haircut." And he easily adhered to it.

Note that nature did not create this standard. Nature did not decree that men must cut their hair short, wear suits and ties, and be called he/him pronouns. If anything, clothing himself in artificial fibers, shortening his hair with man-made metal shears or an electric razor, and, of course, appearing on national television via the internet through metal boxes and devices we call cameras and computers is unnatural—none of these implements or tools are found in nature.

This irony aside, nature has shown us that gender and gender expression come in vastly varied forms. Take a quick stroll through Euro-colonialist history: in King Louis XIV's royal court, the men rivaled the women in their elaborate wigs, high heels, and makeup. Even recent history contradicts what is "normal" today. Up until shortly before World War I, pink was considered a "masculine" color because it was a more "decided and stronger color," while blue was considered "more delicate and dainty" and therefore for a girl.[2] Gender roles are made by humans, not by nature.

And pronouns could not possibly destroy these gender roles.

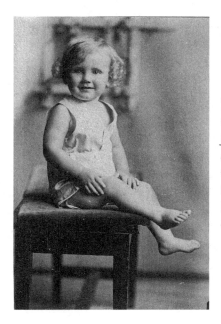

This is my grandfather, a cisgender straight man, when he was a toddler. This photo was framed and hung in my grandparents' home and my brother and I always giggled at how much we thought Grandpa looked like a little girl. "That was how they dressed little boys back then!" Grandpa would explain to us, chuckling as well.

The conversation about pronouns, however, has certainly incited massive anger and pushback—some people lashing out in hatred, many others just not understanding. People often wonder why sharing pronouns is so important: don't people know that Sabrina is a woman and that Jerry is a man? Perhaps Sabrina is a woman, and perhaps Jerry is a man. But that doesn't mean you can always assume what pronouns they use because gender expression—commonly dictated by gender roles—does not always align with gender identity. We cannot always tell someone's identity and pronouns simply by how they look.

Maybe you've heard someone say, "This is ridiculous, why do these Gen Zers care so much about pronouns?" Maybe you've heard people call us "sensitive snowflakes," or maybe you've even had a few similar thoughts yourself.

Well, I hear you. But please don't bail just yet.

Pronouns are not nearly as complicated as they are sometimes made out to be. Pronouns are just words that can replace the subject of a sentence—they are used to refer to people without having to repeat their names, such as "she" and "they." I use he/him pronouns. Someone might refer to me using my name: "Schuyler is transgender." But they could also replace my name with the correct pronoun: "He is transgender."

In English, we use gendered pronouns to refer to individuals, but in many other languages like Korean, Farsi, and spoken Mandarin, pronouns are not gendered. In these languages, there is often a single gender-neutral pronoun. In addition to pronouns causing "a war on nature," Carlson has also claimed that using gender-neutral pronouns makes language "dumber, less precise, and embarrassing." Is Carlson implying that all languages lacking gendered pronouns are dumber, less precise, and embarrassing? Surely, not!

In any case, because English includes gendered pronouns, calling trans people the right pronouns can be a key part of affirming and respecting who we are.

MISGENDERING

The first, simplest, and most effective way to say, "I see you," to a trans person is to call them by the right name and pronouns, always. Referring to someone by the wrong gendered words is called *misgendering* and can often be a very painful experience for a trans person.

"Get over it," I've heard so many people tell us. "It's just a word!" This is true and it also is incomprehensible.

First, I don't know many cisgender men who enjoy being referred to as women or cisgender women who enjoy being called men. In fact, most cisgender people are deeply offended when referred to as the wrong gender—in other words, cisgender people don't like to be misgendered, either!

Secondly, being trans already adds extra layers of difficulty. Many of us have spent our lives not being seen as who we truly are. Many of us experience discrimination, bullying, and taunting as a result of our identities. This makes being called the correct pronouns that much more affirming and being misgendered that much crueler. And because we all live in a transphobic society that concentrates power in the cisgender population, misgendering us only further reinforces this power dynamic and perpetuates systemic oppression against transgender individuals.

For these reasons, many trans folks experience misgendering as an act of violence. Let's lean into this with a simple example: If I am walking with my wife and I accidentally step on my wife's toe and break her toe, it doesn't matter if I meant to or not. Her toe is broken because I stepped on it. If this happened, I would immediately apologize and then take any action I could to remedy the situation—carry her to a nearby place to sit and take her to the nearest hospital or doctor, as necessary. Stepping on her toe was literally violent: it broke her bone! But it doesn't mean that I am a cruel person with violent intentions. It means I made a mistake and caused harm for which I should take responsibility.

In the same vein, misgendering someone can cause them a great deal of pain, regardless of intention. For some folks, unintentional misgendering can be even more painful because it can often come from someone we love or who we assume loves us—whereas intentional misgendering is usually perpetuated by people we've already steeled ourselves against. This unexpected, unintentional misgendering can say more loudly than you'd like: "I don't see you for who you are. I see you for who *I* think you are. I see you under the gender binary that I was taught and not for who you've told me you are."

DEADNAMING

"Why didn't you change your name?" A student from Brookline High School, just outside of Boston, scribbled this on a note card that was handed to me onstage. I read it a few times. *Why didn't I change my name?*

Many trans folks change their names when they learn of their transness and come out. This can be an incredibly affirming and empowering process, a way to declare one's knowing of oneself to the world.

My parents chose the name Schuyler for me before I was born. When I was in middle school and presenting my gender in a very ambiguous way, I was bullied a lot for how I looked and how I acted. Many people would default to gendering me as male, but others were just confused. I was often asked, "So are you a boy or a girl?" More times than I could count, other kids asked me about my genitals as a way of verifying my gender because they didn't believe what I said. So eventually, I stopped answering the question and I'd answer, "I'm just Schuyler." My name felt like the best and most accurate representation of myself at the time. So, having no other words to describe my gender and my gender journey to others, my name was who I was.

For this reason, I have not changed my name, nor have I ever considered doing so. This is not the case for the majority of trans folks, who *do* change their names.[3] Despite not sharing the experience of a changed name, I empathize deeply with the power a name can wield—and the empowerment when we wield the name as truly our own.

Deadname refers to the name someone was given or used before they transitioned and/or discovered their true gender identity. This term is an adjustment to the term *birth name*, because these names are not felt as a birth or a start of anything, but rather an ending. To many trans folks, their old names are dead to them. *Deadname* can also be used as a verb, and for some trans folks, when deadnamed, or called their deadname, a small part of them dies. Some trans folks do refer to their deadnames as *birth names* or *old names*, and I strongly recommend reflecting back the language that a person uses for themselves unless otherwise instructed.

Both misgendering and deadnaming can reignite a history of pain and trauma for trans folks. These are often reminders of living a life as someone we are not, potentially of years of pretending and hiding and not ever feeling known by others.

USING PRONOUNS

"I noticed when you introduced yourself that you said, 'I use he/him pronouns,'" she said, confused. "But you are clearly a man. So why did you do that? I understand that you've, you know…that you're a transgender…person. But you look like a man now! I mean, you *are* a man. Why did you say 'he/him'?"

This question comes in many forms. This particular version is probably of the gentler and more well-meaning variety—albeit stumbling and precarious. A participant at a workshop asked me this a few years ago, and the image stood out in my mind because of how affirming she'd been. She'd begun with profusely complimenting my presentation, and even my appearance. I had thanked her before she'd offered this question.

Sometimes the question comes with strong resistance and anger: "Everyone knows I'm a man! I don't have to tell them my pronouns!"

In short, gendered pronouns and other gendered words are far more nuanced than the strict "this is a boy" and "this is a girl" boxes we were given. Not offering pronouns implies that other folks should either intuit or know your gender simply from how you look. This perpetuates two false assumptions: first, that everyone's social constructions of gender expression are the same and, second, that gender expression always indicates gender identity.

Sharing pronouns not only aims to dismantle both these assumptions, but also creates a safer space for trans and gender nonconforming folks to share our pronouns and be gendered correctly, too.

Gender Expression ≠ Gender Identity

Consider this: no one goes around assuming every person who "looks male" is named Matthew. That is, we don't walk up to every masculine-presenting person and say, "Hi, Matthew!" unless we know their name is Matthew. We usually ask, "What's your name?" We can apply the same logic to pronouns.

Note that these considerations are mostly aimed at cisgender people. If you're trans and/or non-binary and don't know your pronouns yet, or are not comfortable sharing them, or aren't out, that's absolutely okay. Take your time figuring this out. Cis folks, you should be sharing your pronouns. Trans folks, take your time and do what you'd like.

Lastly, recognize that the practice of sharing and respecting pronouns in a gendered language benefits everyone. I know many cisgender people who have gender-neutral names or even names that are traditionally used for a gender they aren't. Including pronouns in one's email signature or Instagram bio can help mitigate being misgendered for anyone.

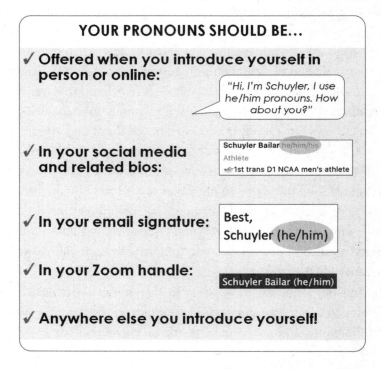

YOUR PRONOUNS SHOULD BE...

✓ **Offered when you introduce yourself in person or online:**

"Hi, I'm Schuyler, I use he/him pronouns. How about you?"

✓ **In your social media and related bios:**

Schuyler Bailar he/him/his
Athlete
1st trans D1 NCAA men's athlete

✓ **In your email signature:**

Best,
Schuyler (he/him)

✓ **In your Zoom handle:**

Schuyler Bailar (he/him)

✓ **Anywhere else you introduce yourself!**

THEY/THEM PRONOUNS

During one of the many speeches I have given over Zoom, a middle-aged person with long wavy brown hair raised a hand to ask a question.

"Thank you for your speech, Schuyler," she started with a smile after sharing her name and pronouns. "So I understand that you are a man now. And—well, people call you that..." She trailed off. I nodded and waited, patiently.

"Well, so, I understand that...you know, people called you 'she' but now 'he.'" She tried again.

"Yes," I said, anticipating the next question.

"But what about people using 'they'? I just find it so *hard*. It's not grammatically correct and I'm from a different generation than you are. So it's hard for me."

This is one of the most common questions I receive.

First, it's extremely likely that you have already used they/them pronouns to refer to a single individual. Consider the following scenario: You're walking down the street and you see a wallet on the ground. What will you say? I bet you will exclaim, "Someone lost their wallet!" using they/them pronouns without hesitation. That "someone" is a *single* person whose gender you do not know. Many people reject using they/them pronouns for a single individual because they believe it to be awkward or grammatically incorrect, failing to see that they likely use they/them pronouns all the time.

Colloquial use aside, using they/them pronouns to refer to a single individual is, actually, grammatically correct. The *Merriam-Webster* dictionary includes three main definitions for *they*. Use case 3d reads, "Used to refer to a single person whose gender identity is nonbinary."[4] *Merriam-Webster* even declared *they* the Word of the Year in 2019.[5–7] This followed the American Dialect Society naming *they* the Word of the Year in 2015[8] and the Word of the Decade for the 2010s.[9] You might be thinking, *So, it's new!* but this is only partially true. According to the *Oxford English Dictionary*, *they* has been used as a singular pronoun since the fourteenth century, about a century after the plural *they* appeared in English.[10]

And even if the singular *they* was brand new, you might consider that updating language is a common practice. Words like *bad*, *sick*, and *wicked* have evolved and expanded in use—once only negative, these are often used to connote positivity. Thousands of other new words and phrases have appeared in the English language and been added into dictionaries, adopted as common vernacular in the past few decades. Just in September of 2022, *Merriam-Webster* added 370 new words—such as *laggy, janky, cringe, metaverse,* and *greenwash.*

That is, while the this-is-new-so-it's-wrong feeling is understandable, newness is not a valid reason to disregard change, and even less a valid reason to disrespect someone. Yes, change is hard, and yes, you can call someone they/them pronouns.

Other new words you might have seen include *ze/zir/zirs, xe/xir/xirs, ze/zim/zis,* or *fae/faer/faers.* These are newer pronouns—hence deemed *neopronouns*—and are used in the same way that other pronouns are used.

"But these are made-up words!" Yes. Every word—literally every single word you use—is made-up. As we've discussed, that is what language is: a conglomeration of sounds (deemed "phonemes" when used to create words) humans have invented and agreed to mean something in order to communicate with each other.

"This is made-up" is not a valid excuse for disrespecting someone's pronouns. Unfamiliarity with a certain convention can explain difficulty adopting it, but discomfort should not prevent you from doing so. You can do hard things.

Similarly, difficulty is not a valid reason to not use neopronouns for someone who uses them. I know people who default to using they/them pronouns for people who use neopronouns and this is no different from deciding to give someone an English name when you find their ethnic name too difficult to pronounce. My brother's name is Jinwon, pronounced like the alcohol "gin" and the number "one." He has encountered numerous people who instead call him "Jinny," or even "John."

Unfortunately, this erasure is common for folks with non-Western names—and this practice is racist and lazy. The same is true for failing to use people's correct pronouns, no matter how new they are to you. Practice and incorporate. If we can learn how to use new words like *retweet* or *FaceTime,* then we can learn to use new pronouns.

Following are a few examples for using gender-neutral pronouns.

Ze/zir/zirs: **Ze** drove **zir** car to the store to buy **zirself** groceries.
Xe/xir/xirs: **Xe** drove **xir** car to the store to buy **xirself** groceries.
Ze/zim/zis: **Ze** drove **zis** car to the store to buy **zimself** groceries.
Fae/faer/faers: **Fae** drove **faer** car to the store to buy **faerself** groceries.

Please note that this is not a comprehensive list of neopronouns. There are many more. If you meet someone who uses a pronoun you've never heard of, spend some time educating yourself on how best to use it.

CORRECTING YOURSELF

I remember a particular moment when I was sitting in the kitchen with my mother who was puttering around. She said something about me and accidentally referred to me as "she," and then realizing her mistake, smacked the table in exasperation and said, "Oh my gosh, *he!*" She paused, a bit dramatically, and then said again, "*He.*" She apologized profusely and tried to explain that she was thinking of me from before and had a different image of me. Her explanation was long and while I understood her intention, I felt very uncomfortable. I just wanted the moment to end and for us to move on.

We were later able to have a more productive conversation wherein I asked her not to make such a big deal when she made a mistake.

"It's okay, I understand that you're going to take time to shift. Just correct yourself quickly, say 'sorry,' and move on, please. I don't need any big apologies or anything," I'd said.

Since then, I've watched many people make similar mistakes: big, dramatic apologies, loud and over-the-top corrections with the correct pronouns, etc. I understand that people believe that they are showing the trans person how bad they feel for misgendering them and how they might not have "meant to" do so, but the intention does not often land in these scenarios. The impact is usually the opposite of the desired effect: this method centers the guilt of the misgenderer and not the pain of the person misgendered. When my mom did this, I felt I had to take care of her and tell her everything was okay and that I was okay and could we please just move on. When people make these extravagant apologies, they make the moment about themselves. Don't do this.

It's also important to note that these types of apologies could draw attention to the misgendering in a public scenario, possibly outing the trans person. In reality, we all flub our words here and there. Cis people misgender cis people by accident, and it's not usually a big deal. If you're in a group, I strongly encourage you to simply correct and move on, unless otherwise instructed by the trans person.

If you find yourself consistently misgendering or deadnaming someone, it's time to practice.

Here are some places to start:

- Write about the five most memorable experiences you've shared with the individual using the correct pronouns.
- Every time you misgender them, gender them correctly three times in three different ways. (E.g., "*He* is going to the store to get *his* groceries because they are necessary to *him*.") Do not do this in the person's presence; do this on your own or in your head.
- Correct yourself in your head, always. Even if that person is not around.
- Do some soul-searching on your own gender. Seeing someone else's gender correctly might require the release or deconstruction of societal constraints, boxes, or expectations of man- or womanhood.
- Investigate why it's hard to call this individual the correct pronouns:
  » You might be embarrassed. If this is the case, read *Daring Greatly* by Brené Brown (she/her) and start to build some shame resilience.
  » You might see this individual only as who you want them to be instead of who they actually are. This is where some of that soul-searching could be beneficial. You might consider talking through your feelings about who you want this person to be or

who you thought they would be with a trusted friend, a therapist, or a family member—but not the individual themselves.

ASKING FOR PRONOUNS

"I understand that pronouns are important. If I don't know someone's pronouns, what is the best way to ask for them?"

When I am asked this question (and I get asked it a lot), I often encourage the question-asker and the audience to reflect a bit: "Whose pronouns do you not know? Whose are you automatically assuming based on how they look? Are you only thinking of asking the one person in the room who 'looks trans,' or whose gender presentation confuses you?"

When asking for pronouns, we should never single out one person who confuses us and ask them. This is othering and inappropriate. And, learning someone's pronouns doesn't have to come only from directly asking. The simplest way to prompt someone for their pronouns is to offer yours.

"Hi, I'm Schuyler. I use he/him pronouns. How about you?" When someone introduces themselves this way, most people will respond by mirroring the information provided. I always encourage people to introduce themselves with their pronouns regardless of whether or not they are trying to figure out a specific individual's pronouns; this normalizes the practice, reminding ourselves and others that we cannot always tell someone's pronouns simply by how they look.

If you've already introduced yourself and/or names are already known, you can still reintroduce with your pronouns. This might sound like, "I don't think I shared my pronouns when I introduced myself. I use he/him. How about you?" or, "Hi! I don't think I caught your pronouns—I use he/him. How about you?" You might choose to do this in a quieter moment and not in the middle of a group so as not to call one person out. I strongly discourage asking for a specific individual's pronouns openly in a group setting. This could be very uncomfortable for that person, and even risks outing them.

If you are unsuccessful in learning someone's pronouns after trying all these methods, I advise avoiding pronouns until you know them and instead use just the person's name.

"THIS VIOLATES FREE SPEECH"

Despite the simplicity of offering pronouns, powerful people have taken a stance against "made-up words" and refuse to use people's proper pronouns as a result. Some of them claim that being "forced" to use an individual's correct pronouns infringes on free speech. This is wildly irresponsible and careless; it is also an inaccurate view of free speech.

When people in the United States reference "free speech," they are usually evoking the First Amendment (whether they know it or not), which states, "Congress shall make no law [...] abridging the freedom of speech." Among many things, freedom of speech includes the right to *not* speak (specifically, the right to not salute the flag), the right to advertise commercial products and professional services (with some restrictions), and the right to engage in symbolic speech (e.g., burning the flag in protest). The Supreme Court has found that freedom of speech does *not* include the right to incite imminent lawless action, to make or distribute obscene materials, or of students to advocate illegal drug use at a school-sponsored event. However, on June 30, 2023, the Supreme Court ruled that a Christian web designer was allowed to refuse LGBTQ+ customers service on the basis of "freedom of speech." For the first time in its history, the Court granted "a business open to the public a constitutional right to refuse to serve members of a protected class."[11] This devastating ruling is the alt-right's continued attempt to pervert "freedom of speech" for power and control, including in the highest court in the country.

In a 2016 debacle that gained international attention, University of Toronto psychology professor Jordan Peterson (he/him) refused to use students' pronouns, claiming that this violated his right to free speech. He continued to spread this message widely and ferociously, certain that this was the government's first steps toward authoritarianism: "I've studied authoritarianism for a very long time," he said. "For 40 years—and they're started by people's attempts to control the ideological and linguistic territory," he told the BBC in a 2016 interview.[12]

Peterson's characterization misses several major facts. First, Canada (along with many other governments with a colonial history) has already oppressed through authoritarianism—and the Indigenous peoples, including their acceptance and reverence of trans people, suffered greatly due to colonial attempts to control Indigenous ideological and linguistic territory. And second, no government's downfall came from demanding people respect one another—if anything, tyrannical governments thrive on active discrimination against a group of people, segmenting community and destroying unity. Third, and perhaps most importantly, the right to say whatever you'd like is always reserved for you at home and in your personal life. When you enter public spaces—or even private spaces that you do not own, such as a university—you must abide by the rules of those spaces. That is not an infringement on free speech; it's a rule in a space you do not own. In Canada, one such "rule" is Bill C-16, which includes gender identity and expression under the protections of the Canadian Human Rights Act, extending hate speech provisions under Canada's criminal code to trans folks.[13]

This dangerous and manipulative twisting of "free speech" has garnered thousands of supporters. But at the heart of free speech rhetoric is one's own agency—they argue that they should be allowed to use the words they want to describe others—isn't that "free speech" after all? No, not exactly—telling someone else who they are through using incorrect pronouns is not about your self-expression, your own identity, or your beliefs. It's about disregarding, demeaning, and controlling another person. In reality, respecting someone else's identity and calling them the pronouns they've requested centers on recognizing another person's self-determination and the ability to self-express—and costs you nothing.

CHAPTER 6

How Do People Know If They're Transgender?

ONE MORNING DURING THE SECOND MONTH OF MY STAY AT the residential eating disorder treatment facility, I was on my way to the therapy center. I was wearing my "man jeans"—the one pair of jeans I had bought from the men's section at the time. They had a tie-dyed pattern of aqua blue and light green. I looked down at my lap and legs as we drove and felt overwhelmingly negative toward my body. I tried to use the coping mechanisms my therapist had taught me about body disconnection and body dissatisfaction.

Why am I feeling this way? I asked myself. I also tried an affirmation, reminding myself that there was nothing wrong with my body. I thought about all that my body does for me and began repeating gratitude statements.

But then a question began burning in the back of my mind. *What if I don't like how I look because I don't look like a man?* And in that moment, my stomach turned and everything sank. I knew.

This knowing was a mapping of language and articulation to feeling—a feeling I'd had for as long as I could remember gender, one that had been nebulous until that moment. If I was honest with myself then, I knew unequivocally that I am transgender.

Over the coming years, I'd realize that this feeling and knowing was not situated in my jeans and how they fit me. Contrary to popular belief about us, being transgender is not solely about one's body and one's physicality. For many, including myself, being transgender is a spiritual, emotional, as well as physical experience.

Of course, realizing that I was transgender in that moment did not immediately translate into words or declaration of identity. It most definitely did not mean I was ready for disclosure or teaching others about my experience. Like most of us, I needed time to let my brain catch up to my heart. In the coming months, I would meet more trans people, go to a few more gender workshops, and spend time digesting what it would mean to claim my truth for myself . . . and then in front of others. In finding community, I would continue to accumulate the language to understand and explain myself—something I am deeply grateful for today.

While some trans people feel that coming out is discovering a completely new part of themselves, for a majority of trans people, "coming out" is less a process of becoming something new than an unearthing of a part of ourselves we've buried, finally finding the words to express who we've always been.

When I came out as transgender, I did not become a new person. I did not become transgender. I did not change who I was. Instead, I found the language, courage, and resources to share who I've always been. I have always been transgender and I've always been a boy. I just haven't always been able to express this to myself and the world.

Usually, when I state this and perhaps go on to explain that my manhood is not defined by my genitals, my mannerisms, or my physical nature, many folks will respond with questions similar to that of the tall, curly-haired man after one of my very first speeches: "Well, what *does* being a man mean to you, then? How do you *know* you're a man?"

When I am teaching, I work diligently to hear curiosity in this question, but it's crucial to understand that while most do not intend malice or invalidation by asking this question, intent does not bar impact.

Asking a trans person to describe their understanding of their gender usually comes across as demanding we *defend* ourselves and is often a microaggression.

A cis person asking a trans person to define their personhood for them can feel incredibly invalidating because it implies, "I don't believe you. Your declaration of yourself and your gender is not enough for me. You must explain and prove to me the validity of your gender."

I have never met a cis person who demands other cis people verify their man- or womanhood. (Except, of course, when they think a cis person is trans and interrogate them as if they were trans.) In contrast, I don't think I've met a single trans person who has *not* been asked to do so. No one asks cis people, "Why are you cisgender?" Meanwhile, trans people are almost never granted the space to know ourselves simply by knowing. Instead, we are repeatedly demanded to explain, prove, and validate something we simply know to be true in our hearts. This is something I encourage cis folks to consider.

Microaggressions also most often reinforce systems of oppression—racialized hierarchies, the gender binary, socioeconomic strata, and so on. Given that cisgender folks are a dominant identity group, a cisgender person demanding a trans person's explanation of the very thing that marginalizes them perpetuates that system of oppression. Though not the "fault" of the cisgender question-asker, the existence of this power dynamic cannot be ignored. It is the responsibility of the cisgender person to recognize it and carefully consider its impact.

When I am asked how I know I am transgender, I employ the same line of questioning as I do when people ask me how I know I am a man without a penis—I just know.

Explaining this further is difficult. In the beginning of my gender-affirmation journey, I had not yet developed a resistance to the transphobic assumptions the world had fed me, and so I decided that I could not truly be transgender if I could not defend my transness well.

I don't know why I am not a girl—I don't know how or what systems have resulted in my being this way, so it must not be real, I told myself. My biology says 'female'—how do I explain what I can't comprehend?

LATE ONE NIGHT in 2014, I found myself on a website filled with information targeting trans men.

"Trans 'men' are really just abused girls with eating disorders who hate their bodies. There is no such thing as trans," the article read. At the time, I lay wide awake in my rehab dorm in my fourth month of eating disorder treatment. Reading this crushed me. *Am I just a "messed up woman"? Am I really a man or do I just "hate my body"?* Almost a decade later, I can still see the web page so clearly in my mind.

For weeks after, I used this logic against myself. Despite not hating my body, I couldn't figure out how to justify my identity in a way that I felt would make sense to the people who wrote that article. So instead, I invalidated myself using everyone else's tools of transphobia. As you might expect, this neither changed how I felt about or what I knew of my identity, nor improved my quality of life.

After several painful months, I realized that maybe it didn't matter.

What if *I* am *just making it all up?* I thought to myself. *And so what? I don't think this is made-up—millions of other people are also transgender—but let's just pretend for a moment that I am. That this isn't real. So what? Who do I hurt?*

This brought me to the most powerful realization of all: It does not matter if I can justify my manhood in words that others will accept. I know that living my life in this way is far better for my mental health, for my very survival, than how I was living before. And in some ways, it's that simple.

As I've continued along my path, I've also learned that my early attempts to justify my manhood used parameters that were already designed to disenfranchise and exclude people whose gender did not conform to the Euro-colonial gender binary: transphobic biology, studies done exclusively by cis people about mostly cis people, through misogynistic and patriarchal lenses.

I know I am transgender because I feel this to be true in my heart—the same way that someone might know that they love the person they have married, or that they love the ocean and the mountains. These are types of intrinsic knowing that no one else can take from me. Allowing myself to realize this, accept it, and then share it with the world demanded the privilege of language and support, as well as perhaps the most crucial factor: trusting myself.

Cisgender folks trust their feelings about their genders so thoroughly that they almost never doubt their gender. They never ask themselves, "Am I actually cisgender?" I encourage cisgender people or those who have never wondered about the validity of their gender to ask yourself this question: *How do I know I am not transgender? How do I know I am the gender I was assigned?*

You need not ask this question with judgment or ire. Ask it with childlike curiosity. How do you know?

Investigating your own gender and reminding yourself that you, too, have a gender and a gender experience are crucial parts of stepping into this journey with us. Here are a few points to help you introspect:

- Remember there is no singular narrative of what it means to be a trans person. Gender (regardless of how society wants to box it) is not binary—it's a spectrum, a continuum.
- Remember that no one else truly has the power to tell you who you are or how you are most comfortable. Only you can know and declare that. This can be scary and difficult. In a world that prescribes us our gender (and a lot of other facets of our identities) without much consent, granting ourselves even a hair of freedom to choose—or even just to wonder—calls for a realm of possibility that many have yet to explore.
- Disrupt your certainty of your own gender—trans people aren't the only people who can question their own identities. Ask yourself: *What if I'm not a man/woman? How do I know I'm a man/woman? What does being a man or woman mean to me? What gendered messaging did I receive as a kid?* You might find that the answer to this last one is either very little or none at all: *What gender-neutral messaging did I receive?*

- Invest in who you are outside of other pressures. Who are you and who do you *want* to be when the lights go off at the end of the day and you're alone with your thoughts in bed? Don't focus only on your body and its shape or your genitals or your hormones. That's only a fraction of this. Ask yourself the questions that pull at your heart, that disturb you: *Who am I inside? What will make me live the happiest, most authentic life? When have I felt the most like myself and what contributed to that feeling? If nothing else could stop me—if other pressures didn't exist, how would I present myself? How would I live my life and carry myself? What would make me happy?* Take your family, your sport, your significant other, your peers, everyone, out of the equation, just for a moment. What would you do just for you? I always imagined myself on an island alone, trying to survive on my own, just as me. Who did I see? I always saw myself as a man. Of course, this line of questioning works for more than just gender, but try to focus on gender for a little while. See what insights emerge.
- Consult your younger self. I always choose my eight-year-old self because I think he knew a lot about who he was, and his knowing wasn't yet hindered by all that the world told him he had to be. Think about who your younger self imagined you to become. Who have you always dreamed of growing up to be? What would your younger self think of you today? Why?
- Remember that the questions are often more important than the answers. This might sound strange, but if you keep asking and wondering about the questions, you'll eventually stumble into the answers. Don't rush. Most of us are taught that chaos and confusion are bad and should quickly be resolved and/or left behind, but unsettled states are actually where we can learn the most. Work to appraise confusion as good—as exploration without judgment.

Ultimately, the singular question you're asking is: *What makes me feel the most like myself and what barriers do I experience to accessing this feeling?*

If you don't know the answers or if your answers waver, that's okay. Take your time. Learning about your own gender—regardless of whether or not you are transgender—can be an exhausting experience.

Liberation from the gender binary in which we've all been placed is challenging and takes time, energy, and a lot of healing.

Gender Dysphoria: Being Transgender Is Not a Mental Illness

I RAN INSIDE WITH THE OTHER BOYS, SWEATY AND PANTING. Though hurrying down the hallway in a sea of kids, I was alone for a moment in my own world of joy from the game. I'd finally earned enough respect as the only "girl" who played football during recess. I'd caught a few tough passes, even scoring my first touchdown and surprising the other guys. I had spent countless recesses over the years never being picked for a team unless our PE teacher forced them to include me. Recently, I'd been picked voluntarily because Riker Samson (he/him) knew I could catch. And this recess I'd finally been picked not-last and even trusted during some important plays.

Caught up in my thoughts, I didn't realize that I wasn't walking alone anymore.

"Are you wearing a bra?" Stella Murphy (she/her) said loudly as she walked in step with me. She stared obviously at my chest. I didn't look down. I knew I didn't want to see what was there.

When I'd noticed with horror that the two little bumps had started growing a few months prior, I hadn't told anyone. I'd just started wearing the tight athletic long-sleeved shirts beneath my T-shirts, no matter the weather. *This'll do until I can get them to stop growing*, I'd thought. Most of the other guys also wore these shirts, they just didn't double layer them. This was far better than telling my mother my breasts were finally growing and having to wear a bra.

"You need to wear a bra," Stella said without letting me answer her original question. I didn't know what to say. I stood, staring at my hands.

"I—I—" I started. "I am wearing this underneath," I tugged at the end of the white long sleeve around my wrist. "It's tight," I offered.

"What? That doesn't work. You need a bra." And with that, she ran off. It was time for class.

I have never forgotten that moment. I can remember the musty smell of the hallway, the sounds of the other kids running inside, the bright windows that looked onto the field where I'd just been happily playing. Most of all, I remember the stomach-dropping feeling her words gave me, and how I stood there, utterly embarrassed and horrified, not knowing how else to proceed.

When I got home that night, I finally told my mother. I cried as I shared that Stella said I needed a bra, but I didn't want one. I didn't want breasts at all.

If I had had the words, I would have said I was experiencing gender dysphoria.

Gender dysphoria is the distress or discomfort that can arise from the incongruence between gender assigned at birth and gender identity. Gender dysphoria, which can be shortened to just *dysphoria*, is often experienced physically with regards to parts of one's body that are traditionally gendered, including chest, voice, hips, facial structure, and body hair.

The first time I noticed my breasts forming is vivid in my memory. For readers who also have breasts that grew during puberty, you might remember them itching and sometimes even hurting as they budded. For me, this pain came with a deep sense of dread—one that I still can feel today when I think of that time. This dread said: *these do not belong here.* They felt foreign and unwanted—a puberty I did not consent to.

Then, I was not able to express why or what exactly it was that I felt. In its rawest form, it was terror. I was so certain I did not want them and yet they still came, my body seemingly betraying me. Late at night, I would press on the little bumps until they hurt. *If I could damage them*, I thought, *maybe they'll stop growing.*

When others ask what gender dysphoria feels like to me, this is my defining memory. However, it's important to understand that not every trans person experiences gender dysphoria, or experiences it in the same manner. People may explain their experiences differently and with varying degrees of intensity. For some, dysphoria causes a sense of disconnection or dissociation from one's body. For others, it's a nagging that can be deeply unsettling when constant.

Here's one analogy: Dysphoria is like a rock in your shoe that's always been there. You get used to it, but it hurts and is bothersome. Something is always off. When that rock is finally removed, it is so relieving. You realize a new baseline: *Ah*, this *is what it's like for others*. This *is what I've been searching for.*

DYSPHORIA—A COMPLICATED DEBATE ROOTED IN TRANSPHOBIA

Some people assert that gender dysphoria is the basis of trans identity— that, in order to be transgender, an individual must experience gender dysphoria. This is referred to as the "trans medicalist" argument—and often also considers transness itself a mental illness or a pathology. Others use the label *trans* to describe themselves but report that they do not experience dysphoria. Over the years, this debate has created tension within the trans community, with people vehemently taking sides.

If you are not trans, you might wonder why people within the trans community have found themselves at a place of division. The answer is transphobia—internalized and systemic. At the core of the trans medicalist argument is the belief that trans people will not receive care if we are not taken seriously in our declaration of our gender and our pain. In order to receive the care that we need as trans individuals, we must be medically diagnosed with gender dysphoria. This is the result of a transphobic system that has repeatedly denied us our rights, our autonomy, and our care, and is perpetuated by doctors who commit acts of transphobia, often seeking to invalidate our struggles. Maltreatment has led many of us to attempt to legitimize our identities using the same tools that are often used against us. In this case: psychiatry and the pathologization of identity.

As previously discussed, I first characterized my transness as many of my peers did: "I was born in the wrong body." I, too, had internalized that dysphoria was necessary to trans identity. Many trans people I interacted with found connection through shared disconnection with their bodies. We found solace together in this misery—figuring out ways to uplift ourselves and each other anyway.

"That shirt makes you look really manly," a friend would tell me.

"Screw dysphoria, we are real men!" we'd tell each other.

This was beautiful—and it was also not a comprehensive story about transness. So when I first met someone who didn't dislike their body, I remember feeling confused. Angry, even.

What do you mean you're trans?! You haven't struggled like me. You haven't experienced the pain I have. You haven't had to fight for affirming medical treatments like we have! The thoughts ran through my mind. *You're not really trans.*

But I quickly realized that these were the same types of discriminatory messages that I had received about my manhood: "You don't match these things that *I* believe make you a man, so you're not a man to me." This understanding allowed me to make more space for people who understood themselves as trans but whose experience did not overlap identically with my own. In the same way that not all trans people understood my particular experience as a transgender athlete or a trans person of color, not every trans person would share my pain in dysphoria and that was okay.

It took a few more years to further intellectualize and digest this understanding. Eventually, I realized that this narrow definition of transness also arose from a scarcity mindset: the belief that there is not enough care for all of us to go around.

I assume it is for reasons like this that those who call themselves "trans medicalists" assert that being trans *is* a mental illness curable through transition, and some seem to fear that our rights will be delegitimized through "allowing" those who do not experience dysphoria to be included in transness.

But I do not find it useful or appropriate to decide what someone else's identity is for them. I strongly encourage others to recognize that it is *no one else's right* to police someone else's gender in any way. We cannot tell someone else who they are. I always reflect on an interaction I had during my childhood when considering this.

"What are you?" the kid asked me.

"What do you mean?" I said, as I always replied, even though I knew what they were asking.

"I mean, you look... Where are you from?" they said.

"I was born in New York City." My mom taught me to answer this way. *You belong here, too. They think all of us are foreigners who don't have a place in this country. They are wrong.*

"No, where are you *really* from?" they pressed, exasperated.

"I'm *really* from NYC. But if you're asking about my ethnicity and ancestry, my mom is Korean."

"What? You're not Korean. You look... not Korean." While demanding explanation about my race and ancestry was quite common, rejecting my answer was not.

"What?!" I said and walked away.

Hopefully you find this interaction as ridiculous as I did. Who was this kid to tell me I wasn't Korean? Why would they even think that and how dare they say that to me? How dare someone tell me I'm not who I say I am!

I invite you to bring this same reaction to the concept of telling someone they are not the gender they say they are. It is ridiculous for someone to attempt to deny me my core identities—as a Korean person, or as a man. And so, in the same vein, it is ridiculous for me to tell someone else they are not trans because I cannot ever know that *for* them. When someone shares their gender with me, I accept their declaration, I value their vulnerability and trust in me, and respect them in whatever ways I can. I encourage others to do the same.

Lastly, receiving treatment for gender dysphoria requires that an individual experiences gender dysphoria. It does not require being transgender—one does not get diagnosed as transgender; one gets diagnosed with gender dysphoria. Being transgender is *not* a medical condition.

WHAT DOES SCIENCE SAY ABOUT DYSPHORIA?

Gender dysphoria is included in the *DSM-5-TR*[*] as a mental disorder and thus the distress gender dysphoria produces is considered clinically significant. However, not everyone is able to access a formal diagnosis of gender dysphoria. Dysphoria is also far more complicated and nuanced than a mental illness diagnosis. Gatekeeping gender-affirming resources through a checklist of dysphoria is not always productive and can exclude individuals that do not fit a narrow definition or presentation of dysphoria.

In many trans-only spaces, I have witnessed folks exchange tips on how best to explain their dysphoria—what to say and what not to say—to their medical and mental health providers so as to receive the care they know they need. This may not seem appropriate, but you must consider that medical professionals have withheld care from trans folks on the basis of incomprehensive and transphobic research for decades. Providers often deny us care because we do not report dysphoria in the exact ways that previous literature affirmed as "enough."

This is not to imply that medical protocol for providing gender-affirming care is not helpful—it can be. But it must be well-informed by trans people, our real-life experiences, and the diversity our community presents.

---

[*] The *DSM* is the *Diagnostical and Statistical Manual of Mental Disorders*, the most widely used resource to diagnose mental illness in the United States. The *DSM-5-TR* is the fifth and most recent version that was released in 2022.

"A NAMELESS TRAGEDY":
A WALK THROUGH THE LITTLE-KNOWN
HISTORY OF TRANS MEDICAL CARE

1868: Magnus Hirschfeld (he/him) is born. Hirschfeld, a gay, Jewish, German physician and sexologist (1868–1935), is credited with coining the term *transsexual* as an identity distinct from those who experienced same-sex attraction. Hirschfeld is a staunch advocate for the decriminalization of homosexuality[1,2] who also believes that a "third sex" exists naturally and proposes the idea of "sexual intermediaries," a term to refer to those who do not conform to cishet norms of the time. Hirschfeld's "sexual intermediaries" also include people he terms (in 1910) *transvestites*— those who choose to wear clothes that are seen as for the "opposite" sex, and who "from the point of view of their character" would like to be perceived as the "opposite" sex. These folks would likely be referred to as *transgender* today.[3]

1919: Hirschfeld founds the Institut für Sexualwissenschaft (Institute for Sexual Research), which opens in Berlin on July 6. The Institute accumulates a large library on sexuality, and Hirschfeld and his team treat patients who wish to transition. Hirschfeld hires psychiatrists for therapy and gynecologists who perform Genitalumwandlung—literally translated: "transformation of genitals." At the time, Hirschfeld's institute provides the most modern gender-affirmation surgeries in the world.[4]

1933: On January 30, Adolf Hitler (he/him) takes power and quickly begins the extermination of those he deems *lebensunwertes Leben*, or "lives unworthy of living." These lebensunwertes Leben include not only millions of Jewish, Roma, Soviet, and Polish citizens, but also transgender and queer individuals of any background.

On May 6, one of the first and largest Nazi book burnings occurs in Berlin. Hirschfeld's institute and library are destroyed. Newsreels of the destruction are well publicized. However, while the incident has been widely reproduced since, rarely has it been named for what it destroyed—it was "a nameless tragedy."[5]

1949: The sexologist David Cauldwell (he/him) publishes an article in which he uses the term *psychopathia transexualis* to describe a patient, Earl, who had requested an operation for "sex transmutation," including breast and ovary removal, a vaginectomy, and a phalloplasty.

Cauldwell seems to be the first to use *transsexual* to refer directly to individuals who wished to or did undergo surgery to "change sex."[6,7] Cauldwell also clearly distinguishes between *biological sex*, which was categorized in accordance with anatomy, and *psychological sex*, which he saw as determined by social conditioning and would be later referred to as *gender identity*.

Cauldwell does not endorse surgical changes for transsexual individuals and instead argues for "psychological rather than physical adjustment." He believes that seeking "mutilative operations" was a sign of "lost... mental equilibrium."[8]

1951: Harry Benjamin (he/him) (1885–1986), a German American endocrinologist and sexologist, performs gender-affirming surgery on Christine Jorgensen (she/her), a WWII veteran. Jorgensen's transition is widely publicized and, as a result, greatly increases the visibility of trans identity itself as well as Benjamin's work.

Although Benjamin exhibits some contradictions in regard to homosexuality, he publicly advocates for gay rights when most American doctors did not and works diligently to meet the needs of his trans clients, not attempting to change their behavior, and instead affirming their identities. Benjamin is an important figure of affirmation during a time when many trans patients reported doctors injecting them with hormones aligned with their assigned gender against their will, submitting them to electroconvulsive therapies without consent, advising carbon dioxide therapy, and even performing lobotomies.[9]

1964: Reed Erickson (he/him), a transgender man who was also a patient of Harry Benjamin, establishes the Erickson Educational Foundation (EEF), which funds research on trans people, and the founding of the Gender Identity Clinic at Johns Hopkins University Hospital a few years later.[10]

1965: Columbia psychiatrist John F. Oliven (he/him) coins the term *transgender* in his reference work *Sexual Hygiene and Pathology*,[11] writing: "[transsexualism] is misleading; actually, 'transgenderism' is meant, because sexuality is not a major factor in primary transvestism." (At this time, he used *transvestism* and *transgenderism* interchangeably.)[12]

1969: The Stonewall Riots occur. Virginia Prince (she/her) uses the term *transgenderal* to refer to herself with the specific aim of distinguishing herself from those who also underwent surgery and, as we'd say today, medically transitioned. "I, at least, know the difference between sex and gender," she writes, "and have simply elected to change the latter and not the former. If a word is necessary, I should be termed a 'transgenderal.'"[13]

1979: The Harry Benjamin International Gender Dysphoria Association is formed. It would later become the World Professional Association for Transgender Health (WPATH)—largely regarded as an international leader for understanding and treating gender dysphoria today.

1980: The professional psychiatric community adopts mention of trans people in the *DSM-III*. The *DSM-III* is the first *DSM* to include transness, but unfortunately does so through including *transsexualism* as a mental disorder. Additionally, the *DSM-III* categorizes trans individuals by sexuality—"homosexual," "heterosexual," and "asexual."

1994: The *DSM-IV* drops *transsexualism* and uses only *gender identity disorder* (GID). Individuals are still categorized by sexuality but in newly named categories: "attracted to males," "attracted to females," "attracted to both," and "attracted to neither." In these classifications, being transgender still causes a person to be considered mentally ill.

2013: The *DSM-5* replaces GID with *gender dysphoria* and stops classifying trans folks by sexuality. This finally removes the pathologization of trans identity and instead considers the distress that some trans folks experience to be clinically significant and therefore a mental illness. This new format aims to separate the distress from the identity of the person, de-pathologizing transness itself. "Gender non-conformity is not in itself a mental disorder," the *DSM-5* explicitly articulates.[14] It also eliminates use of the term *transsexualism*, which has largely become an outdated term.

2013–present: The debate between medical professionals over trans healthcare continues, with the tension lying largely between the medical community and legislative powers. Recent years have seen an onslaught of legislative attacks on gender-affirming healthcare with hundreds of laws attempting to ban and criminalize gender-affirming care for minors (and in 2023, for adults, too), as well as to restrict individuals' ability to change their names and gender markers.

While the *DSM-5* has left some with hopes for more, the official de-pathologizing of trans identity aligns with what many trans activists have fought for—and what research has shown is effective: gender affirmation. The *DSM-5*, along with subsequent guidelines, has encouraged medical and mental health professionals to affirm gender identity instead of attempting to "correct" it. Unfortunately for trans individuals, medical professionals are not given the jurisdiction their expertise should award them. Despite having no inherent medical expertise, many legislative officials have baselessly argued against what all major medical, psychological, and psychiatric organizations support—presumably because transphobia is a more effective and acceptable rallying cry than explicit misogyny, white supremacy, and bigotry.

PART 2

GENDER AND OTHERS

CHAPTER 8

Coming Out . . . or Inviting In

W HEN I WAS ELEVEN YEARS OLD, I REALIZED I HAD A CRUSH on my then-closest friend. At the time, both of us walked the world presenting as girls. That day, I wrote on the edge of a journal page: "Found out I'm gay.—2007." I ripped out the corner and stuffed it into the back of my dresser drawer as if to stuff away the feeling. I hid it so well that I never found that little fragment, despite searching years later.

As soon as I was able to articulate this feeling, a many-months-long stomachache took hold. Its intensity waxed and waned according to how often I thought of my friend and how much time we spent together, but it was ever present, persistent, and lonely.

Later that year, my friend's mother was driving us to the Smithsonian where my mother worked. We were all going to watch my mother give a presentation. In the car, my friend and I sat in the back seat. For a moment, I forgot that this crush felt so forbidden and I was just there, lost in the giggles and fun. But the shame came quickly crashing down when I looked up and saw my friend's mom in the front seat. *What would she do if she knew of my feelings for her kid? She would most definitely think I was gross and probably never let me near again!*

So I shoved my feelings away. I told no one for years. Despite knowing a few adults in my life who were openly gay, I did not know any openly gay students at the time. Even when one of the girls at school came out a few years later in eighth grade, my mom would exclaim, "How would she know that? She's so young!" I had known even younger. *There must be something wrong with me*, I'd concluded.

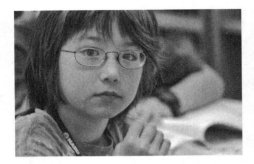
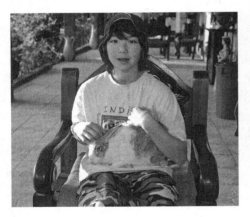
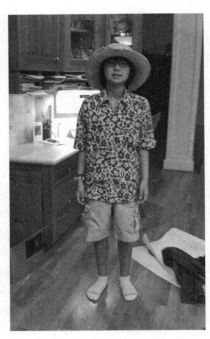

When I got to high school, I decided it was time for a change. I'd been presenting in a stereotypically masculine way for the majority of my life. While this felt comfortable, I was sick of being stared at and harassed in the women's bathroom. I was so tired of feeling like I didn't belong—maybe it was time to become this woman everyone expected me to be.

I decided I'd finally conform.

I grew my hair long and bought tighter, more stereotypically "girly" clothing. For the first time I could remember, I shopped in the girls' clothing section. On my swim team, where I spent most of my social time, I paid attention to what shampoo the girls used and the stores they shopped in and did my best to mimic them. I forced myself to engage in conversation with my girl teammates about boys. I prepared myself for the repetitive question, "So, who do you think is hot?" There were only a few correct answers to this question—all of which were boys.

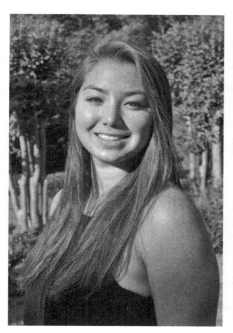
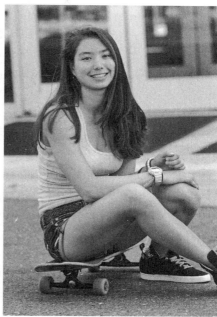

Unfortunately, this shift did not bring about any of the joy or relief I had been seeking; it brought the opposite. It was during this time that my mental health deteriorated and I began struggling with an eating disorder and other mental illness.

The summer before my junior year in high school, the inauthenticity was killing me (quite literally). In the short span of about a week, I decided I had to come out as gay. *This has to be it*, I'd thought to myself. *This has to be the thing I'm struggling over.*

It was a Tuesday morning and I thought I'd tell my parents together, but because my mom left on a business trip, I had to tell them one by one. I chose her first. Maybe a phone call would be easier.

I crushed myself into my closet (the irony lost on me at the time), shut the door, and called her.

"Mom, I have something to tell you."

"Okay, what's the matter?" She was calm but sounded a little worried.

Despite having written myself a little script, I blurted out: "Mom, I'm gay." The words gone from my mouth, I was suddenly in tears.

I think she was more surprised at the circumstances than the declaration itself. She was worried about how upset I was. She said she was more confused that I had to tell her in the first place: "If you just came home with a girl one day, I would have asked you what her name was. No more," she'd said.

My dad responded similarly to my mother. I was not met with hostility or even any kind of challenging of my thoughts. It was all rather anticlimactic, to be honest.

Unfortunately, this was and still is quite a privilege. In a study by True Colors United, some 40 percent of youth experiencing homelessness are LGBTQ+, with the most commonly cited reason being familial rejection due to sexual orientation or gender identity. Fifty percent of LGBTQ+ teens receive a negative reaction from parents and more than a fourth of them are thrown out of their home and family.[1]

My parents never threatened me with finances or my living space. And I am lucky for this.

Over the next few years, I came out to more of my friends at school. I joined my school's LGBTQ+ club and I began dating a friend who came out to me when I came out to her. Together we attended a lesbian affinity group that our classmates had created that year. By the end of high school, it would turn out that a majority of our friend group was queer. I finally had community.

Still, I kept my queerness a secret at the pool. Swimming felt like an impossible place to share my identity. Homophobic slurs echoed off the walls daily, and while I tried desperately to be proud of who I was, I wasn't willing to give up all that I'd worked for. Swimming was my life—every dream and future plan involved being in the pool with these girls. My team had churned out many national champions and even

Olympians. I wanted to be a part of this, and telling anyone on the team about my sexuality felt like a surefire way to lose it all.

"Ew, she was kissing another girl," I remember one of my teammates saying as we sat outside stretching after practice. "It was so gross." In that moment, I'd vowed never to share my identity with them or anyone in swimming. It was too scary.

In many ways, I lived a double life. Because I attended a private school and a majority of my swim friends went to public schools, there was little risk of overlap. At school, I wore clothing I felt expressed my sexuality—neon green jeans, old flannel shirts, and snapback caps—and at swim practice, I talked about boys with my teammates. Sometimes I would even change into a different, "girlier" outfit before I got to the pool.

While difficult, this system was effective for a few years. My sexuality never made its way to swim practice and I continued to be invited to hangouts with the other girls on the team. But despite rarely experiencing much homophobia at school, something still felt incredibly wrong about calling myself a "lesbian." I admitted to a friend that the lesbian affinity group we attended together left me feeling an intense inward disgust, so much so that I often left the meetings before they ended, overwhelmed with nausea.

It would take a few more years for me to find the words to explain why.

During my time at the eating disorder treatment center and the months that followed, I began learning more and more about myself. In a few agonizing months, I realized how well the word *transgender* fit my experiences. Still, I felt that I knew very little about the person I would emerge as when I left that treatment center.

So when my mom visited early in the process, I did not feel certain enough about my identity to share more than the basics.

"Mom, I think I'm transgender," I'd tried while we were driving on U.S. 1. I remember her just nodding—unsure and likely surprised but trying to show me affirmation. "Okay..." she'd responded. When I'd continued on about the potential physical transition and the possibility of not being able to swim anymore, she was a bit more hesitant.

"Okay, well we'll have to talk about that more," she'd said. It was a short conversation. In passing. I know part of the nonchalance came from my mother's unwavering love for me, combined with her desire for me to be okay that stood above any attachments she had to my gender or the way I walked through the world. Part of the nonchalance came from not knowing how serious I was in offering this part of me.

A month or so later I went to a workshop called "A Gender Continuum." It was held at a wonderful little LGBTQ+ education center called the YES Institute.

My therapist had gently nudged me to go several weeks before I'd finally agreed. It wasn't that I didn't think attending would be a good idea—I knew it would be—it was that I was terrified of what it would elicit in me. What truths it would force me to confront. And wow, were my fears confirmed.

I spent much of the two-day workshop in tears. On the first day, four facilitators introduced us to the intricacies of gender, biological sex, and where transness fit among it all. I took avid notes, scrawling with blue pen nearly illegibly into my spiral notebook.

"Jealous of the trans men here," I wrote in between a few facts I'd recorded.

Day two brought in several speakers. I watched as a boy younger than I was sauntered in. His oversize cargo shorts and white tank top over his binder* pulled at something within my chest. *He walks just like me*, I thought to myself, the resemblance striking. There was something about the way he carried himself that felt so familiar. Later, I learned he was a trans boy—fifteen years old.

"How do all these kids know so fucking early??" I wrote in my notebook with an envy that curled my fingers.

The boy had thankfully been able to access gender-affirming hormones after he had attempted to end his life. His mother spoke about the

---

* A binder is an article of clothing that folks may use to reduce or, in many cases, attempt to eliminate the appearance of having breasts. Somewhat a cross between a tight sports bra and camisole, a binder functions by pressing one's chest tissue against one's body to create a flatter, more traditionally masculine-appearing chest.

importance of finding a way to support her child, and he read us a poem about his experience.

"It was like chains caressing my skin," he said as I sobbed, knowing the feeling all too well. "A boy's heart with a girl's body."

"You can't let anyone else rule your life," he read, "because then it's not yours anymore, it's someone else's. And you can't live someone else's life."

"How much happiness have I lost (or gained?) from living my life the way I have?" I wrote, the tears staining the page.

By the end of the workshop, I was in shambles. The second day's page in my journal includes only one line: *So the Gender Continuum class I went to was basically a huge mindfuck.* And by this I meant, I had finally seen my truth. And it was terrifying.

My dad had come to visit and picked me up after the close of the second day. I still had not stopped crying. I ran out to him, sobbing. Wordlessly, he pulled me into a hug and held me tightly as I cried. When I began to quiet, he asked gently, "What's wrong?"

I choked out, "Dad, I'm transgender." He hugged me tighter.

"It's okay, it's all going to be all right," he mumbled as the tears flowed.

*　✳　✳　✳*

SINCE COMING OUT publicly and becoming a speaker and educator, my dad has joined me at numerous conferences and presentations. When asked why or how he was able to support me, he has always replied quite simply:

"When your child is crying and obviously in pain, what do you do?" He always pauses to allow the audience a moment to consider. "You hug them. You hold them. You be there. It's that simple."

It *is* that simple, and it is also not. More than half of trans kids coming out to their parents unfortunately do not share my experience.

I am deeply privileged to have been met with such love. My parents have always been my biggest supporters, and I am lucky to have never doubted how much they love me. I hope you read this sentence and are able to recognize just how low a baseline we've set in society for

LGBTQ+ children—that not doubting our parents' love is lucky: it is a privilege. Parents, please think about this.

Even with this privilege, my journey with my parents was not always easy. We did not always see eye to eye. I could always depend on their love, but not always their understanding.

We had many screaming fights during the year I began my transition. While my parents supported my identity as a transgender man, they were extremely hesitant about my undergoing surgery or taking hormones. Medical changes were scary for them. Top surgery felt rushed and unnecessary.

I left treatment for my eating disorder in October of 2014. At that point, I was certain I needed top surgery and that it was the next step in my journey of self-love and self-affirmation—but without a job or my own health insurance, I needed my parents' help.

My parents' resistance to my transition was bolstered by medical barriers as well. Despite the verbal and psychological support from my therapists at the residential treatment center, none would sign a letter of support for top surgery. The supervising therapist explicitly declared I should *not* proceed with top surgery or any other medical transition step because it was too soon after leaving treatment for my eating disorder. I cycled through three more gender therapists, looking for one who would sign the letter. Each refusal further persuaded my parents that this was a bad idea.

One evening, I found myself on the carpet in my childhood bedroom in pure devastation and defeat, my father standing in my doorway. His resistance and my anger brewed into a fight until we were yelling at each other.

"I don't understand why you have to do this! Why now? Why so fast? I don't understand!" he'd said, upset.

"You don't have to understand! I'm not asking you to!" I'd screamed back. "You're not going to understand, you're not me!" He looked stunned. He didn't say anything.

"I'm just . . ." My scream petered out into a soft plea. ". . . asking you to walk through this with me."

This was a pivotal moment for my dad—and later for both of my parents.

This moment was about realizing that love is so much more important than understanding. My parents spent so much time trying to understand—or preoccupied with the fact that they did not understand—that they were forgetting to actually love me. To trust me. To let me be myself.

Parents, siblings, and friends of trans people are not required to understand us in order to accept, respect, and love us. Sometimes, understanding is one of the last things to emerge, and that is okay. Many parents fail to metabolize this and instead forbid their children from accessing joy that comes from something they do not understand. Letting go of the need to understand requires *trusting your child*. It requires allowing another person to learn for themselves and granting them space to know themselves best.

I would be remiss if I conveyed this fight with my dad to be The Moment everything changed. Very little changed overnight and more disagreements would certainly arise, but in the end, my dad accompanied me to my top surgery. I was required to remain near my doctor for one week after the surgery for a post-op checkup. We stayed at a local transgender surgery recovery center. The center told us that my dad was the first—and at the time only—father to *ever* accompany his transgender son to this center in the several years it had been open, with hundreds of guests staying there each year.

When I cried from happiness upon awakening from top surgery, my dad knew he'd made the right decision to trust me.

In the years that followed, my parents' love would allow them to almost fully understand me and my experience—and to let go when they could not. They have assumed my fight as their own—my dad working as my manager and assistant throughout my career, and my mom shifting to reviewing as many transgender authors' books as she can devour.

While I never want to dismiss the privilege I've had in experiencing this acceptance, I also believe that there are many small and large action items that I and my family took to create this harmony. This is not solely luck; agency is involved. I share this not to aggrandize myself or my family, but rather to communicate: *you have agency, too*. I cannot teach you how to have privilege or how to be lucky but I can share a few things that might help you communicate—whether you are the person inviting others in, or the person being welcomed along.

THINGS TO REMEMBER WHEN SOMEONE INVITES YOU IN

Over the years, I've mentored hundreds of trans and queer people through their disclosure journeys. Before we explore some of my suggestions, it's important to remember that everyone's experience is different and some of these may not work for everyone. These are what worked best for me and those I work with, but if someone tells you they'd prefer otherwise, I encourage you to meet their needs as they ask.

Without further ado, a list of things to remember:

This Is a Privilege

"I am no longer coming *out*," they said with a quiet but firm self-assuredness. "From now on, I am only inviting others *in*." This declaration by an attendee of one of my online LGBTQ+ support groups is one of the most powerful statements I've heard regarding disclosure of trans (or queer) identity.

Their statement aligns with something I have taught cishet people for a long time: when someone shares their trans or LGBTQ+ identity with you, that is a privilege. Treat it as such. It takes great vulnerability and courage to share that we are transgender or queer with others, especially in a world that disenfranchises so many of us. If someone is coming out to you—understand that they are inviting you in to their truth, to a piece of their heart. They are trusting you with intimate information that you are not entitled to. Their disclosure to you is a privilege, not a right. No one is entitled to know our queerness or transness; *we* are entitled to share this with others when and if we want to do so.

I have adopted this language shift because I want to treat my identity like the privilege that it is. I want to respect myself with those boundaries, with that care. This is a way to remind myself and others, "When I share about my identity, I'm welcoming you *in* to my truth. Take off your shoes as you come inside. Be careful as you step into my home. Don't break anything. Be kind, be compassionate. You are welcome here as long as I choose to let you in." In order to be invited in, you need to be someone I would like to welcome.

When trans people choose not to disclose our transness to others, people often grow angry. "They lied to me!" they'll protest. No, I'll respond, you lied to yourself. Cisnormativity has caused you to assume everybody around you is cisgender, and while the existence of cisnormativity is not your fault, it is your responsibility to unpack and dismantle it. And it also certainly does not mean that I've lied to you. (We'll discuss more about this in Chapter 15.)

If someone comes out to you, recognize how sacred, personal, and important that information is. Appreciate that they felt comfortable enough to share their truth with you—that they were compelled by your importance in their life—so express gratitude.

In response, you might try: "Thank you so much for sharing this with me. I'm really glad you trust me with this information. I'm here to support you however I can."

It's Not About You

A trans person's process of self-disclosure is not about anyone else. It is not about other folks' feelings. We don't come out for other people. We come out for ourselves.

Don't complain that someone did not tell you sooner. Don't complain if this person told someone else before you. You're welcome to be upset about both of these things but do not make your feelings the responsibility of the other person. Instead, you may want to interrogate (yourself) about why you weren't told sooner or before someone else. Most often, it is the result of circumstance and convenience—the person just happened to tell others first. Sometimes, the delay has nothing to do with you and it's about the person's own timeline.

And sometimes, it *is* because of you—something you said or did in the past that hurt this person or caused them to fear your reaction. If you find that this is the case, you might consider apologizing for this at some point. I'd recommend reserving an apology for a moment that doesn't take away from their coming out to you. This could be in a later moment during another conversation, or after they've finished sharing. Regardless, ensure that you apologize without centering yourself or your own guilt for causing past harm. Make sure to center their experience and their coming out.

Do not express pain at losing some part of who you perceived us to be. Don't tell a trans man that you will miss his womanhood, or feel like you're losing your sister/girlfriend/mother. Again, these are completely valid and understandable feelings, but they are your responsibility to feel and grieve and heal from, not the other person's.

The point is not to make the moment about you or how you feel about their identity. It's their moment, not yours.

You Don't Have to Understand

Most of us hold a deeply fallible unconscious belief: if we don't understand something, it can't be true/real/valid. But the world is filled with truths that I don't understand. I do not quite understand how planes fly—and yet, they still do. And I trust that science so much, I fly in them all the time. My not understanding how planes fly doesn't somehow make planes *not* fly. My ignorance doesn't invalidate all the theorems that validate the science . . . No, it just means I, Schuyler Bailar, don't get how planes fly.

I don't think being transgender is as complex as the physics of aeronautics, but if you do, that's okay. You still don't have to understand everything about transgender identity or a trans person's experience to love and accept them. Using failure to "get it" as a reason to deny someone their truth, humanity, or autonomy is unkind and invalid.

Coming Out Is Difficult and Terrifying

I've probably spoken with thousands of trans people over my career and I can easily say that while transition is challenging in and of itself, *other people* are the most difficult, daunting, and painful part of the journey for most. As a result, sharing our identities with our loved ones and our communities is often one of the hardest things we do.

Many of us prepare for these moments for months, if not years. To stand up in a cisheteronormative world that tries constantly to erase our very existence, and declare with pride, confidence, and power that this is who we are, takes incredible courage. Due to rampant, and sadly increasing, transphobia, disclosing trans identity is also a large risk—for physical safety, job security, community support, and familial love. Coming out as transgender is often painful, stressful, and anxiety-provoking.

Coming Out Never Ends

Many cishet folks see coming out as a single event. "When did you come out, Schuyler?" they'll ask me.

"Which time?" I'll reply.

It is very rare for someone to come out only once. I can probably count the days I have *not* come out more easily than I can count the times I have. I invite people into my transness every time I make an Instagram post online, every time someone searches for my name and finds my account, every time I give a speech, and with every new friend I make.

Coming out is an ongoing, never-ending process. For many, it can take years of deep and, often, very painful introspection to discover one's identity. And then, it can take years more to gather the courage and support to be able to share that identity with the world—constantly and, for many, forever.

Many queer and trans folks must come out over and over again in order to claim their identities. This can be both exhausting and liberating.

Respect Our Privacy

A trans person telling you they are trans does not provide automatic consent to share this information with others. Disclosing someone's queerness without their consent is called *outing*. When you out someone, not only do you rob them of their agency over their own story and disclosure, you also might potentially put that person in an unsafe situation.

Assume confidentiality unless you are explicitly told otherwise.

If the person has shared a new name and new pronouns with you and you're unsure of where and when to use them, you might say:

"Thank you so much for sharing your name and pronouns with me! Just to confirm, may I begin using these now and in all scenarios? Are there any places where you're not ready to go by these yet? I want to make sure I don't out you when you don't want that!"

Educate Yourself and Be Careful Asking Questions

Although some trans folks will welcome your (appropriately and kindly phrased) questions, many will not, and none *should be obligated to do so*. Your trans friend is not your trans encyclopedia. In addition to burdening them by asking questions, they might also not know all the answers yet. It is your responsibility to educate yourself.

I encourage you to consider the necessity of any questions you choose to ask before you do so. Is there a specific need? Are you actually "just curious" or do you have an alternative motive to your question? That is, are you looking for a specific response or do you truly want to hear their thoughts and answers? Interrogate yourself first. If you find yourself holding a lot of charge or emotion as you consider these questions, take some time to calm before deciding to ask.

Lastly, if you do choose to ask a question and someone refuses to answer or even responds with anger, respect that. Remember, you are not entitled to an explanation just because you are curious. You are allowed to be curious! But curiosity does not necessitate an answer.

What If I'm Also Trans—How Do I Invite People In?

Before you consider coming out, I strongly encourage thinking about if *you* want to. This journey is yours and only *you* should decide when, where, how, and with whom you share your truth. Your identity as a trans and/or queer person does not depend on how many other people you've invited in. Your identity is valid regardless. You do not have to tell everyone as soon as you realize who you are. You do not have to come out ever, unless *you* choose that doing so is right for *you*.

For me, coming out was nonnegotiable. I had fought a battle too long with myself—and yes, I knew that coming out would mean I'd have to fight battles with other people. But I can always walk away from other people. I can never walk away from myself. So I chose to stop fighting that internal battle: to lay down those weapons with which I was harming myself. I chose to let myself express who I really am, to fight the battles with others when I can, and to walk away when I cannot.

If you are not ready to do this, or do not want to—that is okay. Take care of your energy in ways best for you. If you choose this to be your journey as well, here are a few pointers.

Be the Three Cs
Clear

Be direct. Explain as much as you'd like about what it means to be trans or queer or whatever else you are sharing. Be concise—try not to ramble too much because that can be confusing for the listener. Be directive—offer actions the other person can/should do with the new information, such as using the proper pronouns and/or new name.

This might sound like, "I am transgender, which means that while I was assigned female, I am a man. Please call me he/him/his pronouns."

Adding a directive preempts questions—"Okay, so now what? What am I supposed to do?"—that many receivers might have, so tell them clearly what to do with the information. And if you don't want them to do anything or change anything, say that!

These days, when I come out, I'm sharing my gender history. I'm not asking people to change anything. So I add, "You don't need to do anything with this information. Nothing between us needs to change; I just wanted to tell you because it's an important part of who I am."

Compassionate

It took me eighteen years to figure out I'm trans, I can (and want to) give someone more than eighteen seconds to figure out what it means to them. As the process unfolds, recognize that they might not understand, and that's okay. Compassion should also be extended to yourself. If the receiver is not understanding, listening, or respecting you, you might need to set some boundaries. You can still give them the space they need to digest the information you've given them—but you do not need to weather disrespect or discrimination in the meantime.

Confident

How we present ourselves in these scenarios can influence how others receive us. In my experience, the more calm confidence I show, the more likely the person is to receive me with the same confidence in me and my declaration. I recognize this is often far easier said than done, so I recommend practicing beforehand. I wrote letters to many folks I came out to *before* coming out to them to organize and practice what I wanted to say. Sometimes I practiced by reading it aloud to myself or a mirror or a friend. In my most nervous moments, I read the letter aloud to the person when I came out to them.

It's also okay if you can't figure out how to be confident. Just try your best. You can always ask for patience: "This is a really hard conversation for me to have, so bear with me as I get through what I want to say." This invites the listener in and shares a different kind of confidence: vulnerability.

Invite Questions, If You Can

If you feel able to, I encourage inviting others to ask questions if they want to. In my experience, this invitation has been very helpful in creating an environment wherein the receiver can best learn and understand. It allows them to feel like this isn't something strange or a "red-zone"/dangerous topic—it's just another conversation.

Of course, this can also invite invasive questions that could be painful and/or exhausting. Know that not inviting questions is also valid; you have every right to refuse to answer or ask them to refrain from asking. If you do this, I would encourage you to point them to other resources so that they have alternative options to educate themselves elsewhere. See my website for resources you could share.

And if you do allow questions, make sure you feel ready to engage and remember that you can always change your mind. Although I almost always invite questions when I share that I am transgender, this invitation does not mean I want to or will answer every question. It means that I am inviting them to ask.

Disengage when you've met your capacity. This is another reminder to set boundaries, especially when it is clear that no movement is occurring. Boundaries could be leaving the room or not replying when certain topics arise, blocking someone's number, or even cutting this person out of your life. Do not compromise yourself to accommodate someone else's discomfort with your identity. Do not invalidate yourself because they do.

If you are coming out repeatedly, as many trans and queer people must do during their lives, I suggest practicing answers to the common questions people ask so that they do not take as much emotional energy. Valid answers can absolutely include, "I'm not answering that," or simply, powerfully, "No." You might also say, "That's a great question—but I don't have the energy to answer it right now. I'll send you some links!" Or, if the question is, in fact, *not* great: "Hmm, I understand/hear your curiosity, but that's actually quite an inappropriate and invasive question. I don't feel comfortable answering."

The contents of the answer are less important than the ease of providing it. I think this type of practice is key to reducing daily or repetitive social stress as trans people who are constantly interfacing with inappropriate questions.

Remember, You're Not Too Sensitive

"My parents say they're trying to call me the right pronouns, but they only get it right like half the time. I know they love me and care about me, but it just feels like they're not trying hard enough. And it hurts. Am I just being too sensitive?" one of my group attendees recently asked.

A chorus of "No, you're not!" flooded the Zoom chat box and I smiled.

Trans people are often ridiculed as "too sensitive" when we ask that our pronouns, names, and identities be respected. Our pain here is evidence not of sensitivity but rather of universal human emotion. It is not too much to ask to be treated with basic respect and dignity.

WHETHER YOU'RE THE one inviting others in or you're the person being invited in, treat the topic with the respect, compassion, and patience it deserves. Coming out can be a deeply emotional, intimate, and special process for all parties involved. I encourage you to hold the space sacred—because it is.

CHAPTER 9

So You Think You're Not Transphobic?

I'M *NOT* TRANSPHOBIC!" SHE PROTESTED. "I CAN'T BELIEVE HE said that to me. I never want to hurt trans people and it's just so harsh to call me 'transphobic.'"

This acquaintance clearly was upset and offended. I didn't provide much of a response. I just waited.

"It's such an unproductive attack that just shuts down conversation," she continued. I listened as she explained how she felt.

When she was finished, I replied: "I understand why you're feeling upset. It can be really distressing to be called something we perceive as horrible—especially when we didn't mean it," I said, conveying empathy before I shared my opinion. This is emotional hand-holding. A lot of people, particularly those with privileged identities (white, cisgender, straight, etc.), need it when told that they've hurt someone else, albeit accidentally.

"And," I continued, "calling someone transphobic doesn't inherently mean they are a terrible person. It's not a character assault."

She interrupted me, heatedly: "What do you mean? Of course, it's an attack of character! And it feels terrible because that's not who I am!"

"I understand this is how you feel. But that feeling is not the responsibility of the trans person you've offended—that's for *you* to hold."

She didn't seem to like this response, but, to her credit, she didn't argue. She listened, her face contorted with skepticism and frustration.

"Calling something or someone transphobic isn't a condemnation or an erasure of your character. It's a description of an action that that person found harmful. And people need to hear the hurt and the pain they've caused instead of reacting with offense. The proper response to someone calling someone or something transphobic is to listen and be curious about how and why, and then to apologize when necessary."

Our conversation continued and it took some time before the heat dissipated from her voice and her expression. I sat there for nearly two hours discussing transphobia with her.

This is not a unique situation. These conversations—and often confrontations—are common in my life and my work. From these experiences, I draw empathy. I also have made (and will continue to make) my own fair share of mistakes from which I am constantly learning.

"I'M NOT RACIST"

In the summer of 2021, gay Black musician and artist Lil Nas X (he/him) released an album cover in which he is pictured pregnant. Several of my friends sent me the post, asking me to comment publicly on it. I responded with a post titled, "Lil Nas X's Use of Fake Pregnancy Is Insensitive and Transphobic."

While well-received by some, I was also inundated with comments calling me racist and anti-Black. I was stunned and upset.

I am NOT racist! I am not anti-Black! I thought to myself. *I post constantly about Black liberation and Black Lives Matter. I went to all the protests and I talk about systemic racism all the time!* My internal dialogue was fiery, finding all the reasons they were wrong for calling me racist. *You misunderstood my point! I'M NOT RACIST,* I wanted to shout.

Unfortunately, I did the next closest thing. I hastily made another Instagram post wherein I further explained my thoughts. I argued that the "energy attacking me as racist [was] largely misplaced."

As you may expect, this only increased the comments telling me, "You're racist," and, "This is so anti-Black." Thousands of people unfollowed me and I received many more angry and disappointed DMs. News of this made it to Twitter and beyond. This was the closest I'd come to being "canceled."

After my second post clearly was not well-received, I decided to consult with (and compensate) a few consenting Black educators about what had happened and where I'd gone wrong. I educated myself as much as possible. I talked at length with Kayden Coleman (he/him), a gay Black trans man who has birthed two children himself and is also a DEI educator and consultant. Through a public Instagram Live together, I finally understood and accepted that my attacking Lil Nas X in this scenario was, indeed, anti-Black.

Later I synthesized these learnings into a post for my audience: "Plenty of white men have done fake pregnancies and gotten away with it, their whiteness as a shield. Choosing to call out Lil Nas X, and not calling out any other cis men (specifically cis white men) who've faked pregnancy before was rooted in anti-Blackness," I shared.

In this debacle, I had committed a very common error: I asserted myself as an authority on the experience of Black folks and then used that to dismiss Black folks' input. In reality, only Black folks get to tell us what is or is not anti-Black. As a non-Black person, I have no place saying what isn't anti-Black and therefore my statement that their assertions of racism were misplaced was dismissive and wrong.

It would take weeks for this to bubble down—not only publicly but also personally. I was furious with myself for having committed such an obvious error. I knew I should have sat with my feelings after being told my post was racist and invested more time thinking critically about my audience's response. *Why had I jumped the gun and told people they were wrong in calling me racist? Why had I ever thought that was a good idea?* I knew that I knew better.

As I repeatedly combed over the events, I realized the reason I'd dug in my heels: I was so afraid of being seen as racist.

I had felt that being racist—and admitting to it—was the worst accusation in the world, so to be called that necessitated an immediate response that I (supposedly) wasn't racist. In doing so, I had prioritized my own feelings of not wanting to be seen as racist over the actual impact of the anti-Blackness my comments had on others.

From there I was finally able to put into words something that I'd felt but never quite articulated: We *all* harbor anti-Blackness. We *all* harbor homophobia. We *all* harbor transphobia. We are all classist, misogynist, ableist, and so on. Why? Because we live in an anti-Black, homophobic, transphobic, classist, misogynist, ableist society. These biases have been ingrained in us, likely before we could even speak. So, *of course*, we harbor these biases. Denial is not only ignorant and naive but also incredibly harmful because denial prevents an individual from taking responsibility for their actions and working to improve them.

I share this story of my failures and learnings with hopes of inviting you in. Everyone is capable of committing negative actions that stem from systemic oppression because everyone has been steeped in and raised by these systems. Doing good doesn't mean we are void of bias. Doing good means working to become aware of, unpack, and then act in opposition to the bias.

Just because I didn't mean to be anti-Black and didn't believe I was racist for criticizing Lil Nas X doesn't mean I was correct in my assertions. It also doesn't mean that I am committed to being racist, forever entrenched in perpetuating it. It means that I have been raised in the racist world in which most of us were raised, and that I had (and will always have) work to do to unpack my biases.

The same is true for transphobia.

You might be thinking to yourself, *I don't even need to read this chapter. I'm not transphobic! I don't vote for politicians who push these anti-trans laws!* You might have trans friends you love and support. That's wonderful. And, this work is not binary—people trying to do good can still cause harm. Transphobia is not always as obvious as it seems. We can perpetuate transphobia, knowingly or not, when we act in accordance with transphobic biases we must instead unpack and then dismantle.

TRANSPHOBIA: FROM VIOLENT MURDERERS TO QUIET, "INNOCENT" BYSTANDERS

Transphobia is the dislike of, prejudice against, or discrimination toward transgender people based on their transgender identity. Transphobia operates from cissexism—a word you might have seen as well, albeit less frequently.

In short, cissexism is systemic transphobia: a system of beliefs that assumes gender is defined by genitals, that there are only two genders, and that everyone is therefore cisgender. Cissexism also purports (whether unconsciously or consciously) that cisgender bodies and gender identities are more legitimate and natural than those of trans people; that being trans is inherently inferior to being cis.[1-4] Cissexism is the control center from which transphobia acts.

Transphobia itself comes in many forms, both physical and emotional. Transphobia shows up socially as misgendering, deadnaming, verbal or physical harassment for simply existing, and more. Transphobia is evident in many medical settings, workplace environments, at school, at home with family, and beyond.

When we consider transphobia, you might think of an individual who hates trans people—who actively discriminates against us, who commits acts of violence against us, who doesn't believe we are deserving of the same respect as cisgender individuals. And that is not incorrect. These are instances of transphobia—usually considered individual oppression.

Transphobia is also a larger part of systemic oppression in the world. According to the National Equity Project, systemic oppression is "the intentional disadvantaging of groups of people based on their identity while advantaging members of the dominant group (gender, race, class, sexual orientation, language, etc.)."[5] Applied directly to gender identity, then, systemic oppression is the intentional disadvantaging of trans, non-binary, and gender nonconforming individuals while advantaging those who are cisgender. *Intentional?* You might challenge. Yes, intentional.

As you learned earlier, being trans was considered a mental illness until 2013, pathologizing our identities. Gender identity and expression are still not explicitly protected by federal law unless the Equality Act is passed. (The Equality Act passed the House in February 2021, but remains blocked by the Senate.) Several state legislatures have blocked transgender individuals from changing their gender markers on their identification documents, banned the teaching of LGBTQ+ history and related topics in schools, attempted to bar children from exposure to any kind of gender nonconformity, and criminalized doctors who provide gender-affirming healthcare to minors despite the fact that doing so has been approved by every major medical association.[6-18] More than half the states in the country have attempted to block transgender children from playing sports with their friends. Former president Donald Trump reversed the Obama administration's inclusion of transgender soldiers, banning trans people from serving in the military.[19] These are just a few examples of the systemic disenfranchisement of transgender people.

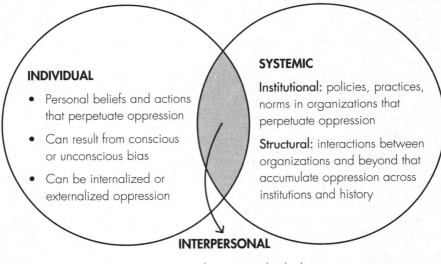

INDIVIDUAL

- Personal beliefs and actions that perpetuate oppression
- Can result from conscious or unconscious bias
- Can be internalized or externalized oppression

SYSTEMIC

Institutional: policies, practices, norms in organizations that perpetuate oppression

Structural: interactions between organizations and beyond that accumulate oppression across institutions and history

INTERPERSONAL

Interactions between individuals that perpetuate oppression

In such an unwelcoming societal landscape, transphobia is also perpetuated interpersonally through relationships and other interactions between individuals. This interpersonal transphobia can create magnified distress, anxiety, and othering of trans individuals, especially when contextualized within the systemic disenfranchisement we already experience.

Violence—such as murdering trans people—is likely the most obvious and extreme version of transphobia. And while murder is a dire issue—2021 witnessed the most anti-trans murders in recorded history[20]—transphobia in all its various forms is prevalent. Due to the inner workings of systemic oppression, most folks are not even aware of the transphobia they perpetuate and might even deny the possibility of ever doing so. But regardless of intention and awareness, many still perpetuate transphobia—albeit accidentally—in the form of microaggressions.

The term *microaggression* can be misleading: labeling the mistake committed as "micro" implies that the impact is also small, which is not often the case. Microaggressions can be more difficult to heal from because they are so insidious that not only does the microaggressor not know or intend to be doing something harmful, but the aggressed also does not always realize exactly why they feel upset or invalidated by what happened.

Microaggressions can also be more difficult to encourage swift and appropriate reformative action because the impact seems less obvious. Recognition and acknowledgment must occur before healing can begin.

For example, I once dated a woman who referred to me as her "little Asian man." She would call me this epithet playfully and, I assumed, lovingly. During that relationship, I received those words without complaint. Because I saw it as something she valued, I even would refer to myself that way from time to time. "I'm your little Asian man!" I'd joke. I understood it was supposed to be cute.

But something always tugged at me—it didn't feel right. Over time, I felt smaller and smaller, especially combined with her other comments: that she would be sad if our children (should we somehow be able to conceive them biologically one day) weren't blond, how Asian folks couldn't drive, and so on.

In hindsight, it's far easier to recognize that these behaviors clearly constituted racial microaggressions. Their impact not only diminished me in an interpersonal environment, but drew from systemic oppression that disenfranchises, emasculates, and devalues Asian men on a larger societal scale.

But I never addressed this with her. Not only did I feel unable to explain how her comments made me feel, I had no idea how to justify why I felt the way I did. *Oh, it's fine, she's just trying to be cute. Don't worry about it, Schuyler. Don't be such a baby.* I would tell myself instead. *Get over it. She's not being racist,* I'd try to calm.

Because of how difficult microaggressions can be to recognize and address, the invalidation of the harm comes internally in addition to externally. The less obvious impact can discourage the harmed person from discussing the issue with others—intimately with partners and friends, or professionally with supervisors, senior leadership, teachers, coaches, and other colleagues—for fear of not being taken seriously. If the individual does choose to speak up about the harm, the ignorance surrounding the microaggressions can result in a great deal of gaslighting of the person(s) who experienced the microaggression.

WHAT SHOULD I DO IF SOMEONE CALLS ME TRANSPHOBIC?

Pause, listen, reflect, apologize.

Let's walk through it.

Pause

Take a moment to collect yourself before you respond. If you find that you are upset, it is crucial that you calm—at least a reasonable amount—before you engage. This is a universal skill, applicable to any moment you feel a surge of negative emotions in conversation with someone. When we feel attacked emotionally, our systems often react as if there is physical danger: elevated heart rate, sweating, rushing thoughts, and more. If you are someone who is generally anxious, you might find this response is more heightened than usual. This all makes sense! It can be scary and distressing to hear something that violates your view of your own character.

So you might be upset, or even angry and offended, when someone calls you transphobic. These emotions are valid and understandable. But you must also remember that the validity of emotions does *not* always validate subsequent actions: *emotions are always valid; actions are not.*

So, pause and collect yourself.

Listen

If the person is sharing how your behavior impacted them and offering an explanation, let them speak—and practice active listening. This means you are not just waiting for your turn to speak or preparing your own defense in your head as they talk.

Try to put aside the defenses of "But that's not what I meant" or "But you didn't understand me," and instead hear how your words or actions have impacted them. If need be, remind yourself that intention, while important, cannot bar or supersede impact. Attempts to explain away someone else's pain or to defend one's original position will likely be received negatively and potentially incite harmful implications.

First, this defensiveness says: "My explanation is more important than how I made you feel," and/or, "You shouldn't feel hurt because I didn't mean it."

If we revisit the simple analogy presented in Chapter 5 when I accidentally stepped on my wife's toe and broke it, you'll recognize that telling her that her toe should not hurt and should not be broken because I hadn't *intended* to step on it would be a ridiculous response. Her toe hurts and is broken regardless of my intent. Similarly, it is not useful, kind, or compassionate to tell someone they shouldn't be hurt or receive transphobia if you didn't intend it.

Second, defensiveness almost immediately questions the authenticity of your allyship. So frequently I've heard people say something along the lines of, "But I'm an ally, how could they possibly call me transphobic?!" Allyship is not a destination where you receive your official Allyship Card. Allyship and true care for people with identities you do not share is a continuous journey of unlearning and mistakes and relearning. I don't believe that an accidental act of transphobia immediately revokes your allyship—but not learning from it certainly does. Staying committed to a title of *ally* instead of actually acting like an ally is not allyship.

Third, defensiveness invalidates the autonomy and self-knowledge of the trans person, saying: "I know you more than you know yourself. I, a cis person, know what hurts trans people more than trans people know what hurts them." Hopefully this sounds wrong to you: not only is it arrogant and incorrect, but it is also an abuse of power that cis people systemically hold over trans people. Cis people do not know more about trans people's experiences than trans people do. I encourage you to grant trans people the autonomy to declare our own pain without qualifying it as understandable to you.

Reflect and Apologize

Instead of defensiveness, communicate empathy and understanding as much as possible as you respond. If you find yourself genuinely confused about the impact of your actions as you reflect, you may ask for clarity, with the understanding that no one is required to answer your questions, especially not when they've just been hurt by something you said or did.

Here are a few samples for how a response might sound:

"Thank you so much for calling me in. I'm sorry for hurting you and I really appreciate you being vulnerable with me and taking the time to tell me how _____ [transphobic action] hurt [or affected] you. I learned a lot from what you shared and will not make the same mistake again. Thank you for educating me! Is there anything I can do to repair harm going forward?"

"I'm really sorry. Thank you for trusting me enough to tell me how you feel. I did not mean to hurt you and I see how I did. I'm grateful for your thoughts and will take them forward with me so I don't repeat my mistakes. I will also do some research on my own about this to make sure I keep learning."

"I'm so sorry for how I've impacted you. I didn't realize _____ [transphobic action] was transphobic. I absolutely hear what you're saying and appreciate you taking the time to share with me. I'm wondering if you feel comfortable or have the capacity to share more so I might not repeat the same mistake."

"Gosh, I had no idea. I'm so sorry. Thank you for sharing how _____ [my words or actions] impacted you. I really appreciate the vulnerability. I'm curious if you have the energy to talk more about this with me because while I understand that ____ is transphobic, I'd love to learn more about how I can do better next time."

Notice how each of these includes doing the following:

- **Apologizing.** It does not matter if you believe you are at fault or not. We can *always* apologize for how our actions made someone feel, even if we are not directly to blame. I've met far too many people who refuse to apologize or empathize with someone's negative emotions (reactions) because "it's not my fault!" This dismissal of culpability is a silly reason to withhold empathy.
- **Giving gratitude.** Disclosing how and why someone has been hurt can take a lot of energy, vulnerability, and risk. Whether done so with calm or in anger, sharing one's pain is an invitation to see them in that state of vulnerability. Join them there.
- **Recognizing.** Summarize what you heard and understood, especially if you plan to ask for clarity. If you skip this step, you risk communicating that you haven't been listening well, even if you think you heard every word. Recognition helps communicate that you're engaged and present. If you truly haven't understood anything, you can still communicate that you understand they are hurting or upset or another emotion word they've used to describe their feelings.
- **Not demanding.** Notice how each of the examples that asks for more clarity also includes recognition of the other individual's consent. I believe this part is crucial. Someone might not have the energy to explain the harm or their experience in depth. They may not have the capacity—or even the desire— to educate you on how to improve in the future. Recognizing this *asks*, ideally gently and compassionately, for education rather than demanding it. This also demonstrates that you know that "no" is a perfectly acceptable answer.
- **Offering to repair.** Offering to pursue action to repair and improve your relationship can communicate your care and suggest

that you intend to continue to act in accordance with your apology. In short, this helps communicate that your apology is not empty words. However, recognize that this offer might not be accepted and could even be rejected with intensity. Depending on the severity of your original impact on the individual, you may or may not be able to repair the harm caused. They may not be open to doing so. They may not have the capacity to. Accept this and continue in your allyship regardless.

This approach is applicable in a variety of scenarios—it works pretty much any time that you are invited to confront an action that causes someone else harm.

WHAT IF SOMEONE ELSE IS BEING TRANSPHOBIC?

It was January and my college teammates and I were gathered for our annual Secret Santa game. This was always more of a roast—you gave a gag gift to a guy whose name you pulled—and told a joke about or story poking fun at the guy when presenting it.

We stood up one at a time, telling stories about each other before revealing in the last line who the "gift" was for. Some were funny and silly. Some were clearly rehearsed. And others were nervous and wobbly. I waited for my own turn, palms sweaty. I had gone over what I was going to say multiple times with a few of the guys in the class above me. Not having been socialized with boys for most of my childhood, I felt that the humor was often lost on me. So I had asked for help.

When it was my turn, I delivered my joke well enough to be received with laughs and applause. Satisfied with my performance, I sat excitedly, waiting for someone to get me.

Aaron (he/him) went last. He was one of my favorite guys on the team—we were in the same training group and often raced together in practice. Unlike the speeches of those who'd preceded him that night, his story was very short.

Aaron stood up and cleared his voice, surveying the room. His eyes landed on me.

"Here're some wieners," he said as he brandished the package of Oscar Mayer hot dogs he held. He threw them to me. "Because it's fun to pretend," he completed his sentence. It all happened so fast. The room was silent. I had no idea what to do. And so, I did what I knew I was expected to. I laughed. The rest of the guys awkwardly followed suit.

Confused, hurt, and feeling deeply alone, I slipped out unnoticed and biked back to my dorm. I don't remember crying; I felt numb. I sat staring at my blank computer screen, stuck in a loop of my thoughts.

Is that how they all saw me? A penis-less man? Just partial-man? Is that how Aaron really saw me? Did I completely misjudge our friendship? No wonder he'd misgendered me the month prior. I was stupid to have trusted him, to have thought that these guys could really see me as one of them!

I spiraled between rejection and the dismissal of my own feelings. Finally, I took to Instagram for community and support. I posted a photo of myself smiling into the camera with the following caption:

Today a friend of mine made a joke about my lack of a penis and I laughed trying to pretend it was okay. "It's just a joke," I told myself. But I know he'd never attack someone for the color of their skin, their womanhood, or any other innate part of their identity. Those wouldn't be "just a joke." But the thing is: neither should my being transgender.

I have fought so hard for who I am—to be seen and heard and respected as myself. And so tonight, of all nights, I will remain smiling because although words can hurt, I refuse to let ignorance or hate drive away the strength & confidence I have built, and the self-love that keeps me alive.

My body is mine and mine alone, and I am proud.

—

To the people judging him: I don't think it's y'all's position to judge him based on this. I think he's a very good person; I just think sometimes people really don't get what being me—being trans—is like. And how could they? Especially when they aren't trans. And getting angry causes alienation not education. So I'm still struggling even as I write this post with whether or not I'm just being too sensitive and should "just take a joke," but I'm just sharing my thoughts here 😳.

—

And yes! Y'all are right! I don't need a penis to be a man—see my earlier posts 😊. I talk about that a lot!

—

#transgender #trans #selflove #selfcare

I hit Post, and went to bed feeling empty and lost.

The messages I received back were supportive.

But before I could feel emboldened or affirmed, I received a text from a senior on the team, apologizing.

"I should have said something. It's not your job as a marginalized person to have to stick up for yourself all the time." Though Nate's (he/him) support was welcome, he also mentioned that some of the guys were upset because they thought I'd "put Aaron on blast" with the Instagram post. Nate said he didn't think they were being fair, but the notice that others were angry about my Instagram post infuriated me. *I couldn't even have that?* Somehow, this made me feel even more alone. As was my go-to at the time, I began writing an email to explain my thoughts.

Before I could finish, Nate texted me again.

"If it's okay with you, I'm going to call a team meeting. You shouldn't have to defend yourself in situations like this. What do you think?"

"Okay, sounds good," I texted back. "Thank you."

"You might want to talk to Aaron before, though, if you can. I understand if you don't want to."

"I will." And I meant it. In a private study room at the library, I explained to Aaron how I'd felt. Try as I might, I couldn't hold back the tears.

"This made me feel like I misjudged our friendship and how you see me," I explained to him. "And I hesitated telling you because I didn't feel like it was valid for me to be upset. I want to be able to joke about myself with others but this crossed a line. This is my identity—one that is constantly pathologized and discredited by the whole world, often times specifically because I don't have a penis. It was so hard to hear it from you, too."

It was clear he'd been thinking about it since he'd done it.

"I'm really sorry, Sky," he began. "I want you to know you didn't misjudge our friendship. I thought that *because* we were close—because I trust you and see you as a close friend—that I could do this. But I understand why I was wrong. You've gone through more than what most of us have and I'm really sorry."

We hugged, both a bit teary.

Later, Nate led a meeting before practice. He reiterated that I shouldn't have to stand up for myself and that we as a team needed to do better. I shared a bit more about how I'd felt. Everyone seemed to listen. Some guys had questions, but all voiced support and empathy.

What began as one of the worst experiences on my swim team became one of the shining moments I'll never forget.

When we got into the pool, three of the upperclassmen thanked me for sharing how I felt. They said they really appreciated it and had learned. Contrasted with the day prior when I felt alone, scared, and hurt, after our team meeting I felt more loved, accepted, and understood than I'd felt with them before.

A FRAMEWORK FOR HANDLING TRANSPHOBIA AS AN ALLY
Say Something

Far more hatred is taught through silence and inaction than active hateful actions. Everyone's silence in response to Aaron's transphobic "gift" condoned the act. Despite the fact that many of the guys *felt* that Aaron had crossed a line, including Aaron himself, no one *said* anything. And this told me that I was alone—that no one would stand up for me and that my pain was insignificant. It even invited me to gaslight myself into believing that I was just being too sensitive.

But one bystander standing up to say, "This is wrong," changed everything. Not only did it embolden other guys to share their disapproval as well, it also made me feel supported. It broke the seal of isolation that I'd previously felt.

Saying something can occur in a variety of forms, depending on the situation and severity of the transphobia. Sometimes this means sending an email or text, and other times, it could mean immediately, and perhaps abruptly, intervening.

Call the Perpetrator In

Calling someone into the conversation when their behavior is transphobic is an excellent way to advance allyship—and this is exactly what Nate did when he called a team meeting. Standing against social direction can be extremely difficult. Doing so can feel lonely, as I imagine Nate might have felt when he first decided to call a team meeting. But we often quickly learn that doing the right thing rarely remains lonely, as demonstrated by the rest of the guys joining him in his quest to make sure I felt like a member of the team.

Use Your Privilege

Nate had social standing with his classmates and the team that I did not. He had access (he lived with his classmates) that I did not. He had energy as a non-trans person to engage that I did not. He used each of these privileges to connect with the other guys to bring us together and allow my voice to be heard and my pain attended to.

Pass the Mic

Do not speak for the person who was hurt unless they indicate this is ideal. Nate offered to stand up for me, but he sought my consent before doing so. He made sure I was comfortable with him calling a team meeting and asked if I was okay with him speaking to the team first.

"I don't want you to have to defend yourself," he'd repeated. "I want to tell them that was messed up, and then if you want to, you can share what you experienced. Does that work?" he'd said. That was perfect.

Assess Your Safety

Productive allyship is nearly impossible if someone is in physical danger. If you decide engagement is reasonable, you have a variety of different avenues to pursue. See Chapter 21 for steps.

CHAPTER 10

Things Not to Say to Trans People

During my sophomore year in college, I was working in the Pepperberg Lab with Irene Pepperberg (she/her) and her two African grey parrots. This was a childhood dream come true—I'd spent hours as a kid mesmerized by Dr. Pepperberg's videos of her and the parrot Alex. I even had a signed copy of her book.

In the lab, I often spent time with volunteers who came for an hour here or there. One day, an older woman I'd never met joined me for the first half of the day. In a quiet moment where we each had a parrot on our shoulder, I sat down to do some work. My laptop was covered with tons of stickers, a few trans-related. She asked me what one of them meant. "What is TTF?" TTF stood for Trans Task Force. As always, I paused and asked myself: *Do I want to share my identity with her? Do I have the energy to have this conversation?*

As previously discussed, coming out is not a onetime show with rainbow cakes and unicorn party hats; for many of us, disclosing transness is a daily consideration or awareness. Outing oneself, even in a low-stakes environment with a co–lab member, can be scary and draining. Sharing my transness with others almost always elicits inappropriate comments and questions at the very least, even transphobia and potential violence at the worst.

In the lab that day, I decided, as I usually do, that it would require more energy for me to manufacture an answer that avoided my truth than to just declare the truth. "I'm transgender," I said plainly. "These stickers show both my own pride about being trans and support for other trans people." She looked stunned, though not in a negative manner.

"Wow, I—I—" she stuttered a bit, clearly searching for the right thing to say. "I never would have known!" she concluded. Then she paused. I knew she was waiting for me to respond or interject. I very intentionally remained quiet, maintaining eye contact with her. I nodded ever so slightly—just to affirm I'd heard her.

"I mean," she continued, realizing I wasn't going to offer anything else. "I couldn't even tell!" She smiled as if this were a compliment.

"Well," I said calmly, "how would you have?" Her eyes widened.

"Well—I—I mean you don't look..." She immediately stumbled, coming to a halt. I waited. "I just mean, you don't look like it," she tried.

As in this scenario, I do not usually tell someone immediately that their comment is a microaggression. Instead, I lead them to conclude that on their own. I often advise other trans folks to do the same if they have the energy—it invites the question-asker to think a bit more critically about what they're implying through their question or comment and arrive at the conclusion on their own.

In order to answer my question, the volunteer was forced to think about what she meant by "looking like it." The honest answer was likely that she thought there is a particular way that trans people look—to which I would have responded, "And what is that?" She'd then have had to share either that she thought trans people have evidence of their transness (i.e., that they "look" like their assigned gender) or that she believed all trans people wore a badge that read, I AM TRANSGENDER. The former is a more common assumption.

When someone tells me in what they believe is a complimentary manner that they don't think I "look" trans, deep down, they usually mean that they cannot see my womanhood—that, to them, I "look like a man" and they cannot tell that I "used to be a woman." They also often mean (and sometimes will explicitly say) that I "look normal" or "good," and therefore do not "look transgender." This is harmful for many reasons, even though many believe they are being affirming. And this is why I usually ask them to consider the implications of what they've said through questioning them.

Other trans folks reading: This is one of the most powerful tools I've learned when confronting microaggressions. I ask, "What do you mean?" with as much genuine curiosity as possible. Sometimes, the response is not what I expect—they've phrased the question wrong and they meant something far less insensitive—but, most often, the answer to "What do you mean" is no longer a subtlety but rather outright bigotry, bias, or discrimination. I've found this line of questioning to be a productive manner of educating folks who would otherwise claim they are not transphobic or bigoted—demanding that they introspect about a supposedly "innocent" thought, question, or even "compliment."

When pressed in this way, most folks will stop themselves before they answer my question because they realize their answer exposes something inappropriate and offensive. And that is why I ask them: this forces them to confront the microaggression on their own when they must explain to me what they mean.

This conversation/questioning might look like this:

Them: "Schuyler, you're, like, more manly than me!" *This is a real comment I've received.*

Me: "What do you mean?" *The question!*

Them: "Well, I mean, you're just . . . more masculine than I ex- pected . . ." *Usually there is some uncertainty with their response at this point.*

Me: "What did you expect?" *Furthering the question.*

Them: "I mean, I expected you to be . . . I guess . . . more feminine."

Me: "Why's that?" *Pressing even further!*

Them: "Well, because . . ." *They will usually grow uncomfortable at this point.* "Because you're transgender."

Me: "I see. Why did you expect me to be more feminine because I'm transgender?" *Outlining it for them a bit.*

Them: "Well you were born . . . I mean you were . . . I mean I was born a boy, so . . ." *They might say something like this.* Or: "I'm not sure . . . I didn't expect trans men to be masculine?" *And sometimes my question will stump them altogether and they won't have an answer. But it's in there.*

Me: "I see. So essentially you harbor a belief that trans men are inherently less masculine than cis men because we are assigned female at birth. Or perhaps you had a belief that trans people look a certain way that I didn't conform to, or that trans men cannot be masculine. These are all fairly harmful misconceptions that you should unpack!"

I encourage use of this line of questioning and dissection for most conversational microaggressions *if you have the energy.* For me, I've found it to be a way to educate a bit more passively. It can lead the microaggressor to the answer more independently, which is less didactic and therefore more likely to be digested and integrated into their future actions.

Misconceptions like in these examples manifest in the form of microaggressions that, especially when accumulated, can be exhausting and painful for trans and other marginalized folks. It might be the first time that lab volunteer said, "Wow, you don't look trans!" but it was far from the first time I'd received that exclamation—and I'm sure it won't be the last.

Before discussing a few more of these misconceptions, I offer a gentle but important note to any other trans individuals that if you are comfortable hearing the following statements or answering these questions, that is absolutely valid. It is your right to respond to questions you are comfortable responding to or to not be offended by certain statements. And I encourage you to remember that just because *you* are comfortable answering these questions does *not* mean that everyone else should also be. The privileges we have (or don't)—such as access to therapy, supportive family and friends, affirming healthcare, etc.—deeply affect our ability to ground ourselves in moments of discrimination. If you're able and willing to receive the following comments, questions, and other misconceptions with calm and kindness, that's great, and I implore you to realize not everyone has this privilege or desire.

Now, let's move into the misconceptions themselves.

In 2021, I asked my followers for things they hoped people would understand not to ask or say to us. Here is that list, compiled directly from hundreds of trans people's responses.

Don't Say, "You don't look transgender!" or, "I never would have known!"

This implies that there is a way to "look" transgender, which is false. "Transgender" is not a look; it is an identity. The belief that you will always be able to "tell" when a person is transgender is misguided at best and toxic at worst. Trans people don't look a certain way; we are not a monolith.

You might also ask yourself, as I usually do, what it means to "look" transgender. Then wonder if cis people also might exhibit these traits. Chances are the answer is yes. Good—keep questioning gender.

Don't Say, "You pass so well!"

Many people also perceive "You pass so well!" as a compliment, but it's not. This is the same as saying: "You fit *my* box of man/womanhood—yay!" This is never appropriate or kind.

Perhaps even more harmful, this implies that it's bad to look transgender. Not only is there not a singular way to "look" transgender, it also assumes that transgender people can't possibly be as attractive as cis people. This is false. Trans people, of course, also exude beauty. Lastly, this statement perpetuates the belief that gender expression (how we look) always equals gender identity (who we are), which is also false.

Don't Ask, "What were you born as?"

You don't need to know what gender anyone was assigned at birth to respect and interact with them. This is an unnecessary and invasive question.

Additionally, the wording of this question implies that trans people have changed gender when we come out, but in reality, many trans people do not report having changed genders, but rather affirmed our true gender. I am a man, and I have always been a man.

If you feel the need to ask this, pause. What insight will you gain from knowing a person's gender assignment at birth? Are you, in fact, really just curious about their genitals? Remember, curiosity is not always a valid reason to ask a question. Sit with your curiosity a bit before you ask—and maybe choose not to ask.

Don't Ask, "What's your *real* name?" or, "What was your name before / birth name?"

First, the names trans people use are our "real" names. Asking this question implies that they are fake or somehow less than valid. The most appropriate term for a name a trans person used prior to transition is *deadname* or *old name* as you learned in Chapter 5. Second, you likely do not need to know this person's deadname. Again, curiosity is absolutely valid, but it does not necessitate asking a question or another person answering the question.

If you are a doctor, lawyer, or another person who must know someone's legal name for some professional or other logistical purpose, make that purpose clear, and recognize the discomfort it may bring the individual: "Because we must interact with your insurance company, I must ask you what your legal name is. I know this can be painful, so I apologize for this discomfort. If you'd like to write it down instead of speaking it, that's totally fine."

Don't Say, "You're so attractive for a transgender person," or, "But why are you more attractive than I am? That's so unfair!"

I have received both of these comments—on Instagram posts, at speeches, and in my personal life.

This supposed "compliment" is usually accompanied by surprise at best, or disgust, jealousy, and anger at worst. This indicates that the commenter believes that trans people are supposed to be less attractive than cisgender people—that, somehow, transness makes us less beautiful. Trans people are not less attractive than cis people. That erroneous belief is harmful and transphobic. Don't add "for a trans person" to a compliment. If you feel the need to do so, ask yourself why. This is your implicit bias against trans people. Unpack it!

Don't Say, "Oh, you're even more masculine/feminine than I am!"

A few classmates and I were walking across the bridge to the pool. Most of the team knew more about me than I did them—at that point, multiple articles about my story had already been published. Everyone knew I was transgender. One of the other guys turned to me as we walked in step with each other.

"Jeez, I keep forgetting you're not just a man like me. You're even more masculine than I am!" He laughed. I had chuckled, not knowing what to say—not only because I didn't feel particularly "more masculine" than him, but also because I knew that this comment reflected some transphobia.

"I mean, why would you assume that you'd be more masculine than I am?" I finally asked, gently. He sputtered a bit before answering.

"I don't know! You're right..." Luckily for both of us, we had arrived at the pool by then and it was time to get changed for practice.

Communicating that you are surprised a trans person exhibits more femininity or masculinity than you do is transphobic because it assumes the following: that trans people are inherently less of whatever gender they are; and that every trans person intends to be masculine or feminine at all, which is not accurate. Holding both masculinity and femininity are not mutually exclusive.

Oftentimes, jealousy or envy comes along with the surprise. I have often felt an undertone of, "Why do you get to be more masculine than me if you're not a real man?" This reaction makes so much sense to me. So much so there's an entire chapter about it. We'll unpack masculinity more in Chapter 18.

Don't Ask, "Did you get *the* surgery?"

As discussed in Chapter 4, asking a trans person if they've gotten "the surgery," is the same as asking what their genitals look like. In addition to being strange, invasive, and inappropriate, it is also irrelevant. The appearance of someone's genitals should have no bearing on your interaction with that person, unless you only interact with folks who have a certain penis length or clitoris size. My sincere hope is that this is not the case.

Still, I understand why some might ask me this question. When I disclose my trans identity, others often assume I am inviting a conversation about my body, and thus my genitalia. But, at least for the large majority of trans people, this is not the case. When we share our transness, we are not inviting questions about our private parts or medical history, we are simply sharing and trusting you with an important part of our identity.

Lastly, do not forget there is no such thing as *the* surgery. There are at least fourteen gender-affirming surgeries trans folks can undergo (or not) in their transition journeys.

Don't Ask, "Are you going to do the *full/complete/whole* transition?"

Characterizing transition as "full," "complete," "whole," or even just "the" implies that there is one way to transition—but transitions are not some sort of prescription you get from a doctor—"Yes, I'll have one full transition, please!" Although, that does sound nice, in theory; in practice, everyone's transition is different because, again, trans people—like cis people—are not a monolith. We don't all want to undergo the same processes. And that's okay. When you use statements like "the transition" and "the full transition," you're unconsciously undermining the agency of the trans individual to define their transition for themselves. Instead, opt for just using "transition" or, even better, not asking this question at all, as it implies that trans people must transition, which is clearly not your decision in any way. Lastly, it is no secret to us trans folks that asking us if we'll get the "full" transition is asking us what's in our pants. Hopefully you understand that is not appropriate or relevant to general interaction with a person—for more, please see Chapter 16.

Don't Ask, "What surgeries are you going to have?" or, "Are you on / will you take hormones?" or, "Do you still have a vagina/penis?" or any other question about our body parts and genitals.

Do you ask any other people in your life to report their medical history and future medical plans to you? Likely you do not.

Not only are these invasive and inappropriate questions, but the information gained should also be irrelevant to most, if not all, interactions with someone. If you don't ask strangers to provide their medical history before speaking to or befriending them, you absolutely should not ask a trans person. If you don't ask strangers what their penises or clitorises look like, you should not ask a trans person about their genitals either. If you do ask strangers this, you might want to reassess your priorities.

"But what about dating?" I know many of my readers are currently wondering. In short, I believe this rhetoric applies to romantic interactions, as well. You don't walk up to someone, pull their pants down, inspect their genitalia, and then fall in love with them. Usually, you start by asking them if and where they'd like to go to dinner. More on this in Chapter 15.

Don't Say, "You need a penis to be a man," or, "You need a vagina to be a woman."

At a speech I gave in late 2018, a middle school student in the second row raised their hand and asked the following question:

"I know you've gotten surgery on your chest, but what about... I mean..." They trailed off, unsure of how to phrase their question. I knew what was coming. "Do you still have *women's* parts?"

I'd smiled. This question is frequently asked and something I have chosen to always welcome when teaching, especially from children. As the audience gets older, the question becomes more and more convoluted as the askers attempt to render an invasive question less offensive. The younger the audience, the more direct they are. Kindergarteners will ask exactly what they mean: "Do you have a penis?"

I began to answer the student's question:

"Well, that's an interesting question! In short, I have not gotten surgery in any other locations for gender reasons. So I still have the parts I was born with. But I want to talk to you about language. I know you called them 'women's parts,' but I am a man. And my parts are mine. So just by the way grammar works, my parts are a man's parts. Does this mean that every man has the same parts as I do? No. And I understand that. But that doesn't mean that my parts are any less a man's."

The student nodded in understanding.

Fortunately, this is usually quite simple for children to grasp. They haven't yet been inundated with messaging that sex is completely binary and that gender must be dictated by sex. They have a far more fluid understanding of the world and my example of my own penis-less manhood is not as shocking to them. The more we can share that bodies and genders show up in many different combinations, the more we can dismantle the Euro-colonial gender binary that restricts not only trans people but also cis people.

In short, genitals do not dictate gender. If you understand your gender through your genitals, it's high time you began asking yourself more about your gender.

Don't Ask, "When did you *choose/decide* to be transgender?"

When I am asked when I "chose" to be transgender, I reply: "When did you choose not to be?"

Most people will quickly grow flustered, sometimes even frustrated.

"I didn't choose! I just am not!" They might protest.

"Me, too!" I will nod.

I chose to affirm my transness. I chose to tell people about it. But I did not choose to *be* transgender.

Being transgender is not something that anyone decided or chose. Just like *not* being transgender is not something someone decided or chose. Someone *can* decide to come out. Someone can *choose* to accept our own transness and *choose* to tell others we are transgender. Trans people can *choose* labels that feel applicable to them and best explain their experiences. In places where and for people for whom gender-affirming healthcare is accessible, we can *choose* to transition.

But being transgender itself is just an identity. No one has to *do* anything to be transgender. Nothing happened to *make* someone trans. Someone just *is* transgender.

You also might consider how difficult it is to be openly transgender—it is unlikely that anyone would simply "choose" this without strong conviction that it is right for them.

Lastly, it's worth noting that *even if* transness were a choice...so what? Would that be so bad? Who does it hurt if someone chooses not to conform to the gender they were assigned at birth and discards that box?

Some trans people I know have challenged me to consider that if we don't make space for the potential that someone could choose to be trans, we might imply that being trans is something horrible. When, in reality, every trans person I interviewed for this book told me that they love being trans. I agree. Being trans is one of the most beautiful lenses through which I live.

Don't Say, "This is so hard for *me*," or, "I'm just so used to your deadname / old pronouns so it's hard to change."

Parents and family members, I'm talking to you. Although none of this is about you, it is allowed to feel hard for you. That *feeling* is valid. *Feelings* are always valid. Actions because of those feelings are *not* always valid.

Just because a task is hard does not mean you shouldn't or cannot do it. You absolutely can, and should, do hard things, especially for your children. Of course, recognize that mistakes happen. It's not the absence of mistakes that makes you kind, it's how you deal with them that matters. Apologize and correct yourself. Remember that habit and history can explain but are not valid excuses. And, as time progresses, tolerance for mistakes will likely decrease—and rightly so.

If you find that someone else's transition is difficult for you and/or stirs something within you, seek community and help but do not hold the trans person accountable for your reaction. Attend a community support group; communicate with a therapist or a spouse or friend; or research more resources online.

Don't Say, "But you were such a pretty girl/handsome man!"
or, "Why are you destroying your man/womanhood?"
or, "You're ruining your body."

These types of comments were probably the most common responses from supposedly well-meaning people that I received in the beginning of my transition. Everyone was so disappointed that I would leave behind my beauty and my suppposedly exemplary womanhood.

These comments are based on a few misconceptions. First, I found that a concerning number of people believed transition to be a result of "failing" at one's assigned gender; people assumed that I felt like I was not a good enough woman, and therefore wanted to be a man. This often drags with it Eurocentric beauty standards, size standards and fatphobia, and even racism and misogyny. I do not believe that one can "fail" their gender—gender is not a test. I did not fail womanhood. I gave womanhood a well-thought-out try. Transition and my manhood are not about "failed womanhood," but rather my intrinsic knowledge of my own gender identity.

Second, these comments imply that beauty alone could bring happiness in one's gender. This is so far from the truth—not only for transgender people, but also for cisgender people. Trans people don't transition because we were ugly; we do not transition to be beautiful. We transition to be happy. We transition to live.

My transition was *not* to make others comfortable or content, to fit into others' standards of manhood, to be attractive in the eyes of others, to be beautiful in the eyes of others, or to garner approval of my physical appearance from others. My transition was not for anyone else. My transition was for me.

Don't Ask, "Can I see a before picture?"

Over the years, I have repeatedly shared images from all parts of my life, ranging from baby photos with my enormous chipmunk cheeks, to photos of middle school me sporting khaki shorts and my Justin Bieber haircut, to photos of me in my prom dress, to me now. Most often, I share these for other trans people. I never imagined that my own future could look as it does today. I never imagined I could one day feel as aligned with myself as I do. For the countless other trans folks who also do not see themselves in the future, I share myself in different iterations to prove possibility and instill hope. *There is more out here in the world for you than you might imagine*, I want them to hear.

But while I am comfortable sharing these, no one—especially not trans folks—owes you photos of their journey to arrive in front of you today. Not only can this feel invasive and painful—many trans folks do not like looking at old pictures of themselves because this brings back trauma and dysphoria—but it also can be very reductive of our humanity. Our journeys are often sensationalized through images, reduced to the perceived juxtaposition between who we are and who we once appeared to be.

Trans people do not exist to exhibit shocking transformations. We are not girl-then-boy, or boy-then-girl. Again, most of us do not characterize our transitions as having changed genders, and asking for photos further legitimizes the gender binary and unnecessarily underscores the importance of our appearance. We are people with rich histories and nuanced stories. We are not a before and after. We are all a during and during.

Don't Ask, "Do you think you are just going through a phase?" or, "Does a part of you think this might be coming up now because it's trendy?"

While some might ask these questions with good intention—they don't want a friend to make decisions they might regret or they worry their friend might be too influenced by the media instead of their internal selves—it is *highly unlikely* that being trans is a phase or some sort of result of a trend. Trans people are not "just confused" or "trying to get attention." For most folks, coming out can be quite difficult and even painful—not something someone tries out on a Saturday because they saw it on TikTok. Because of persistent and violent transphobia, most of us think critically and for long periods of time before sharing our identities with the world.

If anything is a phase for us queer folks, it's cisness and straightness. I spent years trying desperately to be straight and cis to avoid the pain and discrimination that accepting and declaring my transness might cause. In the end, I chose to claim my identity so that I was able to live in my own truth, even with all the hatred that has come with it. Trans people don't come out because it's trendy or silly or fun, we declare our identities as survival on our journeys to pursuing fulfillment and joy.

I sometimes will offer an alternative line of thinking: Maybe it is a phase—*and so what if it is?* Everyone goes through numerous phases in their lives, be it a passion, or a job, or a relationship that doesn't last. Many of these "phases" have long-lasting, even lifelong effects, and that is okay. Though being trans is almost never "just a phase" (or maybe it's just the longest "phase" most people will have in their lives), it's also okay if someone realizes over time that they aren't actually trans. True resilience comes from the trust we have in ourselves to make the best decisions we can and, when some of those decisions inevitably don't yield the expected or desired results, we trust ourselves to figure that out, too.

Don't Say, "You're too masculine/feminine,"
or, "You're too tall/short,"
or, "Your voice is too high/low."

These variations were some of the most common responses my Instagram followers shared. I was devastated, and sadly unsurprised, to hear how many trans folks have been told that they couldn't possibly be who they are because of some particular facet of their body. This is transphobic, mean, and ridiculous.

Most people would not walk up to a cis man and tell him he's too short to be a man. Sure, he might be ridiculed and bullied for his height, but people rarely deny his very manhood. That would be absurd. He's a man; his height cannot take away from that.

The same should be applied to trans people. Our bodies do not define our genders. Our bodies are not to be judged and boxed; no one's bodies are.

I encourage us all to move away from this culture of body-shaming, body-judging, and all-around body-focusing. Remember that everyone—including trans people—is more than their body. Don't reduce trans people to our bodies and how they look to you.

Don't Ask, "Have you thought this through?"

When people asked me this in the early days of my gender affirmation, I had to resist the urge to curse. "Yes, of-fucking-course I have," I wanted to spit. I have not yet let this response escape audibly, and usually opt for a curt, "Yes. Of course."

No person randomly comes to the conclusion one minute that they are trans, having never considered it before, and then spouts it to the next person who will listen. Most people have spent months, if not years, thinking this through, crying themselves to sleep at night, agonizing over how and when and what to say about their identities. Many trans people have already spent years trying to stuff down their truth, trying to mask it, or even trying to trick themselves into believing they were wrong. This heavily internalized gaslighting that we have learned from society can slowly, but surely, degrade our sense of self, and many trans people consider ceasing to exist before sharing their identity with their loved ones and the world.

So yes, we have thought this through. Our transness is not a whim or an afterthought or a trend. It is not impulsive or poorly considered. It is serious and important—and accepting it can be lifesaving.

Don't Say, "This came out of nowhere, what do you mean you're trans? You've always liked being a girl/boy."

Some trans people have known they were trans from a very young age. Some trans kids are able to articulate their identity as early as they can talk—at three, four, or five years old. But not everyone finds the words this quickly. Not everyone is able to unpack and unlearn all the cisnormativity in which they've been raised.

Additionally, when someone says, "You've always liked being a girl/boy," what do they actually mean? When I've pressed people on this question, they often express that the child did not explicitly exhibit desires to assume the stereotypical roles of another gender—for example, someone assigned female at birth like me who did not reject dresses, dolls, or the color pink; someone who maybe even enjoyed wearing makeup and doing traditionally "feminine" activities. It's crucial to remember that femininity and masculinity are not necessarily predictors of gender identity. There are many boys who like to dress up and wear makeup. There are plenty of girls who reject these things.

It's important to separate gender expression from gender identity and allow someone to claim their gender identity with their own agency instead of attempting to box them by the gender rules you understand.

Don't Ask, "Wait...aren't you just gay?"

Gender identity is not the same as sexual orientation:

> Gender identity = who you are.
> Sexual orientation = to whom you are attracted.

Most often, when someone transitions, sexuality does not shift. When sexuality does shift through transition, as previously discussed, this is often because people feel more comfortable expressing themselves and their true sexuality through finding authenticity in transition.

When we transition, the label for a person's sexuality could change to reflect the person's gender identity. As I mentioned in Chapter 1, I've always dated women. Before I transitioned, I called myself *gay* because at the time, I thought I was a woman and didn't know I was transgender. When I came out as a trans man, I began to call myself *straight* because I am not a *woman* attracted to women; I am a *man* attracted to women, and the word we use for that is *straight*.

Still, in the years since I've come out, I've begun to use the label *queer* for my sexuality, despite still having only seriously dated women.

Straight has come to feel reductive of my identity and my history through gender. *Queerness* encompasses more of what I know to be true about myself and my journey.

Don't Say, "You're not a real man/woman."

While this is blatantly transphobic and unkind, it is all too common. In the beginning, it was easy to react to comments like this with pain and self-consciousness. I would recoil, feeling small, and unable to claim my own story. But over time, I've realized that other individuals do not have the power to tell me who I am—even if they are more systemically empowered than I am. They can never take from me what I know about myself.

I've learned to employ the same indignance when told I'm not Korean, or not American, or not some other inherent part of my identity. I remind myself that denying my gender is just as absurd as someone attempting to deny my race or nationality.

How dare they try to tell me who I am! How ridiculous it is that they think they know me better than I know myself! How insignificant their opinions are in the face of the truth of my identity!

If you find yourself thinking that trans people are not "real men" or "real women," I encourage you to ask yourself why that is. Be curious! What do you find when you dig into this question? Is gender truly defined by your genitals? Does your man- or womanhood depend on the appearance of your genitalia? Maybe it does. Likely, it does not. Regardless, it is worthwhile to consider that others may not define their gender the same way you do—and their genders are no less valid or real.

Don't Say, "So . . . I can't talk to trans people about anything?!"

If not asking invasive and inappropriate questions of trans people means you cannot talk to us about anything, you might want to take a step back. There are many more things to talk about with trans people than our private medical history, surgery plans, and genitals. I am confident you do not approach random cishet strangers or even your cishet friends and ask them, "When did you know you were cisgender?" or, "You're straight, how did you tell your parents?" or, "Are you comfortable with your genitals and their size?" Why? Because that's rude, strange, and unacceptable behavior.

You should have the same respect for trans folks.

A great first line when meeting a trans person can always be "Hi, how are you?"—just like with any other person you meet.

PART 3

GENDER AND SOCIETY

CHAPTER 11

What Kids Teach Us About Gender

WHEN I WOKE UP FROM TOP SURGERY, I BEGAN TO SOB AS soon as I looked down at my chest. Even though I was covered in thick bandaging, my chest was now flatter than it had been in a long time. As I cried, my chest tight on the inside, too, the nurses scrambled to reassure me that everything was okay. They thought I was crying because they'd lost my earring.

"I'm crying because I'm so happy," I told them through my tears. They laughed in relief.

Though my family had been supportive of my identity, they'd struggled with the concept of medical transition. Everyone was nervous about surgery. In addition to both parents' uncertainty about going against what the therapists had suggested for me, my mom didn't understand why I wanted to cut off a part of my body that was completely, theoretically "healthy." But *I* knew top surgery was right for me. Despite the medical guidelines at the time that instructed beginning with hormone therapy, I was certain I first wanted top surgery.

When my dad watched me break down in the recovery room, he relaxed. He saw me joyful for the first time in years. Since then, he's told me that was a pivotal moment for him. He was able to see my peace and

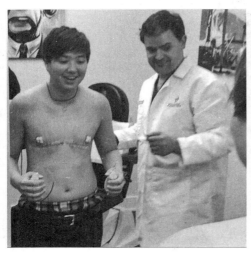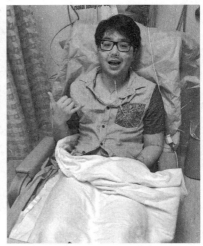

joy—to realize that trusting me in my decisions about my own body had been the right call.

"That joy was enough for me," he told me. "It was so clear this was right for you."

To this day, my mom laments her ignorance surrounding trans experiences and trans healthcare. She has told me numerous times, sometimes in tears, that she wishes desperately that she could have provided me with those resources so I could have transitioned earlier. And that I could have been spared the pain that resulted from not living my gender from an early age.

I do not blame my parents for what they didn't know or understand; I am well aware that education about being trans is lacking. Most people have no clue what they are talking about when we discuss trans issues, especially concerning care for trans children.

In February 2022, Texas governor Greg Abbott (he/him) declared that providing gender-affirming healthcare to a trans child would be deemed child abuse, and that Texas Child Protective Services would investigate families of trans children, effective immediately. That week, some families were broken apart, with trans children separated from parents and removed from their homes. In March 2023, a Florida Republican followed suit, introducing a bill that would allow the courts to remove children from homes where a parent or sibling is undergoing any medical care related to gender affirmation, as well as trans children from supportive parents. Such legislation is bolstered through claiming that providing kids with gender-affirming healthcare hurts or damages the child.

In reality, the exact opposite is true: denying care is abuse; denying care contributes to a number of negative mental health outcomes for children, including self-harm, depression, and suicide. This is backed up by peer-reviewed research, as well as by leading medical authorities.[1–20]

Unfortunately, Governor Abbott, like Florida's governor Ron DeSantis (he/him) and many others, irresponsibly ignores experts. Despite the fact that every major medical, psychological, and psychiatric association agrees gender-affirming healthcare is necessary, appropriate, and can be lifesaving, these state officials have arrogantly decided they know better. Abbott and DeSantis are far from unique. In the age of disinformation, right-wing politicians no longer refer to science. Instead, they rely on transphobia, lies, and fearmongering.

So, let's talk about the science.

CAN KIDS REALLY KNOW THAT THEY'RE TRANSGENDER SO YOUNG?

Throughout my career, I have had numerous parents of transgender kids approach me with a confusing combination of respect and inability to extend the same respect to their own children. I frequently receive the following question from adults:

"Well, I understand you know who *you* are, Schuyler. You seem very articulate and mature, but you transitioned after you were a kid. At eighteen, right? What about the kids who are deciding this so young? Their brains haven't even developed yet! Aren't they too young to make this decision?"

Usually the asker is a nervous parent who desperately wants the best for their child and is terrified that affirming the child's transness will cause the child harm in the future. I have a great deal of empathy for this panic; I know that my mom struggled with this even though I was technically no longer a child when I came out.

Kids are absolutely capable of knowing their gender identity; this is supported by a few key facts:

First, according to major medical associations like the Mayo Clinic, gender identity forms as early as three to five years old.[21] Gender identity is usually established long before sexual orientation, but because many people confuse these, they assume that gender cannot be known prior to adolescence or adulthood. This is false. As soon as a child is able to verbalize their identity, they are capable of knowing it.

Of course, this does not mean that every kid realizes that they are transgender as a toddler. Social and parental pressures as well as societal stereotypes of gender, which are often rigidly enforced at school and at home (and everywhere else), can cause many transgender individuals to remain presenting as the gender they were assigned at birth for many years—some unaware of the reasons behind any disconnect, some unaware of their transness altogether.

Let's not ignore that if a child who is *not* transgender never wavers in their identity in their childhood, no one claims that they are too young to know they are *not* transgender. No one is telling little cisgender boys or cisgender girls that they are too young to know they are boys and girls, respectively. Cisgender children are trusted to know their gender from birth. Transgender children deserve the same self-actualization, autonomy, and dignity.

Second, gender identity is not a decision. Trans children do not *decide* they are transgender, they decide to *tell you*. And what immense courage that often requires, especially in a world rife with violent transphobia and strict gender stereotypes and expectations. I spent nearly five years harboring and hiding my sexuality, and even longer holding my gender identity. Many kids will have spent months or years crying alone and laboring over how to share themselves with us.

Third, when people refer to children's "brains not being fully developed," they are referring to the prefrontal cortex, or PFC. This is largely regarded as the control center of the brain—it is the most recently evolved part of the brain and controls executive function. The claim that the PFC is not fully developed in kids is accurate: executive functioning does not mature until early adulthood. Executive function is often referred to as cognitive or self-control and includes the following three skills: cognitive flexibility, working memory, and inhibitory control, collectively contributing to rule-following and moderating social behavior.[22–25]

Let's focus on inhibitory control for a moment. Inhibition includes the ability to hone attention and focus, ignore distractions, and regulate or control base emotions and impulses. While inhibition is often very useful and allows us to adhere to social rules and therefore function appropriately in society, it also allows us to inhibit ourselves—our very identities.

If you're an adult, you've likely experienced this. Everyone inhibits (or hides, avoids, doesn't show) pieces of themselves for various reasons when they interact with others, especially in social settings.

But as stated by the question-asker, kids do not have mature inhibitory control—they do not have the mature neurological pathways in the PFC yet to enact it. As a result, kids have a unique ability to express themselves exactly as they are, because that is all they have. They have not grown up to learn who they are supposed to be, so they are just who they are.

Mature executive function (from a fully developed PFC) can actually *reduce* the ability for a person to be able to openly speak their mind and express their authenticity because mature executive function allows for a heightened ability to inhibit oneself—and potentially could allow a trans person to inhibit their expression of self due to fear or some other hesitation. An underdeveloped PFC might actually allow kids to declare their identities with more clarity than an adult.

Lastly, the question posed inserts a comparison between me and other trans people that is often elitist, ageist, and sometimes even racist. Confused? Read on.

"You're so articulate" and "You seem so mature" are handed to me as compliments but are followed with "and my child is not." The parent or adult then will often explain why they doubt the validity of a young child's transness or ability to know oneself. This is dangerous reasoning because it declares: *Since my child does not appear as articulate or mature as you are, I do not believe they deserve the same rights or trust that you do.*

This sounds harsh. Because it is. This is what a child will internalize when they share themselves and are met with doubt and rejection. Many parents believe that it is their responsibility to lead the child to somewhere positive, but I firmly believe it is the opposite. The parent must allow the child to lead, and the parent's duty is to hold the child's hand, to be backup, to provide support, especially in matters of identity and self-determination.

Invalidating a child's understanding of themselves not only indicates to the child that they cannot trust you with declarations of self, but that the child should also learn to doubt themselves. This disruption of learning to trust oneself can become deeply rooted, disturbing the child's very sense of self. Numerous studies have shown that invalidating childhood environments are hotbeds for the production of serious mental illness such as depression, eating disorders, and even personality disorders like borderline personality disorder and dissociative identity disorder.[26–28]

The answer for our question-asker is: Children *are* capable of knowing their gender identity as toddlers and are neurologically better equipped to declare their gender identity at a young age due to immature inhibitory brain structures. Children, regardless of their ability to articulate perfectly their identities, should be respected and affirmed for who they are.

CHAPTER 12

Gender-Affirming Care

I'M TRANSGENDER, TOO," HE WHISPERED, HIS HAND CUPPED around my ear. I smiled.

"That's awesome," I answered carefully, aware that too much excitement might be inappropriate and too little would fall flat.

"Yeah, I told my mom and dad that I was a boy when I was really little, and now I don't tell many people I'm trans. I'll be eleven"—he pauses, looking at the ceiling—"in eight days!"

"Wow! Happy early birthday. I'm so excited you get to just be you," I said, a lump forming in my throat. He grinned, waiting for me to continue. Not knowing what to say, I tried something generic. "How is everything at school, how are you doing?"

"I'm good. I like being me," he answered, nodding to himself. "I liked meeting you and hearing your story, too. I like seeing other people like me."

It was all I could do not to cry.

People often ask me where I find the ability to remain hopeful or optimistic and the answer is always trans children and their joy. That kid was just living his life, and happily so. We met at his school during a small meeting the administrators had put together with only their trans and queer students. We had continued chatting and he shared that he'd been on puberty blockers for a few years and was eager to start on testosterone soon.

"I'll start when the rest of the boys start puberty." He grinned, a twinkle in his eyes.

⚜   ⚜   ⚜

IT'S BEEN A while since I met that kid—he must be a high school student now, and he's probably started on testosterone. I've held on to the image of him standing there talking to me, hoping to take some of his trans joy with me, an antidote to the horrible, incorrect ways people characterize our healthcare.

"You're mutilating your body!" is an extremely common allegation. "Why are you destroying what God gave you?!" they'll demand.

And unfortunately, these types of accusations are not relegated to the uninformed commenter on social media; they have made their ways into news articles and out of the mouths of powerful individuals.

I've read countless media pieces on gender-affirming care, and even the very best of them rarely begin with defining the term. But knowing exactly what gender-affirming care entails for whom and at what ages is crucial to understanding what gender-affirming care means. This is imperative when considering banning access to it for youth.

According to the World Health Organization, "Gender-affirmative health care can include any single or combination of a number of social, psychological, behavioural or medical (including hormonal treatment or surgery) interventions designed to support and affirm an individual's gender identity."[1]

Widely agreed upon by all major medical, psychological, and psychiatric associations, gender-affirming care is medically necessary and appropriate, evidence-based healthcare. Gender-affirming care honors the gender identity of the patient through a multidisciplinary approach to allow the patient to assert their gender identity in healthcare.

Gender-affirming care does *not* try to force the individual to align with the gender they were assigned at birth; gender-affirming care believes the trans person and facilitates that person's journey to embody their most authentic self; and gender-affirming care can look different for different individuals.

Gender-affirming care means having providers who refer to us with accurately gendered vocabulary, use our correct names, and who do not pathologize our trans identities. It includes affirming and inclusive intake forms, as well as understanding that a person's routine healthcare might not always fit into a box of cis man or cis woman. For example, as someone who has a cervix, I must have a pap smear every few years. Gender-affirming care is aware of this and provides the necessary services without incorrectly gendering me—e.g., sending me to a "women's clinic" or telling me I need "female care."

Gender-affirming care can include . . .

* Hormones (testosterone, estrogen, puberty blockers)
* Surgical procedures
* Correct pronouns and name, regardless of legal designations
* Affirmations of the trans person's gender identity (and no attempts to change the trans person's gender to what they were assigned) regardless of steps taken in medical transition
* Affirming intake forms:

INSTEAD OF...	TRY THIS...	BECAUSE...
Sex: M / F or Biological sex: M / F	Gender assigned at birth: Gender identity: Pronouns:	Asking for sex in this way is reductive and does not always provide the information salient to providers. On its own, this can seem transphobic, or at least, excluding of trans people. Asking for gender identity and pronouns makes space for trans folks. Make sure to actually use the pronouns asked for!
Name:	Legal name: Preferred name, if different:	Many trans people use a name that is different from their legal name—asking for both and ensuring that the preferred name is actually used is inclusive, affirming, and kind.

INSTEAD OF…	TRY THIS…	BECAUSE…
FOR WOMEN ONLY: [questions about menstruation and pregnancy]	Questions about menstruation and pregnancy. Skip if these do not apply to you.	Not everyone who menstruates / can get pregnant is a woman, and not every woman can get pregnant and/or menstruate. So there's no need to specify "for women." Simply ask the questions about pregnancy and menstruation to attain the information necessary! People who cannot get pregnant or do not menstruate will skip.

WHAT ABOUT GENDER-AFFIRMING CARE FOR KIDS?

Though many people immediately jump to thoughts of surgery, gender-affirming care for children rarely includes going into the operating room. As with adults, gender-affirming care can differ from child to child. Most gender affirmation before puberty includes no medical interventions at all. If a five-year-old child declares he is transgender—"Mom, I'm actually a boy!"—he might get a different haircut, new clothes, and perhaps use a new name and pronouns. No gender-affirming surgery is performed on a five-year-old. No hormones are provided at that age.

When a trans child nears puberty, some medical steps can be taken. Children can take puberty blockers, which block the effects of sex hormones like testosterone and estrogen (usually released in increasing amounts during puberty).[2] As St. Louis Children's Hospital explains, puberty blockers are like "hitting a pause button" on puberty. This allows the child more time to figure out what is best for them, without undergoing a puberty that could potentially cause detrimental mental health outcomes.

Depending on the doctor, location, and local laws, puberty blockers are usually provided at about ten to eleven years old, around what's called "Tanner Stage 2" of puberty, which marks the beginning of physical development when hormones begin to increase.[3] Some providers and guidelines mandate that the child must exhibit some visible effects of puberty (such as budding of the breasts, or enlargement of the testicles) before blockers are provided, while others allow individuals to access blockers before puberty begins.

When children reach puberty, they are able to take cross hormones if they desire. (As a reminder, cross hormones are hormones that are not usually produced in high quantities during puberty—e.g., for a trans man like me, cross hormones are testosterone.) Though rare, if a child decides they would like puberty to ensue without intervention, they are also able to do so. Puberty blockers can be removed and natal puberty will commence. In all U.S. states that allow blockers and/or cross hormone treatment for minors, the child must also attain parental consent.

In short, most gender-affirming healthcare practices for children involve little to no medical interventions before puberty. As puberty approaches, reversible, safe puberty blockers at or right before puberty's onset and hormone treatment during puberty become options. Surgery for minors is incredibly rare and most doctors do not provide such at this time.

Now that you understand what gender-affirming care entails, let's dive into the common arguments—or, rather, as they are more accurately described, propaganda tools.

COMMON MISCONCEPTIONS

Myth: *Transgender advocates want your children to be trans! They're going to make everyone transgender!*

Truth: No one wants anyone's cis kids to be trans. The goal is to let trans kids be trans; or rather, to be *accepted* for being trans. We don't want to turn cis kids into trans kids. We want to make sure trans kids can grow into healthy, happy, and alive trans adults. The fear that providing accessible gender-affirming healthcare is going to make everyone transgender is not only unfounded, but also divisive and manipulative.

"Just keep it to yourself," I've heard so many people say about trans identity and its widespread notoriety. "Don't push it on little kids!" This rhetoric has been used to paint trans and queer educators as "groomers,"* claiming that people like me are harmful to children.

Defenders of Florida's infamous 2022 "Don't Say Gay" bill, which forbade teachers from teaching about LGBTQ+ history and related topics, referred to the legislation as the "anti-grooming bill." This suggested the deeply homophobic idea that the only instance in which an adult would speak about queer and trans topics with a child was in order to groom them for (sexual) abuse.[4] The fact that a significant portion of actual sexual abuse in the United States is perpetrated by white, cis, male family members seems to have been ignored.[5–9]

Hypocrisy prevails: Of the two major political parties, more Republican officials have engaged in numerous sexual abuse incidents, specifically with minors and young students.[10] Take a moment to read the citation if you'd like, but let's peruse some recent facts:

- Former Florida U.S. representative Mark Foley (he/him) was forced to resign in 2006 after news broke that he'd sent sexually explicit messages to teenage pages.
- Illinois U.S. representative Dennis Hastert (he/him) pleaded guilty in 2015 to charges of illegally paying off the high school wrestlers he'd coached and sexually abused decades before.
- Supreme Court justice Brett Kavanaugh (he/him) was accused of sexual assault during his 2018 nomination hearings.
- Alabama Senate candidate Roy Moore (he/him) was accused of preying on girls fourteen and sixteen years old in 2018 and was even banned from a local mall as a result.
- Florida U.S. representative Matt Gaetz (he/him) was investigated for sex-trafficking.

The list goes on.

---

* In the newest use of the word, a groomer is, according to *Urban Dictionary*, "someone who builds a relationship, trust and emotional connection with a child or young person so they can manipulate, exploit and abuse them."

How ironic that those inciting moral panic by accusing queer and trans people, who are simply living openly, of being groomers are often cis men who are *actually* grooming and abusing young people.

Teaching LGBTQ+ history to children in schools is not harmful, abusive, or dangerous. No studies or reports exist proving any correlation between teaching LGBTQ+ history and increased likelihood of committing sexual assault.

No, the only "groomers" here are the (majority white, cis) men who are abusing young people.

Myth: *We shouldn't be letting kids get irreversible surgeries!*

Truth: Most kids are not receiving gender-affirming surgeries because most doctors will not provide surgery to anyone under eighteen, and none do so before adolescence.

The anti-trans rhetoric wants to convince you that toddlers are getting gender-affirming surgery to change their genitals, but this simply is not the case. The only genital surgery that is done on children is nonconsensual genital mutilation wrongfully performed on intersex babies—often without even the parents' consent. Of course, bills banning gender-affirming care have specific carveouts to *permit* intersex genital mutilation—further reinforcing that this is about controlling bodies, not saving kids; about protecting cisnormativity, not protecting children.

The World Professional Association for Transgender Health (WPATH) Standards of Care recommend gender-affirming surgery be available per desire beginning at eighteen. Accordingly, accessing gender-affirming surgery—on genitals or otherwise—is incredibly rare for anyone under eighteen. Those who are able to get surgery before becoming an adult still do so later in their teens—usually at sixteen or seventeen, and only after living in their affirmed gender for extended periods of time as well as many layers of approval, including parental consent, medical review, and even ethical review boards.

There is no such thing as gender-affirming surgery for transgender children—that's a dog whistle from the right. Gender affirmation in children is entirely social, involving support from the people around them and things like hair and clothing changes. There isn't even really medical affirmation in children until they start to undergo puberty, at which point some transgender children may be able to access puberty blockers—drugs that have been used to halt precocious puberty in cisgender kids for decades. Some adolescents who have been affirmed in their gender for a long time may be able to access surgery, after going through extensive evaluation processes and with the consent of their parents, but it's not common. It's also worth noting that cisgender adolescents also get surgeries that affirm their gender—breast reductions and procedures for gynecomastia, nose jobs, and the like. But gender affirmation for children is just loving them and supporting them and giving them the ability to be themselves.

—Dr. Elizabeth Boskey (she/her), Phd, MPH, MSSW, social worker and researcher focusing in trans health[11]

"Cisgender children aren't asking for life-altering procedures, transgender children shouldn't, either!" you might be thinking. And you'd be wrong. Cisgender children absolutely undergo life-changing surgical procedures. And in some cases, they aren't even asking for them; they're being forced into them.

In 2013, the most common cosmetic surgeries performed on (cis) patients thirteen to nineteen years old included breast augmentation, rhinoplasty, breast reduction, otoplasty, and liposuction.[12,13] While the FDA's guidelines approve breast augmentation for individuals eighteen and older, some surgeons still perform them on minors.[14] Rhinoplasty is the most requested aesthetic surgical procedure in teenagers and can be performed as early as thirteen. Otoplasty (ear pinning) can be done as early as five or six.[15] Despite the numerous health and emotional risks presented with these surgeries, opposition to these surgeries—political or otherwise—has been minimal if at all.

Myth: *We have no research on puberty blockers and hormones; they're not safe!*

Truth: This is false on both accounts. Puberty blockers are safe, and research supports that. Decreases in gender dysphoria, improvements in body image, reductions in depression and suicidality, and decreases in overall psychological distress are associated with not only access to puberty blockers, but also the timing of access to puberty blockers. Those who have access to puberty blockers earlier in puberty (as opposed to later when more effects of puberty have occurred) are even more likely to experience positive outcomes, including lower rates of suicidality.[16–35]

Puberty blockers and hormones such as estrogen and testosterone have been used on cisgender people for far longer than on transgender folks. The argument that puberty blockers are unsafe completely ignores the existing data that they have been used safely on cisgender children who experience early onset puberty for *decades* without issue. If puberty blockers are safe for cisgender kids, they are safe for trans kids.

Put simply: trans people experience better mental health outcomes when they are able to access gender-affirming hormones in adolescence than if they only can access them in adulthood.

If you're interested in the research, please see my website for more information.

Myth: *There are bad side effects of puberty blockers! They are risky!*

Truth: The "side effects" most people refer to include weight gain, hot flashes, and mood swings—all of which have been found to be completely reversible[36] and are also all symptoms that every child has the potential to experience when going through natal puberty.

The final "side effect" that most people refer to when fearmongering about puberty blockers is a supposed decrease in bone density.

However, the research that suggested trans women could experience lower bone density as a result of puberty blockers in early puberty[37] was later debunked by a study that found that low exercise, specifically in transgender girls, was a primary factor in low bone density.[38] This makes sense: trans girls are most affected by anti-trans sports legislation and bullying and, as a result, many are unable and/or unwilling to participate in team sports or other exercise activities. Put simply: it is likely that lower bone density is not a result of puberty blockers, but rather transphobia.

The term *side effects* is often used to incite a feeling of danger surrounding puberty blockers, when many of these effects would happen with natal puberty as well. The primary difference is that natal puberty is not reversible, puberty blockers are. Puberty blockers are safe; natal puberty for trans kids might not be.

But even with the research and science in mind, many parents will still approach me with fear. I always think of a certain worried mother when I think of trans children and the necessity for access to care. She had pulled me aside after a speech in Pittsburgh and told me about her child.

"She—she—he—he's trans, like you. He told me a few months ago after he . . ." It was clear she was trying to suppress her tears. Unsuccessful, she wiped her eyes as her voice broke. "She—he! *He* was in the hospital. Suicide attempt. He's only eleven . . . And I don't know what to do." The last sentence came out between choked sobs.

"May I give you a hug?" I asked. She nodded. I leaned in and squeezed her tightly. Conscious of her ability to feel my body against hers, I breathed as evenly as I could, holding back my own tears. After a few moments, I pulled away. "This is so hard. I'm so sorry he's struggling so much." I waited as she regained her composure.

"I don't know what to do," she repeated. "He says he wants puberty blockers. But I don't know if they're safe! I've read about all these side effects—and I just want him to be okay!"

"That makes so much sense," I nodded. "You care so deeply for your kiddo; that is plain to see. I'm so grateful for how much you love him—and I'm sure he is, too—"

"I'm just so worried he'll regret it, what if he's wrong?" she interrupted me.

"Oh, but what if he is right." This was more of a statement than a question.

"What if they're wrong?" is one of the most common fearmongering tactics that anti-trans rhetoric relies on—because it is highly effective, engaging and employing the parents' worry about their child's safety to blind them to the more important question: *What if the child is right?*

"What do you mean?" she asked, puzzled.

"What if he is right about who he is? What if he is right that he needs puberty blockers?"

"I'm not sure," she stumbled.

"That's okay!" I offered, gently. "If he is right, then he gets a chance to live his life the way he wants to—the way that aligns with him. If he's right, he's far more likely to stick around in this world with lifesaving medical care. If he's right, it's likely you'll get to keep your child around." She nodded, digesting what I'd said.

"I understand your concern for your child's well-being, and I am so glad he has such a thoughtful mother. And I worry that you're worrying more about what could go wrong than what could go right. Both should be taken into account. Most of the research shows no negative effects of puberty blockers, but even if there were a few, the negative effects of not providing gender-affirming healthcare are far more dire."

"I didn't think about it that way," she said, nodding. "You're right."

Trans children experience up to five times higher rates of depression, self-harm, suicidal thoughts, and suicide attempts than cisgender children their same age.[39] Some 82 percent of trans people have contemplated suicide and approximately 40 percent of us have attempted at least once,[40] with transgender *youth* exhibiting even higher rates: 86 percent of trans youth contemplate suicide and 56 percent actually attempt it.[41]

Trans youth are already at risk, especially in mental health, and research has found that trans children who are forced to undergo natal puberty experience mental distress, including depression, self-harm, and suicidality.[42] Research has also found that access to puberty blockers in adolescence is associated with lower rates of suicidal ideation across one's *lifetime*.[43]

In the bluntest terms: Trans kids who want and get puberty blockers when they are adolescents will be less likely to kill themselves. And suicidality is far more dangerous than any possible negative side effect puberty blockers could ever cause.

We are missing out on the key question, which is not, "What if the puberty blockers have a negative side effect?" (Of course, as you now know, the research says they do not.) Instead, we must ask, "What if *not* providing puberty blockers has a negative side effect?" In this situation, the latter question is far more important because, yes, research indicates that *not* providing them can have extreme—even deadly—consequences.

Myth: *Most children who say they are trans don't end up staying trans!*

Truth: Yes, they do.

Denial of persistent trans identity is one of the most common rebuttals I receive when I talk about the need for providing gender-affirming healthcare for children who need it.

In December 2022, I gave a virtual keynote at a GSA Forum in New Jersey. After the speech, I opened for questions as usual. The fourth question was asked by a younger kid who told me that he was a sophomore, and also transgender.

"My mom keeps sending me articles about people who've transitioned who...aren't happy. Who are still miserable after they transition. She's afraid transitioning won't help. And I don't know what to tell her. So..." He trailed off, the tears beginning. "You're a transgender adult. So...I wanted to ask you...Are you happy?" He choked into his sobs before he finished. I could feel mine lumping in my throat. I swallowed and took an audibly deep breath before I replied.

"Thank you for this question," I began. "The answer is yes, absolutely. I am a happy, thriving, fulfilled transgender adult. And there are so many more of us than your mom probably has found. Unfortunately, parents are prone to reading the case studies—anecdotal and often sensationalized pieces that cover one or a handful of individuals—instead of peer-reviewed research studies. And that can skew their view." He nodded, wiping his tears.

"I know so many other happy trans adults—but they're often not as visible as the ones who are struggling or still others who are loud about their regret and/or de-transition. This is actually key to recognize: the trans people who are out there just living their lives, well, they're just living their lives."

"That makes sense," he said.

"Are there trans people who still struggle after their transitions? Sure. But that's not because their transitions didn't 'work.' It's because of transphobia. We live in a world that is pretty mean to trans people and even self-grounding can't protect against the pain we experience at the hands of discrimination. I still experience transphobia—but I'm certainly happier dealing with other people's dislike of me than my own. I can easily answer your question that my transition has brought so much happiness, fulfillment, and, most importantly, peace to my life."

Either in fear or denial, many folks will dive into referring to sensationalized media that demonizes transition. Some will even try to cite a study, claiming that "the research" or "studies" show that kids "grow out of it." Though most do not actually know what sources they are citing, a few studies from 2011 and 2012 did suggest childhood gender dysphoria did not persist into adulthood.[44,45] Of course, these studies are more than a decade old, methodologically questionable, and, in some cases, directly debunked later by reexamining the data and finding that the opposite was true: gender dysphoria does persist.[46]

In 2018, several researchers published a review of these older studies, and found that the older research was limited and substandard: "Some of the earliest research on young gender-expansive youth is methodologically questionable," they wrote.[47] Research was not done with enough participants (one study reviewed only twenty-five individuals compared to more recent studies that review thousands) and much of this early research has not been replicated. This greatly decreases the results' veracity and reliability.

Reading these studies makes obvious that the researchers were not in the least bit affirming of trans people's transness. Their language and terminology are outdated and often wildly transphobic—even for 2011 or 2012—and focus primarily on sexuality, as opposed to gender identity. One study referred to participants exclusively by the gender they were assigned.[48] More recent research with methodological integrity clearly indicates that trans identity persists: most kids who claim they are trans continue to identify as such. Trans kids are who they say they are.

In 2021, researchers at Harvard Medical School studied thousands of people (17,151 to be exact) who had socially transitioned at some point in their lives. An overwhelming majority of people (86.9 percent) persisted in their gender identity—and what researchers discovered about the 13.1 percent who de-transitioned is even more illuminating. It's not just that people do not de-transition often; it's that when they do, it's not because they're not trans, it's because of transphobia and related social/interpersonal pressure. *And*, most people who de-transitioned did not get surgery or take hormones; those who are able to access medical affirmation are far less likely (by nearly eight times) to de-transition.

Here's a breakdown of the data:

- **De-transition is most often a result of transphobia, not because someone isn't trans.** 82.5 percent of de-transitioners de-transitioned because of at least one external factor, such as family and societal stigma. Only a small fraction (15.9 percent of de-transitioners) de-transitioned because of at least one *internal* factor, such as uncertainty regarding their gender. In short: most people don't de-transition because they aren't trans. Most people de-transitioned because of societal pressure; because of transphobia.[49]
- **De-transition most often occurs due to pressure from our loved ones.** Younger folks who de-transitioned were more likely

to do so because of pressure from parents, community, society, friends, or roommates, while older participants' reasoning was more likely to be caregiving responsibilities, or pressure from a spouse/partner.[50]

- **De-transition is rare, and it's even rarer for those who've medically transitioned.** Only 2.1 percent of individuals who'd ever pursued gender affirmation (those who had "transitioned") de-transitioned due to an internal reason such as uncertainty about their gender or transness, meaning that people who medically transitioned were nearly *eight times* less likely to de-transition than those who had only socially transitioned.[51]

- **De-transition usually occurs before age ten, before medical steps are taken.** Remember, most children are not old enough for surgery, hormones, or even puberty blockers. Gender affirmation for most kids includes a haircut, name change, pronoun shifts, and a trip to a clothing store.[52]

Though 86.9 percent is an overwhelming majority, it's also worth noting that a more recent study, specifically following trans youth, found an

FREQUENCY OF AND REASONS FOR DE-TRANSITION

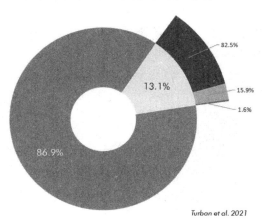

- People who do NOT de-transition
- People who DO de-transition
  - People who de-transition because of at least one external factor (e.g., transphobia, lack of support, stigma)
  - People who de-transition because of at least one internal factor (e.g., uncertainty about gender)
  - People who de-transition for uncategorized reasons

82.5%

13.1%

15.9%

1.6%

86.9%

Turban et al. 2021

FREQUENCY OF DE-TRANSITION AFTER MEDICAL TRANSITION

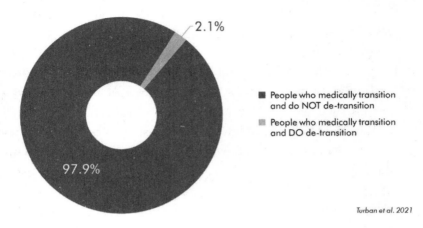

Turban et al. 2021

even lower rate of de-transitioning: only 2.5 percent of children reverted back to a cisgender identity after a five-year period.[53]

I've read and heard many irresponsible and ignorant politicians cite the (fake) statistic of "98 percent of kids who say they're trans realize they're not!" Of course, when pressed they cannot back up this claim with citations or data, because quite the opposite is true. Research

FREQUENCY OF DE-TRANSITION

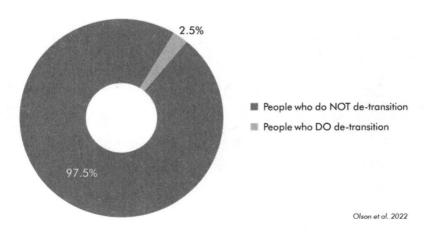

Olson et al. 2022

reinforces that transness is a persistent identity, not a passing phase or something children will outgrow. The problem is not transness but, rather, transphobia.

Myth: *Regret is likely and therefore children should wait until they're eighteen to make these decisions.*

Truth: Regret is possible, but extremely unlikely. And fear of regret should not stop us from making important decisions that could improve our lives.

But what if they regret it?! Some people regret it! Yes, some people do! But as we have seen from the data, this occurs a very small percentage of the time.

I have often been accused of erasing the stories of de-transitioners. I want to be clear: Noting the low prevalence of de-transition does not discredit or invalidate the stories and struggles of those who de-transition. Their experiences are valid, *and* advocating for access to gender affirmation because most people do not regret gender affirmation does not erase the existence of de-transition. It advocates for access.

"You know what most people fail to notice about de-transitioners?" my friend, activist, and media personality Ashlee Marie Preston (she/her) asked me once. "They're almost always white."

De-transition demands that one has actually had access to transition. You've got to have a doctor that believes you need hormones and will provide them for you. You've got to have healthcare or cash to pay for the treatment. You've got to have a doctor or psychologist approve you for surgery and then you have to actually pay thousands of dollars to get the surgery. Contrary to the assertions that doctors are just doling out hormones and surgery like candy, gender-affirming healthcare is actually extremely difficult for most people to access.

When gender-affirming surgery is brought up by participants in my monthly support groups, most of the time it's because they've endured years of waiting to gain approval. *Years.* For many trans folks—especially those who experience intersectional marginalization—hearing stories of "too easy access" can be confusing and even angering. Most trans folks I know have fought tooth and nail for their hormones or surgery. Even I struggled, going through a canceled top surgery because no doctor or therapist of mine would sign my letter approving the procedure. If I, as someone with the benefit of supportive parents, financial resources, and accessible healthcare, struggled to do this, imagine how much more difficult the experience may be for someone less privileged.

Black and brown folks, for example, already experience high levels of medical discrimination. People of color are not only less likely to be insured, but also less likely to receive adequate and appropriate healthcare compared to their white counterparts.[54–57] Medical racism combined with transphobia can result in an even more difficult time for Black and brown trans folks to access gender-affirming care. That most de-transitioners are white could be because they've had the most access to care. And no, this does *not* mean we need to reduce access to care—but it does mean that there will always be patients for which certain treatments are not effective, and there will always be doctors who misjudge or misdiagnose.

In accounts of de-transition, disgruntled parents will claim that their child received care hastily from their doctors, that their doctors were too quick to provide gender affirmation and didn't take the proper steps to understand the patient's struggles. If these are all true, they do not indicate that gender-affirming care should be criminalized or that access should be restricted—we should not punish the patients for medical malpractice. Instead, these indicate a necessity for trans-competent training for medical professionals; we need better trans-informed medical care.

Lastly, do not miss perhaps the most important part of this: de-transitioners most often live to tell the tale. With nearly a 40 percent rate of suicide directly increased by familial rejection and blocked access to gender-affirming hormones, trans kids who were rejected or refused care too often *do not stay alive.*

As for "what if they de-transition?", research suggests that if they're well supported, they'll be fine.[58] When youth are affirmed throughout their process, even reverting back to presenting as the gender they were assigned at birth is not harmful, but rather a healthy and accepted part of their identity exploration.

Most fearmongers ask the question: "What if they're wrong about being trans and they regret gender affirmation?" I urge you to explore the reverse: "What if they are *right* about being trans and regret *not* attaining gender affirmation?"

Myth: *Children are too young to make these life-altering decisions!*

Truth: Children—and their parents on their behalf—make life-altering decisions all the time.

My parents chose to put me in year-round competitive swimming when I was eight years old. By twelve, I was going to practices at four o'clock in the morning so that I could go to two practices a day, before and after school. I spent all my free time during middle and high school underwater; I spent countless weekends at all-day swim competitions; I missed more school than any of my peers to attend travel meets…And I'd go on to get recruited to swim at Harvard, Yale, Columbia, Princeton, and Dartmouth. Putting me in swimming was a life-altering, life-charting decision; I could not even begin to imagine what my life would have been and would be now without that decision in my youth.

I could count many more decisions that I made or that my parents made for me that were life-altering. But you don't see nationwide attempts to ban parents putting their kids in sports (except trans kids, of course, but that's a different story), sending their kids to specific colleges, or choosing classes or other extracurriculars for their kids. Why? Because these are personal decisions that should be made by individuals.

But it's not surgery! Well, as aforementioned, cisgender children do receive cosmetic elective surgeries, many doing so even younger than those who receive gender-affirmation surgeries. And yet, there is no nationwide brigade against doing so even though the rate of regret for cosmetic surgery is significantly higher than for gender affirmation.[59]

If we avoided doing important things for fear of regret, we'd rarely do anything. Certainly we need to consider our decisions with intention, care, and, when appropriate, the consultation of experts. After that, the individual must take a leap of faith with the confidence that if the decision yields an unfavorable or unexpected result, they will be able to figure out the next step.

If you are a parent or another adult close to a trans child, keep reading—the next chapter delves further into facing doubt, fear, and apprehension regarding our transitions.

CHAPTER 13

What I've Learned About
Being Trans . . . from Kids!

A FTER INTRODUCING HIMSELF WITH HIS NAME AND PRONOUNS as I'd asked, he said, "I have a question . . . Do you like cheese?" The crowd at a small middle school in Western Massachusetts erupted with laughter. This particular question-asker was a sixth grader who'd stood up when I'd called on him. He wore a quarter-zip sweater and khaki pants. Even standing up, he was shorter than most of his classmates who were seated.

"No, I'm serious," he said with a straight face as his peers giggled. "Do you? Because I do."

"Yes, I do, actually, I love cheese," I started, trying not to laugh as well.

"What kind? I like muenster."

"That's actually a favorite of mine, too! I also like pepper jack."

"Cool!" He giggled and sat down, passing the mic off to the teacher near him.

Remembering moments like this makes me smile. Younger audiences ask me why I chose to swim instead of skateboard, what my favorite cereal is, what it felt like when people were mean to me, what my favorite color or Marvel movie is, and more. They do not shy away from asking about my transness, but they rarely focus on it, and when they do ask, their questions are surprisingly insightful and pure. I have found my eyes welling with tears far more often in reaction to a child's question than an adult's.

Here are a few examples of real questions and comments from elementary school students:

If you didn't feel comfortable in the girls' bathroom, why did you use it? A kindergartner asked me this at my third speech. It gave me great pause. I sat there, on the floor with nine kids cross-legged in front of me waiting for my answer. I thought about it. *If it was uncomfortable for you, why did you do it?* What an honest question. I wish more of us asked ourselves this.

If you were both afraid and excited to swim on the men's team, does that mean you felt "ambivalent"?

Do people make fun of you?

At my school, we don't make fun of people who look different. Anyone can use the bathroom. It's just a bathroom.

My favorite stroke is butterfly! What's yours?

Girls and boys have longer hair. Girls and boys have short hair. It's okay for people to look different!

Why do people think being transgender is bad?

Older audiences—such as parents, working professionals, coaches, administrators—ask questions almost exclusively about my experience as a trans or queer person. But, as the audience gets younger, the questions become less and less focused on my gender or sexuality and instead are about who I am as a whole. Kids are far more able to see all of me—as well as to care about me as I relate to them—than adults are. And I think we can all learn from this.

When I travel to schools, adults are often nervous to discuss gender and gender identity with children. "But this trans thing will just confuse them!" parents and teachers fear. "Wait until their brains are ready for this information."

Well, given that gender identity solidifies in childhood—between three and five years old and, therefore, their brains *are* ready around that age—we should absolutely begin talking about gender in childhood, as early as kindergarten!

My younger cousins were four and nine years old at the time I was coming out as transgender. While coming out to my aunt and uncle was rather uneventful, I was quite nervous to talk about my identity with the kids, especially with the four-year-old. What words would I use? Would he even understand the concept?

When it came down to it, telling them both about my gender was surprisingly simple—for them. Neither kid got particularly stuck on anything I said, and they switched pronouns faster than any of the adults.

In the years I've done this work, I found this ease of reception to be consistent among younger kids. Based on my experiences of speaking in dozens of primary schools, I've learned children need far less complicated and lengthy explanations of gender.

When I talk to younger children, this is how I explain I am transgender:

When a baby is born, the doctors look at the baby and say, "This is a little girl!" or, "This is a little boy!" And sometimes, the doctor gets that wrong. So, when I was born, the doctor looked at me and said, "This is a little girl!" And so, everybody thought that I was a little girl. But when I got older, I realized, "Wait! That's not who I am!" and when I was able to tell people, I said, "I'm not actually a little girl, I'm a boy!" And that means I am transgender—that the person everybody told me I was isn't actually who I am. There's nothing wrong with being transgender. I just have to explain that to people.

If non-binary is also on the list, I'll add:

Sometimes, people aren't boys or girls. They don't fall into these little categories of boy and girl, and that's totally okay! Sometimes people are in between, or they're neither boy nor girl, or they're a combination, and that's called non-binary. *And there's nothing wrong with being non-binary, either!*

It is rare for kids—especially younger ones—to have many questions following these explanations. Usually, they nod in understanding and are ready for the next question. Sometimes, they'll excitedly engage with me to share about their own gender experience and how it relates to what I've said. It's quite beautiful.

We often forget that kids are wonderful at emotions. They live in emotion. Humans are neurologically "programmed" to connect; kids are not born hateful. They are taught to hate over time. Kids are actually born with an immense capacity to love.

But you'll confuse the kids! Yes, maybe we will! And maybe that's okay. It *definitely* is okay.

Unfortunately, confusion and chaos are most often appraised as bad, unwanted, or something to remedy. But confusion and not knowing are exactly where we grow and learn about ourselves. The U.S. school system has a lot of shortcomings but one of the gravest is the lack of space for children to learn about themselves, their emotions, and their identities. But if we can appraise their confusion as positive—as exploration—it might not be as scary for the child. Confusion becomes another tool for discovery.

I've found that most parents are far more frightened of the world than their children are. While I have a great deal of empathy for this fear, I also want to remind any parents that it should not ever be the responsibility of the child to mitigate and hold their parents' fears. That is a parent's responsibility as a parent. I have watched in devastation as parents teach their fears to their previously courageous, bold, proud trans child. Teaching a child caution and realistic expectations is important—for their safety and for their ability to navigate the world—but teaching them to fear the world because a parent does is harmful.

After a speech I gave at a school in central Pennsylvania, a mother came up to me to talk about her child.

"He's just so bold and the other kids are going to make fun of him," she told me. "I'm so worried about his safety. He doesn't seem to care that he doesn't do what the other kids do. I mean . . . he's going to school in dresses and he wants to wear makeup . . . I don't know what to do!"

"I'm so glad you're sharing your concerns," I began.

"I don't know what to do! He shouldn't dress like that, what if he gets hurt?" She interjected before I could continue.

"I hear you," I said gently. "I know it's such a difficult place to be in. You're afraid for your kid's well-being and that's so important. I can tell how much you care about him. That love is crystal clear to me. And I know you want to protect him as much as possible."

"I do!"

"I understand. I know you are afraid. But it sounds like he hasn't adopted that fear yet. That's also okay. There's a difference between teaching him fear and teaching him awareness. One will cause him to draw inward, the other will allow him to walk the world with educated courage. So teach him to be mindful. Teach him to be careful. Teach him to understand his surroundings and his positionality in the world. But don't teach him his identity is something to fear, something he should worry about. Teaching a child to fear being themself is not going to bring them joy or emotional safety; it'll likely bring the opposite. The best thing you can do is create safety at home—the world is going to be mean and scary no matter what. I know you want to be a safe place for him."

"Of course, I do! But what about other parents . . . they'll say mean things and I am sick of being judged! I don't want them to make fun of him!" It was as if she were pleading with me.

"That is so valid. And, at the end of the day, you can't control what other parents do. You can only control what you do. If you want your child to adjust how he is presenting himself to make other people more comfortable, then you are prioritizing other people's judgments and your fear of those judgments *over* the freedom of expression and the well-being of your child." She was silent, thinking.

"I know you don't want to do that. I know, from how you've talked about your child, that you love him dearly and you want the best for him. The way to do that is to let him be himself—to trust him to figure that part out. Don't make him change to fit in."

It's also important to remember that creating space for kids to wonder about their gender and the expansiveness of their identities is a beautiful privilege—an opportunity for them to explore and discover more about who they are. If I confuse a cisgender child by presenting my own transness and the diversity and possibility of gender, that child gets a privilege that most cisgender people never do. Most cisgender adults have *never* questioned their gender.

Lastly, as usual, I encourage folks to ask themselves the reverse-risk question. Most often, we ask, "What if we confuse the kids by talking about transness?" And I ask, "What if we don't give those kids access to language that allows them to describe themselves by not talking about transness?" In the first scenario, the worst we risk is a little confusion, while also gaining a great deal of self-discovery. In the second, we risk losing children's lives. The choice is clear.

CHAPTER 14

Peeing in Peace: Trans People and Bathrooms

ONE HOT DC SUMMER WHEN I WAS TEN YEARS OLD, I WENT to a weeklong summer camp at the National Zoo. Animals were my biggest passion and interest then, and I was very excited to spend a whole week with them. Unfortunately, camp also meant something that I dreaded: interfacing with people who didn't know I was supposed to be a girl, which really meant having to tell people, "I'm a girl."

Back then, everyone gendered me as male if they weren't told otherwise. I hadn't yet hit puberty. I had a short "boys'" haircut and wore almost exclusively cargo pants and T-shirts, so I looked just like most of my male peers.

Still, not having discovered the word or identity *transgender*, I called myself a girl. Not without distress, I felt compelled to correct others when they thought I was a boy.

One particular camp counselor decided it would be her mission to make my week miserable. Despite me informing her numerous times that I was, in fact, a girl, she constantly harassed me in the bathroom.

The first few days, she sneered at me in a tone that made me want to fade away: "Are you *sure* you're *really* a girl?"

"Yes," I replied before quickly locking myself into a stall to relieve myself.

On the third day, I tried drinking less water and holding my bladder as long as I could. In the muggy DC summer, this was a terrible idea. But luckily, I'd made a friend. And Seo-yeon (she/her) wouldn't stand for this.

"I'm going with you," she declared on the third day, linking her arm into mine. "Let's go."

She marched us into the women's bathroom, her head held high.

"No *boys* allowed in here," the same camp counselor taunted on cue.

"She *is* a girl," Seo-yeon said loudly. "You don't know what you're talking about. Shut up and leave us alone." Stunned, the counselor said nothing. Seo-yeon proudly tugged me over to the stalls.

I'm not sure what facial expression I'd worn, but inside I felt warm. It didn't matter that "girl" still didn't feel like it fit me. It was so nice to have someone stand up for me. I felt protected.

For the rest of camp, Seo-yeon and I went to the bathroom together. If anyone said anything to me, she screamed at them until they left me alone. Seriously, she *screamed*.

Unfortunately, I didn't have Seo-yeon to accompany me to bathrooms for the rest of middle school. Even though my classmates and peers knew that I was supposed to be a girl, I was constantly berated in the girls' bathroom at school.

"What are you doing in here? This is the *girls'* room," they'd say to me in a nasty tone. Nothing made me feel smaller.

"I am a girl." I was always barely audible in my response—not even sure of the statement myself.

Going to the bathroom became a terrifying experience. Most of the time, I tried to just hold it, but when I couldn't, I'd run to the other end of the school where the single-stall teachers' bathroom was. It was far better to risk getting in trouble for using the teachers' bathroom than it was to be scorned by all the girls at school.

When I had no choice but to use the girls' room, I would wait until I was certain no one else was around. I felt like I was sneaking in—I'd walk up to the door and press it open slowly. If I saw someone inside, their face usually terrified by my boy-ness, I would yelp, "Sorry! Wrong bathroom!" and keep walking down the hall as if I'd made a mistake. I'd then have to try again later.

I've never forgotten the sound of the heavy bathroom doors whooshing open and the rapid pace of my heart as I tried to use the bathroom in peace during middle school.

The fear instilled in me carried beyond school—to the grocery store bathrooms, airport restrooms, and the pool locker room. At public restrooms, women would yell not only at me but also at my mother.

"How dare you bring your *son* into the women's room, he's clearly too old," they'd sneer at her.

"This is my *daughter*," she'd bark back. I would cower.

Eventually, I would refuse to use the bathroom in public altogether. When flying, I would wait until we boarded the plane to use the single-stall, ungendered airplane bathroom. At the pool, I learned that if I changed into my swimsuit in the car that I could use this as a symbol of my belonging in the girls' locker room. I'd hop down from our bright green car with my similarly neon green backpack. About fifteen paces from the entrance to the girls' locker room, I would shift the backpack to one shoulder and remove my T-shirt, exposing the women's swimsuit. This was my ticket to entering the bathroom without harassment.

So, years later when someone finally asked me for the first time which bathroom I wanted to use, I immediately said the men's. I can't remember many women's bathrooms I have *not* been harassed in. The men's bathroom in contrast—in its disgusting, pee-soaked glory—has been an odd haven for me, at long last.

Trans people and our right to use the bathroom of our choice has been a lightning-rod topic for years. The controversy regarding allowing trans people to use the bathrooms that align with our gender identity was arguably the first major legislative attack that inaugurated the series of multiplying anti-trans bills.

But, of course, trans people are far more likely to experience harm, as I did, in the bathrooms than to cause it. Unfortunately, this is not the message that most people receive, so let's spend some time myth busting this propaganda.

Myth: *Allowing transgender people to use bathrooms is a threat to public safety.*
Fact: The twenty-two states and more than three hundred cities in the U.S. that include LGBTQ+ people in their nondiscrimination protections in public accommodations have seen no increase in public safety incidents as a result of their nondiscrimination policies.[1,2]

Myth: *Letting trans people into bathrooms will result in more sexual assault, particularly of women in the women's bathroom.*
Fact: Nondiscrimination laws have not increased assaults in bathrooms. A study by the Williams Institute in 2019 found no correlation between passage of nondiscrimination laws (such as those that protect trans people's right to use the bathrooms of our choice) and the number or frequency of criminal incidents in bathrooms, locker rooms, or dressing rooms.[3]

Myth: *Allowing trans students to use the bathrooms aligned with their gender identity prioritizes trans students over cis students and their safety.*
Fact: Not only are trans students more likely to be assaulted than cisgender students, but a recent study shows that trans students are at even greater risk of sexual assault in schools where they are prevented from using the bathroom that aligns with their gender identity (35 percent) than students at schools where they are permitted to use their aligned bathroom (26 percent).[4–6]

Inciting panic regarding bathrooms and supposed threats to the safety of cis women and girls was first employed by Republicans in 2014 in Houston, Texas. The city council had passed the Houston Equal Rights Ordinance (HERO), which would have prohibited discrimination in the workplace, housing, and other public accommodations, based on several characteristics, including gender identity and sexuality. HERO's goal was to improve LGBTQ+ protections because it was—and still is—legal to fire people for being queer or trans in at least eighteen states.[7–9] Note that status has not changed at the time of this writing. In forty states,

LGBTQ+ Americans do not receive a full compliment of protections: in eighteen states, employers can legally fire an employee for being trans; in twenty states, landlords can reject tenants for being trans; in thirty states, students can legally experience discrimination for being trans; in forty states, jury selection may discriminate based on gender identity.[10]

HERO was doing very well until Republicans "began scaring people about bathrooms."[11] They argued that this nondiscrimination policy would result in trans people using bathrooms aligned with their gender identity, thus opening the floodgates for nefarious, deviant individuals who would take advantage of the law to hurt women. The argument was that (cis) men would disguise themselves as trans women so that they could gain access to women through the women's bathroom, with the goal to sexually assault women.

Let's take a deep breath. This gets heavy quickly—and that is why this scare tactic is so effective.

Bathroom bans became a unique focus in 2016 when Republicans repeated these techniques to pass HB2 in North Carolina, a bill that restricted access to public bathrooms so that one must use the bathroom corresponding with the gender marker on their birth certificate—with the explicit aim of banning trans people from using bathrooms consistent with our gender identities. They used the same arguments to bolster their case: *if we let trans people use the bathrooms of their choice, cis men (posing as women) are going to abuse this and harm women!* Cis men!

The irony would be laughable if it weren't so harmful. Trans people are far more likely to be assaulted in bathrooms, and yet these arguments are crafted around painting trans or otherwise gender nonconforming individuals as the likely perpetrators of violence.

These arguments forget such a crucial, glaring point: regardless of who commits sexual assault and where, *sexual assault is still illegal and wrong!* These criminals are not going to care what is or isn't illegal—do we really think they are considering the law as they decide to sexually assault someone? "Oh, now it's more legal for me to enter the women's bathroom, so let me legally enter so I can engage in one of the most heinous illegal actions."

Terry Kogan (he/him), a law researcher at the University of Utah who has done extensive research about the history of gender-segregated bathrooms, helpfully reminds that these predators "are not waiting for permission to dress up like a woman to go into bathrooms."[12] Kogan also notes an important piece of history: gender-segregated bathrooms arose out of the sexist belief that women needed to stay at home, were weaker, and were in need of protection from the "harsh realities of the public sphere."[13] Even the original purpose of gender-segregated bathrooms is rooted in patriarchy and misogyny.

The bathroom frenzy seeks to align trans people with deviance—an intentional and manipulative tactic to further demonize us in the public eye, to paint us as other, as nefarious, as dangerous. Of course, in reality, no evidence points to trans people ever being significant perpetrators of sexual violence—or any violence for that matter. The precise opposite is true: in comparison to cis people, trans individuals are more likely to experience sexual assault.[14] One in three (presumably cis[*]) women and one in four (presumably cis) men will experience sexual assault[15] while one in two trans people will experience sexual assault.[16–19]

You might have noticed that panic about bathrooms was incited by right-wing politicians—who statistically are more likely to be sexual assaulters themselves (recall Chapter 12). This fabricated panic dismisses the root of the fear they are instilling: If you are afraid of men—presumably cis men—masquerading as women in order to assault them, you are afraid of toxic, predatory cis men. You are not afraid of trans women. The very men perpetuating patriarchy are causing widespread panic about patriarchy by villainizing trans people, when they themselves are the true perpetrators.

Cis men's fear of their own despicable behavior is explicit: In May 2023 when the Illinois House passed a bill allowing businesses to create all-gender bathrooms, Republican state senator Neil Anderson (he/him) said he would "beat the living piss" out of any man in the bathroom with his daughter, declaring, "it's going to cause violence from dads like me."[20]

---

[*] General research in the population disproportionately measures the cis population. For this reason, while these statistics do not explicitly cite "cis women" and "cis men," it is likely that the collected data was largely from cis people.

If you are someone who has feared for the safety of the women and girls you love at the hands of trans people, it's imperative to recognize that trans people are not an inherent threat.

In reality, the facts show that the most likely person to assault your daughter or child is someone they already know or even a family member. Ninety to 93 percent of child sexual assault victims know their offender—with a third to a half of the perpetrators being family members.[21,22] Only about 7 percent of perpetrators are strangers. Eighty-eight percent of perpetrators are male.

So let's put that all together in the plainest words: the people who are most likely to sexually abuse your child are the cis men already in their life—their father, their stepfather, their grandfather, their uncle, their brother, their mom's boyfriend, or other male friends.

If we were to apply the same fearmongering to this data, then we should ban all cis men from the homes of women and children. This is not only impossible but clearly unreasonable.

We *must* cease punishing marginalized groups for the toxic behavior of cis men. It is valid to fear cis men—patriarchy has caused the most harm to the most people for the longest period of time. But the solution is not to remove the rights of trans people because cis men might abuse the law. The solution is to teach men to be better.

Well I don't care how someone identifies, I don't want someone with a penis in the bathroom with my daughter!

Unfortunately, this is also something I've heard quite frequently. First, this assumes that all trans women you run into in the bathroom will have a penis, which is false. Second, regardless of someone's genitals, if you are concerned with what genitals another person is peeing with, that is not their problem; it's yours.

We do not have mandatory genital inspections for everyone who enters a gendered bathroom—and if we did, that would be a complete violation of privacy. You do not know what every woman's genitals look like in the bathroom, nor should you. They are called private parts for a reason.

Some folks will share that they have experienced harm at the hands of someone with a penis and that is the reason for their fear. Of course, this pain is incredibly valid. And it does not mean we should discriminate against trans women or investigate the genitals of others around us. That is, if someone was assaulted by an Asian man and develops a fear of Asian men or men who might resemble the assailant, it does not mean that all Asian men should then need to vacate the streets. That is not fair. And it also doesn't mean that the individual who was harmed is invalid for fearing or feeling triggered. The feelings make sense but should be dealt with in therapy, not by banning everyone who resembles the person who harmed them.

Allowing trans people to pee in peace does *not* threaten others.

CHAPTER 15

Trans People and Dating

"THERE'S LOTS OF TYPES OF DATING," I BEGAN ANSWERING THE question.

"There's long, long-term dating—like my parents, who have been married almost forty years. There's shorter than that, of course, like a few years, or even a few months." The audience was following, although mostly unsure of where I was going.

"And then, there's really short-term dating. Maybe a few weeks, or a few days . . . or, maybe even a few hours . . . or minutes depending on how long you—" They had erupted in laughter at this point.

"Okay, okay." I grinned. "You get it. We're on the same page. Awesome. So, lots of different kinds of dating. How people navigate dating often depends on the situation and type of dating."

This is a practiced answer I've given hundreds of times because one of the most common questions I've received onstage is about dating: if I date, how I date, what dating is like, if I'm in a relationship, if I have sex, how I have sex, and what sex for trans people is like. Of course, these are generally very invasive questions to ask cis and trans people alike. But I do believe they are important in conversations about trans people, so I understand why people are curious.

Before we dive into the answers, I must first remind you that not all trans people will engage with questions like these. Most will not: you should expect trans people will not answer these kinds of questions. I imagine you don't ask random cisgender individuals how they date or what sex positions they enjoy because doing so would be wildly inappropriate, rude, invasive, and strange. Please extend the same grace and respect to trans folks.

The short answer to the series of questions is that I have dated, I have had sex, and I am now married. I have been in a variety of relationships, mostly longer term. In these relationships, I've experienced a variety of transphobic remarks, from a girlfriend telling me that they'd dreamed of me with different genitals, to another discarding me altogether because I am transgender, and still another declaring that my parts were not very masculine.

I engaged in very few short-term relationships—one-night stands or otherwise—and it is difficult for me to discern if I would have explored this more if I were not transgender. Regardless, I am certain that being transgender contributed to my nervousness and hesitancy to pursue anything short-term or specifically sexual in nature when I was not in long-term relationships.

Though I am transgender, I am often assumed to be cisgender, and at college parties or other situations in which hooking up was a common practice, I feared for the moment I'd have to disclose my transness. Would someone be angry or violent? The latter was unlikely given two truths: First, I am a transgender man, and not a trans woman. Trans women are far more likely than trans men to encounter violence (sometimes fatal) when dating cisgender individuals. Second, I have mostly dated women and, statistically, women are far less likely to enact violence in interpersonal relationships.

Still, I never knew how the moment would go—and most often I was neither eager nor even ready to find out. Rather than risk being in environments in which I'd interact with strangers, for dating I tended to lean into spaces where my transness was already disclosed. This included pre-existing friendships and online dating apps.

From my experience mentoring and interacting with other trans individuals, my experience is neither unique nor uncommon. Unfortunately, I've found that a majority of trans people have encountered difficulty navigating dating, mostly due to fear of rejection and subsequent consequences, including violence. This transphobia—and yes, I believe it is transphobia—can have painful and deep repercussions on a trans person's self-esteem and sense of belonging in the world.

Most of my trans clients have told me that their parents have said something about their child not finding a loving partner because of their transness. A devastating amount of trans people have heard a parent tell them, "If you come out as trans, no one will ever love you." Numerous parents even voice this concern directly to me: "I'm so afraid no one will ever love my child." This tells me that these fears come from a place of love, but unfortunately, love is not what is communicated. Instead, the child feels exiled and worthless.

When I talk with parents, I remind them that creating a space of love at home is of utmost importance to fighting external transphobia—that replicating transphobia at home will never heal or protect the child. Then, we dive into the deeper implications this transphobia enforces—in dating and in life.

"NOT WANTING TO DATE TRANS PEOPLE IS NOT TRANSPHOBIC; IT'S JUST A PREFERENCE!"

In March 2021, a video describing a "new sexuality" went viral on TikTok. In it, a boy claims that he has come up with "super straight," a sexuality that excludes trans people because he was tired of being called transphobic. When asked about dating trans women, the TikToker says in his video, "She's not a real woman to me. I want a real woman. [. . .] So now I'm a super straight. [. . .] You can't say I'm transphobic because that's just my sexuality, you know?"[1] The TikToker's account was eventually removed for violating community guidelines.

But sadly, the movement continued. A disappointing number of individuals piled on the trend, declaring their own "super straightness." Thousands of people joined a subreddit for "super straight," unveiling their deep-seated transphobia. Some even claimed they were dealing with "superphobia," describing the "oppression" they were experiencing for their supposed sexuality. The Reddit has since been banned for "promoting hate."[2]

While the label "super straight" was explicitly intended to exclude trans people on the basis of our transness—and is therefore, by definition, transphobic—the argument that it's "just a preference," is still, by far, the most common argument I've heard attempting to validate rejecting trans people on the basis of transness.

It's just *preference*. Unfortunately, it's not that simple.

At the most granular level, "preference" here usually refers to genital preference: some people claim they prefer dating men with a penis, others prefer women without one. "Super straight" and similar ideologies then utilize this "preference" to declare they would not date trans people, based on the assumption that trans men do not have penises and trans women do. But even this base assumption is false: some trans men have penises and some trans women do not.

Beyond this inaccuracy, even the concept of genital "preference" is reductive. If we lived in a perfect world free of transphobia, then yes, being attracted only to certain genitals could be "just a preference." But the thing is: *we don't live in that ideal world*. We live in a racist, sexist, misogynist, homophobic, and very transphobic world. Our preferences were not formed in a social vacuum. Our preferences are born in and of a world fraught with systemic oppression and massive identity-based injustice. Given this, I believe it's impossible to extricate "just a preference" from systemic oppression—in this case, transphobia—present in our everyday lives.

Consider the same excuses that are frequently given about race: "I'm not racist, I just don't like Black women," or, "I'm not anti-Asian, I just don't date Asian men," and so on. While no one should ever force you to date someone you don't want to date, these "preferences" are still inherently racist. They are born of and contribute to a system of oppression that continues to discriminate against and disenfranchise Black and other people of color. The same goes with the choice not to date trans folks.

Someone can absolutely choose not to date us, *and* that choice can still be transphobic.

If a trans man doesn't have a penis, it is for one reason: because he is transgender. If a trans woman has a penis, she has it for one reason: because she is transgender. Rejection of a trans person based on their genitalia is thus inherently a rejection based on their transness.

Beyond definitions, I urge you to consider sex and dating for people who are not transgender. As mentioned earlier, most cisgender people don't inspect the genitalia of prospective partners before deciding whether or not to date them. While sexual chemistry is important to many people in relationships, most figure it out as they go. People buy what they don't have. They learn what the other person likes. And they discontinue what doesn't vibe.

The "genital preference" argument also ignores that cisgender people experience genital variations as well. The belief that another genital presentation is unacceptable or unlikable cannot be extricated from the transphobia that our society imparts upon us.

> Never okay to murder anyone over this, at all. One question I do have that seems to be extremely mixed even among trans individuals is whether or not they have an obligation to disclose their genitals or status as transgender in the event of a sexual encounter. If the person's genitals do not match up to the expectations of the partner, does the partner have legitimate grounds to withdraw consent, or is that transphobic? I personally think you should always be allowed to withdraw consent and that it's not necessarily transphobic to not have a sexual desire for certain genitals, as not everyone experiences arousal from viewing certain genitals, but I've heard arguments that this is not a legitimate reason to stop a sexual encounter and that doing so is transphobic. I'm not sure tho, honestly looking for feedback or an opinion on this.
>
> 1d　21 likes　Reply　Message

pinkmantaray ✚

in short, my answer is yes to both of your questions. Yes, someone's genitalia not meeting expectations is absolutely a legitimate reason to withdraw consent— because ANY reason is legitimate!! Anyone can withdraw consent for any reason at any time. AND yes, the reason for that withdrawal can still be transphobic, (or, in other scenarios, racist, classist, ableist, etc.) So, in this case, in my opinion, it is both legitimate and transphobic to withdraw consent due to a trans person's genitals. (Consider the definition of transphobia: discrimination based upon one's transness. If someone decides to reject someone because their genitals are not what they expected because they are trans, then that person is rejecting someone due to their transness—the definition of transphobia. I will offer that acting transphobic is an act. It is not always a definition of character. And it is not a sentencing to hell or horrible person-ness. But it is, in my understanding, by definition, transphobic.)

23h   33 likes   Reply

"BUT I WANT TO HAVE CHILDREN AND TRANS PEOPLE CAN'T! MY REJECTION ISN'T TRANSPHOBIC!"

This one is complicated. In short, assuming that a trans person cannot have a biological child is not always correct—many trans people are capable of birthing or contributing to birthing children. Additionally, 9–17 percent of the world population have experienced fertility problems.[3,4] This is many times more than the number of trans people in the world. Whenever you date someone, you are risking that either you or your partner will be infertile or have other difficulties with conceiving a child with your own bodies. As a result, plenty of cisgender couples access other ways of having and raising children. Denying a trans person—or any person, regardless of gender history—solely on their childbearing capacity seems unkind and unreasonable.

⸻ ⸻ ⸻

IF YOU ARE feeling defensive or even angry because you think your preferences are not transphobic, take a moment to pause. You might need to revisit Chapter 9 and review those steps. Breathe. This is not an attack or a degradation of your character. Your mind might be shouting, "I'm not a bad person for not wanting to date a trans person!" No, you're not a bad person. You are a person who's been steeped in a transphobic world *and* your "preferences" are inextricable from this world. Labeling an action as transphobic does not inherently mean that you're a horrible person, or even forbid you from continuing with that action. That is, people can act transphobic and also not be terrible people who hate all trans people.

I'll bet most people—including trans folks ourselves!—hold (often unconscious) transphobic biases. Why? Because we all live in a transphobic world! We all need to at least recognize that (un)conscious bias is our starting point.

"THIS IS FORCING PEOPLE TO HAVE SEX WITH TRANS PEOPLE!"

In the several times I've talked about this issue online or in person, I've received comments like this, claiming that by declaring "genital preference" inherently transphobic, I am denying another person their agency to consent. That is not only far from the truth but another manipulative tactic to demonize trans people and reinforce the narrative trans people are inherently deviant predators.

I cannot stress this enough: Calling an act transphobic (or racist, classist, ableist, or any other type of bigotry) *does not* deny someone's agency or ability to consent. Calling an act transphobic is calling an act transphobic. That's it. Perhaps it also could entail encouraging that person to investigate their unconscious biases and untangle themselves from the systemic transphobia they've unknowingly and perhaps unwillingly digested. But regardless, anyone can withdraw consent for any reason and at any time, and that withdrawal should always be respected. *And* that withdrawal can still be due to transphobia and transphobic bias!

so, let me get this straight. If a trans woman who hasn't undergone a genital change willingly omits the fact that she still has a dick and lets the guy she's with bring her to bed, knowing his expectations and her willingness to follow along with it,, it's still the guy's fault when he finds out they have the same genitalia and doesn't want to go through with it? Let me know if I got that right

1d   8 likes   Reply

pinkmantaray ✪   it's not at all about if he wants to have sex with her. Anyone is welcome to revoke consent at any time for any reason. No one is saying that people must have sex with people after they disclose they're trans. Read my post. This is about how no one should be angry or MURDEROUS when they learn of our identities.

1d   164 likes   Reply

"IF I'M INTERESTED IN DATING A TRANS PERSON, WHEN SHOULD I ASK THEM ABOUT THEIR GENITALS?"

I hope you read this question and immediately realize how invasive and ridiculous it sounds. If you are truly interested in a person for who they are, it should not matter what their genitals look like. If you are interested in them just for their genitalia, that's not dating and you probably should not be seeking a relationship; you might be fetishizing and/or in need of some priority reevaluation. Remember that it is not a standard or accepted practice to demand information about someone's genitals on the first date.

Still, I know many folks will still wonder if, when, and how it is appropriate to ask a trans person they're dating or might be interested in dating about their genitals, so here is my answer: let them tell you. If you are interested in them for more than their genitalia, then the answer should not matter.

CHAPTER 16

"You Lied to Me"—
Trans People and Disclosure

T HE FOLLOWING IS AN EMAIL I RECEIVED FROM A FOLLOWER A few years ago.

On 8/20/20, 1:39 PM, "Redacted" <Redacted@Redacted.com> wrote:

Hi there,

I've been following your page for about a month or two in an effort to learn how to be a better ally.

I recently put a post in my story that said "BLACK TRANS LIVES MATTER." Someone I know responded saying that I should just say "Black Lives Matter." My responses said that we needed to remind people that Black Trans Lives Matter because they are often killed for being who they are. His response was that Trans women are often killed because they try to trick men. There was some other vile stuff.

I wanted to know if there was somewhere I could find some good ways to answer when people say this crap? I felt like I needed more ammunition.

Much love

Unfortunately, this topic was neither new nor surprising to me.

I feel like you lied to me.

Why didn't you tell me?

You've been pretending this whole time?

Surprise, disdain, and betrayal are all seemingly common reactions that trans people—especially trans women—experience when they choose to disclose their transness and were previously assumed to be cisgender. Many people choose not to disclose their transness for a myriad of reasons, but most frequently for safety and ease.

Living one's life intentionally not disclosing transness is often referred to as *living in stealth*, sometimes *being* or *going stealth*. The term *stealth* evokes complex feelings in the trans community. While many approve of using it, many do not. *Stealth* can further associate trans people with intentional deception, trickery, or deviance, when in reality, trans people who live in stealth are not trying to trick or deceive, but rather just survive. I rarely choose to use this word but do not believe it is my place to police other trans folks' use of it.

Even after eight years of being a public figure and wearing my transness as obviously as I possibly could—nearly naked in my Speedo for much of my time in college—I am still afraid to share that I am transgender at times. We never know how others will react or how extreme the rejection might be. The 2015 U.S. Transgender Survey found that nearly half of the respondents were verbally harassed in the last year due to being trans, and nearly 10 percent were physically attacked due to being trans.[1] In many cases, trans people are afraid of sharing that we are trans, and validly so.

Some of us choose not to deal with these risks on a daily basis and decide not to disclose our transness. In all honesty, I have often felt jealous of the peace I know my friends who do not disclose their transness experience. They deal with far fewer inappropriate questions, verbal harassment, tokenization at work, and other aggressive, threatening behaviors.

I strongly believe trans people do not owe anyone else our identities. If a trans person does not tell you they're trans, they are not "tricking" you.

This statement has incited much controversy each and every time I share it. Pushback ranges from attacking the integrity of trans individuals, calling us liars and fakes, to accusing trans individuals of rape for choosing not to disclose their identities in romantic situations, to still more extreme attitudes: believing trans people deserve to be murdered for not disclosing.

Let's address these accusations one at a time.

"YOU'VE LIED TO ME!" OR "YOU'VE BEEN FAKING IT!"

"Faking what? Lying about what?" I might ask. There are only a few logical answers: "Faking being a ('real') man," which immediately discloses the transphobia in assuming that trans men are not also real, valid men, or, "Lying about being cisgender," which is false. I have never claimed to be cisgender—nor have most trans folks. We might "look" cisgender to the viewer, but that is not our fault or responsibility to unpack. If I "look" cisgender to you and you assume I am as a result, that's cisnormativity you need to unpack. The anger or feeling of betrayal in response to learning someone is not actually cisgender is transphobia.

Consider this in the context of race: For a majority of my childhood, people assumed I was Chinese. The assumption that I was Chinese could have been based on the knowledge that there are more Chinese than there are Korean people in the world, so, from a statistical standpoint, assuming I'm Chinese is reasonable. But if someone were to get angry when I explain that I am not Chinese, but rather Korean, that wouldn't make much sense. It would only be angering and upsetting if there were some sort of perceived discrepancy between the two options: that being Korean was inferior to being Chinese. For example, if someone liked Chinese people significantly more than Koreans, that might explain anger upon learning that I am Korean instead of the assumed Chinese. This would be considered prejudice against Korean people, and their reaction of anger a result of that internalized prejudice. Because most people do not have a strong preference between the two, I have never experienced someone being angry at my Koreanness, but when we transfer this paradigm back to gender, anger is very common. Therein lies the transphobia: society biases us against trans people and toward cis people.

"THIS IS RAPE BY DECEPTION!"

I have heard so many variations of this statement. Some have likened the lack of disclosure of transness to lack of disclosure of sexually transmitted infections and diseases or to lying about having had a vasectomy. Calling lack of disclosure "rape by deception" immediately identifies intimacy or contact with transness as harmful or bad. Court cases in which individuals have been convicted for rape by deception include men pretending to be another man's spouse or significant other in order to gain consent and a man masquerading as a government official in Israel, promising state benefits to persuade women to have sex with him.[2]

Each of these results in significant negative consequences that, individually, are also crimes. Not disclosing STIs or STDs can result in the contraction of said STI or STD. Lying about having a vasectomy or removing/poking holes in a condom without a partner's consent can result in forced impregnation. And pretending to be someone you're not in order to gain access to really anything is not usually legal, either.

Again, herein lies the transphobia: *But you're pretending you're a real man/woman!*

I will repeat myself: Trans people are not pretending to be real. We *are* real. If you don't want to date a trans person, say so. The expectation that every trans person is going to feel comfortable disclosing their gender history, as well as potentially their medical history, is unrealistic and unkind.

Even if we were to conclude that lack of disclosure was somehow deceptive and someone felt deceived, it is still no grounds for violence or murder. As Ashlee Marie Preston put it, "Insinuating that Black trans women play a role in our own murders instead of examining the spiritual sickness involved in taking another person's life is symptomatic of a society devoid of empathy."[3]

"TRANS PEOPLE SHOULD JUST BE HONEST."

I love authenticity—and I would bet that most trans people do, as well. The majority of us come out as transgender and transition because we want to be authentic and honest with ourselves and others. But the comment that we "should just be honest" is not often said in good faith.

If pressed by asking, "Honest about what?" the answers range in explicitness of transphobia, but the undertones are always there: "Honest that they're trans," or, "Honest that they're not a real man/woman," or, "Honest about who they *really* are."

Being honest and disclosing every detail about ourselves that is important and relevant to someone else are not the same thing.

No one is capable of disclosing every detail about themselves that is important and relevant to another person—not in daily life or in romantic interactions. For example, as I've mentioned, I have a history with an eating disorder. In the beginning of my recovery, I resolved that I would not date another person with an eating disorder because I expected it would be too much for me to handle and I'd risk my own relapse. Expecting every potential partner to immediately disclose their mental health history and journey with me before or during the first date and without my directly asking would have been massively invasive and unreasonable. Instead, I should communicate that boundary upfront to any potential partners and then allow them to disclose if they felt comfortable.

I want to be clear that I liken disclosing eating disorder history to disclosing transness not because they are both mental illnesses (they are not; while an eating disorder is a mental illness, transness, as we've discussed, is not), but rather because both disclosure of eating disorder history and disclosure of transness can be sensitive, vulnerable, and private.

Putting this back into the frame of gender: if you won't date a trans person, it's up to you to communicate and maintain that boundary—not the trans person. Assuming that transness should always make the list of important identities or truths to disclose implies either that transness is notable to everyone, which is not always the case, or that transness is inherently negative and worth disclosing in confession, which definitely should not be the case. The latter is a more common expectation and enforces the transphobic idea that trans people are somehow less-than, imitation versions of men and women who only certain people would be okay dating.

Just be honest is a code for transphobia; if society were to see transness as positive—or even just neutral—few people would demand the disclosure of our identities as if they were some kind of disease.

"TRANS PEOPLE SHOULD DISCLOSE FOR THEIR OWN SAFETY."

A few years ago, a Twitter reply to "Trans women should disclose they're trans" went viral. It read: "Cis men should disclose that they'll murder a woman if she's trans."

Trans people are not responsible for the actions and intentions of their murderers, regardless of disclosure. Trans people should not have to worry that disclosure of our identities could result in being a victim of violence or murder. Trans people should not be held responsible for the murderous actions of anyone else.

But in a world wherein the possibility of violence is all too real, safety is, of course, paramount. The urge to disclose for safety comes from within and beyond the trans community. When anyone has come to me to discuss issues of disclosure, I always encourage them to include safety in their priorities. *Where are you going to tell them? How? Who else will be there? Do you feel safe? Do you have an exit plan, if necessary?* It is each individual's prerogative to decide when and how and if they disclose, and safety should always be taken into consideration.

As the pop recording artivist and trans woman Mila Jam (she/her) says,

> *I've done all of them. I've been candid, I've been shy, I've been "I'm going to tell you," "I'm going to retract." Now, I prefer to let them know as soon as possible, at the best comfortable moment. Before there are plans made. It's about survival. I would not want to be attacked by a partner. I think people should disclose [their identities], but they don't have to. [...] If someone would have told me that I could have whatever genitalia I have and someone will love me regardless... that would have been even more affirming.*[4]

I agree that disclosure can protect against potential negative interactions—and that is only the case because there are individuals in society who will harm and/or murder us for being trans—not because there is anything wrong with being trans. And I know many trans people who have experienced benefits in disclosing their transness further into a relationship (of any kind).

I am one of these people. I have several friends who I know would not have befriended me if they'd known of my transness prior, and who, after getting to know me, were able to accept my transness later. Society's transphobia can make it difficult for cisgender individuals to make their own judgments about trans people. Without a cloud of this preexisting transphobia, some individuals are able to see a person despite the prevalent hateful rhetoric and their empathy can shine.

Ultimately, there's no trickery or deceit on the part of a trans person; the decision of whether or not to disclose one's transness early in an interaction is up to the trans person. It is no one else's decision.

CHAPTER 17

Trans Athletes and Sports

"HAT'S A MAN!" THE LADY SCREAMS AT ME. "HOW CAN ANYONE think this is fair?!"

I'm sitting in the stands closest to the edge of the pool. This lady has been watching me cheer for Lia Thomas (she/her), a transgender woman who is currently competing at the 2022 NCAA Women's Swimming Championships. I stand up as they announce her name.

"Go Lia!" I shout. I am wearing a black polo with a trans flag embroidered on the chest. The flag is overlaid with text that reads, TRANS ATH-LETES BELONG IN SPORT.

The lady is sitting in the row behind me, continuing to jeer at me and Lia.

"That man is a cheat!" she yells.

I feel my blood begin to boil. The lady is part of a larger group of people who wear shirts that read, WOMAN: ADULT HUMAN FEMALE, and, NO MALES IN FEMALE SPORT. They are specifically here to protest the participation of Lia Thomas in the women's category. This comes on the heels of thousands of media articles focusing on Lia, with many powerful people expressing their outrage at her inclusion, perceiving her as a competitive threat.

The debate over the inclusion of trans athletes in sports has gained international attention over the years, usually focusing on select athletes who are competing in the women's category: Laurel Hubbard (she/her) of New Zealand, the first openly transgender woman to compete in the Olympics (weightlifting); CeCé Telfer (she/her), the NCAA D2 national champion (track and field); Andraya Yearwood (she/her) and Terry Miller (she/her), two high school runners in Connecticut; plus a handful of others.

Each time, the media erupts with controversy over and vicious attacks against these women. Usually, people who know nothing about sports begin to offer their extremely biased and misinformed opinions. Detractors like Donald Trump Jr. (he/him) and Florida governor Ron DeSantis abuse their power and platforms to spread transphobic narratives. The questions and comments become a bitter refrain.

What about the biological advantages?

Trans women are actually biological male!

If we let trans women play, they will dominate and destroy women's sports!

And of course, *I am not transphobic! I just care about fairness. Protect women's sports!*

This topic is textured and multilayered, and, at the core, not truly about transgender people. The arguments against the inclusion of trans athletes remain fairly consistent, so we'll dissect those. But first, let's look at some recent history.

A BRIEF HISTORY

Contrary to public belief, transgender athletes have existed in sports for a long time. We haven't come out of nowhere in the last few years. Consider some highlights:

1976: Tennis player Renée Richards (she/her), wins a women's tournament in La Jolla, California. As a result, the United States Tennis Association begins requiring genetic screening for female players. Richards files a lawsuit against USTA.

1977: The New York Supreme Court rules in Richards's favor—a landmark case for trans rights.[1] Richards competes in women's tennis for a few years, becoming the first known trans woman to do so in pro sports, before retiring to a private life.[2]

2003: The International Olympic Committee (IOC) convenes the Stockholm Consensus, officially permitting trans athletes to compete in the Olympics category aligned with their gender, given a few, albeit very strict, stipulations: genital surgery, including gonadectomy (removal of the gonads), legal recognition of gender, and hormone therapy for at least two years following the gonadectomy.[3]

2008: Hammer thrower Keelin Godsey (he/him) becomes the first openly transgender person to compete in Olympic Trials. He places fifth in women's hammer throw, just missing a spot on the Olympic team.[4]

2011: Transgender man Kye Allums (he/him) plays basketball for George Washington University, becoming the first openly transgender athlete to compete in the NCAA in any sport.[5]

That same year the NCAA releases their policy, the NCAA Inclusion of Transgender Student-Athletes, allowing trans athletes to compete for the teams aligned with their gender identity. Unlike the 2003 IOC policy, the NCAA's does not require surgery, but requires at least one year of testosterone suppression for trans women.[6]

2013: Fallon Fox (she/her) becomes the first openly transgender MMA fighter, garnering widespread attention and unfortunately becoming the target of bigotry from many notable public figures.[7]

2015: Chris Mosier (he/him) qualifies for the men's duathlon world championship and successfully challenges the IOC's restrictive policies from 2003, removing any surgery requirements altogether and reducing the required duration for hormone suppression to twelve months in place of two years.[8,9]

Later that year, I become the first openly transgender athlete to compete for a D1 men's team in the NCAA in any sport, beginning my four years on Harvard men's swim team.

2016: Chris Mosier becomes the first openly transgender man on Team USA, becoming the first transgender athlete to compete internationally under the IOC's new policy.[10]

2017: Transgender high school students Andraya Yearwood and Terry Miller place first and second in Connecticut's Interscholastic Athletic Conference, garnering international attention.[11] Three families of girls that lost to Andraya and Terry sue the state, arguing their girls are unable to win against trans athletes. In 2021, the court dismissed the case.[12]

2018: Patricio Manuel (he/him) becomes the first openly transgender boxer to compete in a professional fight.[13]

2019: CeCé Telfer, student-athlete at Franklin Pierce University, becomes the first openly transgender person to claim an NCAA championship title, winning the 400-meter hurdles at the NCAA D2 Championships.[14]

2020: In another first, Chris Mosier becomes the first trans athlete to qualify for and compete in a category other than the category of the gender assigned at birth at the U.S. Olympic Trials, racing in the 2020 Olympic Trials for racewalking.[15]

2021: New Zealand weightlifter Laurel Hubbard becomes the first openly transgender woman to compete in the women's category in the Olympics. She is joined by three other trans and non-binary athletes at the Tokyo Olympics—Quinn (they/them)[16], a non-binary trans masculine athlete who competes for Canada's women's soccer and is the first openly trans athlete to win an Olympic gold medal; Chelsea Wolfe (she/her), a trans woman who is an alternate for the U.S. BMX team; and Alana Smith (they/them), a non-binary trans masculine skateboarder who competes for the U.S. women's skateboarding team.[17]

Following the Olympics, in the fall of 2021, the IOC releases updated guidelines in a six-page, ten-principle framework titled, "IOC Framework on Fairness, Inclusion and Non-Discrimination on the Basis of Gender Identity and Sex Variations." This framework removes the explicit hormone regulations on transgender athletes and emphasizes nondiscrimination, the well-being (both physical and mental), and privacy of athletes who are transgender or have sex variations.[18]

This same fall, Lia Thomas begins competing for the University of Pennsylvania's women's swim team. After breaking a local pool record at a small mid-season invitational meet, an international media storm ensues, quickly centering her in the tension surrounding the participation of trans athletes in sports.

2022: The NCAA releases updated guidelines, allowing the national governing bodies to put forth rules for each individual sport instead of the NCAA. This supposedly mirrors the IOC's newest guidelines; however, the NCAA guidelines deviate in a few dangerous ways. They include *no* safeguards against harmful, invasive procedures or treatment (such as mandatory surgeries or visual inspections of athletes' genitalia); continue to place the burden on college athletes to prove they do not have unfair advantages simply because of who they are; do *not* comply with the World Professional Association for Transgender Health's most recent Standards of Care; and do not pursue engagement with transgender and non-binary athletes themselves.[19]

This same year, Lia Thomas becomes the first openly transgender athlete to win an NCAA D1 championship title, placing first in the women's 500-yard freestyle, raising international outrage never seen before.

This is not a comprehensive history—for that, I'd need to write a book only about transgender athletes. But these examples are crucial to helping recognize that trans athletes, while we have existed as long as athletics have, have been excluded far more than we have been included. And there are far fewer of us than most people suspect. There are more people creating rules about us than trans athletes who have ever competed at elite levels.

I have worked with several of these governing bodies, including the NCAA, USA Swimming, World Aquatics (formerly FINA), USA Water Polo, and World Athletics (formerly the IAAF), and I'm certain rules will continue to evolve.

TRANS MASCULINE ATHLETES

After my first video profile in 2016 on CBS's *60 Minutes*, I made the mistake of reading the comments on Facebook. "Beautiful competitive woman turned into ugly mediocre guy," someone had written. At the time, that comment deeply impacted me. I can still feel my hands dampen with anxiety, sitting on my bed in my freshman dorm. I was partially disturbed by the attack on my appearance, but even more so, I felt angry and indignant: I was not mediocre.

My experience highlights one of the primary arguments against trans masculine folks competing against cis men:

Trans men will always lose, there's no point in including them in men's sports. They can't compete with cis men.

The belief that those assigned female at birth are by default athletically inferior to those assigned male at birth is misogynist and unfounded—here's some proof:

- I competed in one of the most objective sports in existence: you're either faster, or you're not. There is no ability to argue with the results. At the end of my college career, I was ranked 443rd of 2,983 men in men's 100-yard breaststroke in the NCAA and 557th of 4,006 men in men's 100-yard butterfly in NCAA. This means that I beat 85 percent and 86 percent of all men in the NCAA who competed in my two best events. Keep in mind that only about 7 percent of high school athletes go on to compete in the NCAA and only 2 percent compete on a D1 varsity team.[20]

- Duathlete and trans man Chris Mosier has qualified for Team USA six times in his career. He has won numerous national championships. He is faster than nearly all other men in the U.S. in his events.
- In 2018, the professional boxer Pat Manuel won his first professional fight against a cis man. He won his second fight in March of 2023, remaining undefeated in the men's category.[21]

Here's another common complaint: *You're doping, so it's unfair.*

I've received this argument at approximately the same frequency as the first. And it's equally baseless. My testosterone levels were strictly regulated as mandated by the NCAA rules at the time. I was required to apply for a waiver that permitted me to take testosterone while competing on the men's team. I was also required to submit lab work testing my hormone levels multiple times per season, every season, to prove that my testosterone levels were within average (cis) male ranges. I maintained hormone levels in the bottom half—usually bottom quarter—of that range, well below the average men's athlete's levels, which are usually higher than the average cis man's.

Some folks have asked me why I kept them low; if I was permitted to exist within the full range, why not be closer to the high end? Wouldn't that be beneficial for athletics? Maybe. But I was not taking testosterone for sports. Testosterone's function was gender affirmation, not athletic performance. This is crucial to recognize. Trans people don't transition to play sports. We transition to live—and some of us also happen to be athletes.

You might also consider that although the NCAA requires that all athletes consent to random drug and hormone testing, most of my teammates (and most NCAA athletes) are never tested for their levels. I submitted my labs about three times each season. My hormone levels were more regulated than probably all other guys I competed against.

Attempting to argue against trans masculine inclusion due to hormone advantages is, again, arguing against numbers and facts.

TRANS FEMININE ATHLETES

Now this is where things can get heated. Some of the discussion points and arguments are similar to those regarding trans masculine athletes, so let's start there—the hormone question:

"Trans women have higher levels of testosterone!"

This is usually one of the first semithoughtful arguments against trans women in sports. However, in all elite-level sports in which trans feminine athletes are permitted to compete in the women's category, testosterone levels are regulated in trans women athletes.

Trans women athletes I know have testosterone levels far below average cis women.

Additionally, various studies have suggested that testosterone is not always a crucial factor in speed or athletic ability. It is only one of many factors, and testosterone alone will not make anyone a champion athlete.

"Even if testosterone levels are regulated, trans women still have gone through testosterone-driven puberty and are taller, bigger, and stronger, and that's an advantage."

In 2019, I gave a speech at a college in North Carolina. The audience was mainly athletic teams who were required to attend. Someone asked, as someone always does, about the inclusion of trans athletes in the women's category.

"Thank you for this question," I began. "Can I have all women athletes stand up, please?" It was noisy as about half the room shuffled to stand.

"Great, now sit back down if you are under five feet four." Less than a third sat down, leaving about one hundred women standing. "All right, all of you still standing are above average height. Makes sense; you're athletes. Cool. If you're shorter than five feet eight, sit down." Another handful sat down. About half the original population remained.

"Shorter than five feet ten." Thirty or so athletes were still standing. As I continued, more women sat down. I got to six feet four before the entire auditorium was sitting again.

"I'll assume that none of you are trans—not only because it's unlikely but also because I know most of the trans athletes competing right now." I chuckled as did the audience. "Great, so most of you are taller than average. Many of you are considerably taller than average. And about fifteen of you were still standing when I got past six feet." I gestured to the area where women's basketball was sitting, "I can imagine that many of you have been commended for your height and playing basketball, right? 'She's so tall,' they'll say. 'She was made for basketball! Look how tall she is, look how big her hands are... She's made for basketball!' Right?"

Many of the women nodded.

"Well, let's imagine a six-foot trans woman athlete. Society will immediately say that's unfair. The reality is this accusation is often transphobic, sexist, and misogynist. Trans women's gender expression is often policed and accused of being 'too masculine' or 'manly'—a hallmark of misogyny in policing the womanhood of women."

The comparison resonated with the audience—I could see heads nodding as people understood what I was saying.

The accusation is also racist in practice: many of the trans women who have been attacked are Black and brown trans women. This is not a coincidence and this is also not new. Black and brown women's bodies have a long history of being policed, especially in sports.

Consider this comparison:

Michael Phelps, the winningest Olympian of all time, exhibits several biological features that provide unique advantages in swimming. Phelps's torso is abnormally long and his legs short. His wingspan is four inches longer than his height.[22,23] Additionally, Phelps's lung capacity is twice the average—do you think this might prove an advantage in a sport where you hold your breath? You bet it does! Lastly, his body produces half the levels of lactic acid as the average athlete. Lower levels of lactic acid production mean shorter recovery periods and therefore a higher capacity for athletic labor.[24,25] Do these pose athletic advantages? Surely, they do, and surely they are genetic and biological!

When Michael Phelps's lactic acid levels were tested by the IOC, he was praised as genetically superior. Numerous reports were released about his amazing biological advantages—all in praise and celebration. "What an incredible athlete!" everyone said.

On the other hand, no such jubilation awaited Caster Semenya (she/her) when she won the women's 800 meter in the 2016 Olympics. When Caster Semenya was tested, her medals were taken from her and she was barred from competition unless she artificially lowered her testosterone levels.

Both athletes have biological differences resulting presumably from genetics—or at the very least, an intrinsic factor not altered by any exogenous factors—that could advantageously impact sport. Michael Phelps was praised. Caster Semenya was defamed and prevented from competition.

Michael Phelps is a white straight man. Caster Semenya is a Black queer woman who is often accused of appearing "masculine." Unfortunately, Caster is not the only Black woman to have been excluded based on sex variations. Silver medalist at the 2016 Olympics Francine Niyonsaba (she/her) of Burundi and bronze medalist Margaret Wambui (she/her) of Kenya were both barred from competing in the Tokyo 2020 Games due to genetic hyperandrogenism, or higher levels of testosterone.

Remember that testosterone is just one factor that can impact athletics—why should athletes like Semenya, Niyonsaba, and Wambui be excluded on the basis of supposed biological advantage while athletes like Michael Phelps are praised and permitted to dominate for nearly two decades, collecting over twenty gold medals (more than any other athlete in history) using their biological advantages?

The reality is that biological differences (and even clear advantages) have always been undeniably present in all sports. In many ways, that's the whole point of competitive sports! In every category, bodies are different. Among cis athletes, this is usually understood and accepted. People don't say that the tall (white) cis girl should be excluded from playing basketball. They don't say that's unfair. But when stigmatized, racialized, and other gender identities are involved, people call these differences "unfair."

Biological differences are especially accepted—and even celebrated on men's teams. The shortest guy on my swim team was five feet six. The tallest guy was six feet seven. That means the shortest guy was more than a *foot* shorter than that tallest guy. Does the taller guy have the bio-logical advantage of height? Sure, he does! But is it unfair and meriting disqualification? Of course not! It's just a biological difference. (It's also worth noting that guy who was five feet six was one of the fastest swim-mers we had, and was voted team captain his senior year.)

So yes, trans women absolutely can exhibit biological diversity...just like everyone else! Cisgender women exhibit biological diversity, as well. And what might appear a biological advantage might not translate into athletic superiority: plenty of very tall people are terrible at sports; plenty of short people excel in competition.

"We need rules for children, too! We need to protect young girls."

Nearly all legislative attacks on trans athletes at the state level—the hundreds of bills that have been proposed in over half the states in the United States—target children. Ten-year-olds who want to kick a soccer ball around with their friends or run track after school. Seven-year-olds who want to play volleyball or tennis. These bills are not about the Olym-pics, the NCAA, or even professional sports. Local legislatures have no jurisdiction over most elite athletics. This is about kids.

And historically, most children's sports do not mandate hormone restrictions or other regulatory practices. This, unfortunately, began changing in 2021 as states began filing and passing laws excluding trans children from playing sports with their peers.

This is crucial, not only ideologically, but also biologically: there are no significant biological differences that impact sports in children. The only notable biological difference between kids assigned female at birth and those assigned male at birth is the presence or absence of a penis. You might wonder why I've even included this note. Many states' anti-trans sports bills include proposals for genital exams in order to "ver-ify gender" of children. These are incredibly invasive, inappropriate, irrel-evant, and pedophilic. No one plays sports with their penis—and if they do, that is a very different problem.

As they do with adult trans athletes, most naysayers get hung up on testosterone. Besides the fact that testosterone is still only one factor that can contribute to athletic ability, there are usually no differences in testosterone between those assigned male at birth and those assigned female before the age of twelve or thirteen.[26]

Beyond this, most people are *not* Olympic athletes. Most folks are not even *elite* athletes. Most kids will not compete at international, national, or even regional competitions. I say this simply to remind us that most people don't play sports because they win all the time. More than chasing victory, most kids play sports just to have fun.

Barring kids from playing sports is a way to disconnect from and rob them of their bodies. This, combined with other attacks on bodily autonomy, particularly for trans youth, is an intentional violation of freedom. Kids should not have their bodies invasively examined under the guise of verifying their gender (assignment) just to play sports. If—and only if—the child arrives at an elite level where biological differences might be more relevant, governing regulations will await them there.

Additionally, this alleged fight for "fairness in women's sports" creates an impossible situation. In June 2022, World Aquatics (formerly FINA), the international federation recognized by the IOC for administering international competitions in water sports, banned trans women from the women's category unless they transitioned before twelve. But the United Kingdom and the U.S. have multiple laws banning (even criminalizing) the ability to transition before eighteen. World Athletics followed suit with a similar policy in April 2023. The astounding contradictions reinforce this is not about fairness or about kids' well-being. This is about trying to stop trans kids from thriving and becoming trans adults.

"Biological males are taking real women's spots!
Trans women will steal all the scholarship spots from cis women!"

Let's revisit language: when a trans woman is on a women's team, there are still *no* men on that team. Trans women are women, and it's both inaccurate and transphobic to refer to them as "biological males." Trans women are not "biological men." Biological sex is not binary; there is no such thing as a "biological man" or "biological woman." If you need to differentiate trans and cis women, say that: trans and cis women. If you need to talk about folks with higher levels of testosterone, say that. If you need to talk about reproductive biology, say that.

Next, the claim that trans women are "stealing" cis women's scholarships in college has zero data to support it: as of 2022, not a single out trans woman has ever received an athletic scholarship for a women's sport in the NCAA.

Remember Andraya Yearwood and Terry Miller, the two Black trans girls who placed first and second at a state championship in Connecticut? The three girls whose families sued against Andraya and Terry's wins each received scholarships to prestigious universities. Neither Andraya nor Terry received a single offer—and neither continued running in college.

This is a result of discrimination that trans people experience. Trans women are not getting off easy or breezing through life. Thousands of cis women receive athletic scholarships every year and trans women receive exactly none. Attempting to denigrate trans women on the basis of supposed "stolen" scholarships is yet another example of the hate, misinformation, and lies intended to incite panic about trans people.

Similarly, trans women are not "stealing" spots from cis women in the Olympics. In fact, trans folks are vastly underrepresented in elite-level sports. In 2016, 5,059 women competed in the Olympics. Approximately 1 percent of the population is transgender, so if trans women were accurately represented, fifty or so trans women should have competed in the Olympics. In 2020, one—and *only one*—did: New Zealand weightlifter Laurel Hubbard.

When trans women compete and succeed, they are not stealing anything. They are reaping the rewards of their hard work and determination, just as any other athlete does when they succeed.

"I totally care about trans rights, but we have to protect
women and women's rights! I'm not transphobic,
we just can't have biological males in women's sport!"

Before we dive into these comments, I will remind you of language. I cannot count how many people have professed their non-transphobia to me while simultaneously misgendering trans people and reducing us to our genitalia. If you're truly not transphobic, you will call trans women what they are: women. I understand there are differences between trans and cis women, but as mentioned previously, we can describe differences between people without inciting transphobia. Review the terminology section if you're in need of a couple pointers.

Trans exclusionary radical "feminists" ("TERFs")* have pushed the narrative that excluding trans women from women's sports is "feminist." This argument has been quite successful in creating moral panic, encouraging people to vote for draconian bills that further oppress all women and people who are not cishet white men.

Those who believe trans women threaten women's rights have been tricked by anti-trans rhetoric that uses the guise of "feminism" to manipulate people into supporting them. It's an appetizer, a hook, to get you in the door. It's a devastatingly effective method to divide, and then more importantly, control a population. Consider banning trans athletes an appetizer to the next oppression—because it is: in order to exclude trans femme athletes, the policing of *all* women in women's sports is required. Trans athlete bans do not affect only trans girls. They affect all girls.

Most people miss that in order to exclude transgender women and girls from participating in women's and girls' sports, sports governing bodies need to know which athletes are transgender. We cannot

---

* First coined by the activist Viv Smythe (she/they) to describe a "trans-hostile" movement she saw strengthening in Britain, the term *TERF* ("trans exclusionary radical 'feminist'") in and of itself is misleading as feminism does not exclude trans people. The term can describe supposed feminists who rejected that trans women are women. Some so-called TERFs find the acronym derogatory in nature, while others proudly describe themselves as such. In either case, those who exclude trans people while simultaneously considering themselves "feminists" are usually awarded this label. In truth, TERF ideology is more accurately described as "trans exclusionary radical ideology," and aligns itself often with white feminism—another realm of supposed "feminism" that also excludes women, Black women, namely, but also many other marginalized women who do not fit white standards of womanhood. It seems that most TERFs are employing a method of exclusion that is unsurprisingly patriarchal, misogynist, and racist in nature—and not only results in excluding trans women but also any cis woman whose body does not function in the way that TERF ideology (read: patriarchy) demands that it should.

simply look around the field, point someone out, and claim, "You're trans, get out." That is profiling, which is illegal, not to mention ridiculously unfair. Instead, a method of checking or verifying transness is necessary—through medical and legal record investigation, genotyping, hormone evaluations, and even visual genital exams.

There are two ways to enforce this: (1) check every single athlete who participates before deeming them eligible or not, and (2) accusation-based testing, which would entail testing an athlete who has been accused of being transgender.

The first option is logistically and financially impossible, nor would every parent consent to having their child's medical and legal records exposed, much less their genitals examined so that they can kick a soccer ball around with their friends after school.

The second not only demonizes and weaponizes transness, but also endangers all girls and women. Stay with me.

Allowing a governing body and, in this case, the government, to "check" women and girls to see if they are transgender, once accused, means that any athlete accused of being transgender can be checked. Read that again. *Any girl*, regardless of whether she is cis or transgender, could have her gender investigated if she is accused of being transgender. And don't forget to consider that, in most states, almost anyone could accuse any athlete of being transgender for any reason.

This threatens all women—and women's sports as a whole. At what point is a girl "too good" to be cisgender and therefore likely to be accused of being transgender? When is a woman "too masculine," or "too tall," or "too fast," or "too strong," to be cisgender and thus accused of being transgender?

Unfortunately, this policing of women's bodies—proving what is considered "woman enough"—has persisted for as long as women's sports have existed. And those who suffer the most from attacks on the validity of their womanhood are already marginalized women—Black women, most especially.

Serena Williams (she/her) has been repeatedly ridiculed, attacked, and degraded in sports. A Russian tennis official, who was later sanctioned, once called her and her sister Venus (she/her) "the Williams

Brothers."[27] Doubt over and attacks on Serena's womanhood have been so prevalent that a documentary titled *Irrefutable Proof That Serena Williams Is a Man* was released in 2014.[28]

Serena's not the only one. Add the track and field sprinter Sha'Carri Richardson (she/her). And the gymnast Simone Biles (she/her), who was also attacked for supposedly having an unfair advantage because she was able to complete the Yurchenko double pike vault, which was supposedly "too dangerous" for other athletes.

> *In other words, on a technical and cultural level, Biles, a young Black woman, is being punished and subjected to undeniably racist and sexist double standards for her greatness. After all, we've seen some form of this before, for other Black women athletes—Caster Semenya, a South African two-time Olympic champion runner, was literally barred from competing in women's sports last year unless she agreed to take medication to lower her naturally higher levels of testosterone. When Black women athletes work hard and go above and beyond, they're treated with suspicion, as if they're somehow being dishonest, or as if their success is a detriment to others that should be punished, restricted and prevented rather than encouraged. From Semenya to Biles, they and other Black women athletes face the same, intertwined racism and misogyny.*[29]
>
> —KYLIE CHEUNG (she/her) writing for *Salon*

These anti-trans bills build upon already strong social norms of policing Black and brown women's bodies, paving the way for the *legal* policing of all women's bodies. Anti–trans athlete bills legitimize incredibly patriarchal, racist, misogynistic, and transphobic conceptions of womanhood, solidifying womanhood as only what is seen as "woman" by patriarchy and white supremacy.

In 2022, following the passing of one anti-trans athlete law in Utah, a young cisgender girl athlete was accused of being transgender because she "outclassed" the other athletes.[30] Subsequently, she had her gender history investigated by officials who reviewed her records all the way back to kindergarten to verify that she was not transgender. She was not. Reports indicated that she was not the first to experience this invasive check; she most likely will not be the last.

Excluding trans women will bring destruction to women's sports by policing all women's bodies and reducing them to a very narrow view of what their bodies look like, how they can perform, and who women are.

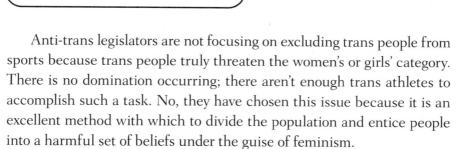

UTAH:
- 75,000 high school athletes in the state
- 4 transgender athletes in the entire state
- 1 transgender kid playing girls' sports

ARIZONA:
- 170,000 high school athletes in the state
- 16 trans kids attained waivers to play with the team aligned with gender identity since 2017

OKLAHOMA:
- Trans inclusive policy in place since 2015
- As of 2022, no request ever made to use the policy because no trans girls ever competed in OK

Anti-trans legislators are not focusing on excluding trans people from sports because trans people truly threaten the women's or girls' category. There is no domination occurring; there aren't enough trans athletes to accomplish such a task. No, they have chosen this issue because it is an excellent method with which to divide the population and entice people into a harmful set of beliefs under the guise of feminism.

If fairness is truly the central crusade, then let's focus on fairness.

In the Women's Sports Foundation 2020 report, "Chasing Equity," regarding barriers to sport for women, the inclusion of trans women is not mentioned once. Trans women do not threaten the fabric of women's sports. Excluding and attacking trans women does.

The reality is that most folks do not care about women's sports until a trans woman wants to play. And then, suddenly, they are massive sports fans and fairness advocates. But are they out protesting against the rampant sexual abuse girls experience in sport? Were they fighting alongside Megan Rapinoe (she/her) and other professional women's soccer players to attain equal pay? Are they ensuring that Title IX requirements are met in all schools? (The answer is largely no, they are not.)

If folks truly want to bring fairness to the forefront, then they should fight against the main barriers to access for sports: socioeconomic disparity, often intertwined with systemic oppression such as racism.

Remember that some 64 percent of Black children don't know how to swim, compared to 40 percent of white children who can't swim.[31] Why is this the case? Contrary to popular (racist) stereotypes, this isn't because Black people cannot swim by nature. It's because of segregation: Historically, Black folks didn't have access to recreational pools, much less lessons or classes to learn how to swim. Up until the 1960s and 1970s, pools were still segregated into "whites only" and "colored."

If we want to talk about fairness, let's talk about *access* to sports. If we truly care about equity and justice in sports, we need to focus on uplifting marginalized groups, not on attacking them.

YES, WE'LL TALK ABOUT LIA THOMAS

Although trans women are disproportionately underrepresented in women's sports, and only twenty or so trans women have won a national or international competition in women's sports, the hatred and vitriol each high-profile trans woman has received is always extreme. Fallon Fox, Andraya Yearwood and Terry Miller, and now Lia Thomas have drawn immense attention, each a recipient of the tired and overused transphobic arguments, "it's unfair," "so-and-so is a man," "they're cheating!" among even crueler accusations I don't care to repeat. Because Lia is a friend of mine, and probably the most hotly debated trans athlete, I want to talk in depth about what happened to her so that we can truly dissect (and hopefully eventually lay down) the biased obsession with trans women in sports.

Lia Thomas is an American swimmer who competed for the University of Pennsylvania. In February 2022, Lia won the 500-yard freestyle at D1 Championships and became the first openly transgender D1 champion in any sport.

Lia began her collegiate career on the men's team, where she competed for three years before transitioning. After a gap year during the pandemic, Lia began swimming on the women's team in the fall of 2021. When Lia broke a few local pool records at a mid-season competition, the world erupted in response. Protests occurred outside the pool, despite Lia having satisfied all NCAA regulations required to compete in the women's category at the time. Lia had taken suppressants to reduce her testosterone levels to average (cis) female levels, and had done so for over two years, nearly tripling the required period by the time she competed at championships.

At nearly every speech I gave prior to Lia's coming out, I was asked what would happen when someone "did the opposite." *Would they receive the same support that I did?* I always answered the question bluntly: "No, absolutely not. Whoever she is, she will be a target of misogyny and transphobia, and if she's a person of color, racism, too." And sadly, I was right: Though Lia had the clear support of her family, friends, coaches, and many of her teammates, she also received immense hatred and backlash from the media and world at large. The viciousness with which the world received her was devastating, as well as a striking reflection of the darkness still harbored in our society.

Whenever I present this topic onstage, or even one-on-one, I encourage the person on the receiving end to take a few deep breaths. I find that people quickly become angry and upset. These knee-jerk reactions aren't surprising given what we've been taught. Yes, some might not feel that it is fair for Lia to compete. I understand why they might feel that way. I, too, once struggled with understanding these topics. I, too, grew up in a world that privileges cisgender individuals over transgender people at all turns. I, too, was taught that biology was binary and that "boys are better at sports than girls."

That is the legacy of growing up and living in a transphobic world. Committing to this work demands questioning and dismantling that learned transphobia.

Lastly, let's not forget to recognize Lia's humanity. We are not discussing "The Lia Thomas Issue" or "The Lia Thomas Problem." We are talking about a person—a human being like you and me and everyone else we know. *She* is not an issue or a problem—the considerations and tensions surrounding her participation in sports are.

LIA'S STORY

I sat across from Lia in a nice Italian restaurant in Atlanta. It was one of those modern-type decors, industrial with black metal piping and big exposed wooden beams. Her mother, father, and a few of her friends joined us at the table. Everybody ordered a drink—Lia had just finished her final session at NCAA D1 Championships. Although that night she'd placed eighth, a few days earlier, she'd solidified her position as the first openly trans D1 champion.

"How are you feeling?" I asked her after everyone had received their beverage.

"I'm so tired," she laughed. "But happy."

I spent dinner periodically fighting back tears, as I witnessed Lia's ease and joy—so different from how she had been when I'd first met her years earlier. Her misery then had been crystal clear. I remembered fearing for her path on the women's team, knowing the world was not likely to meet her with kindness, but feeling more terrified of the consequences if she chose not to prioritize her authenticity.

Here she sat, though, laughing and living. Her happiness in authenticity was obvious. During that dinner, all the hatred, the media, and the protesters were irrelevant. During that dinner, Lia could just be a proud champion athlete.

Lia first messaged me on Facebook Messenger in June 2018 after a friend connected us. She'd realized she was transgender a week and a half before she began college but had not been ready to confront it. "I can't deal with this right now; this is too much," she told me she'd thought to herself back then. But as she finished her first year at Penn, her identity had solidified in her mind: "Trans woman—that's who I am, that's me!" she recalled.

"Coming out was one of the hardest things I've done," she wrote to me that first day. "But it was nice to be able to talk to somebody about it." Lia had come out to a close friend of hers and she shared that she was planning on coming out to her brother soon, hopeful he'd be accepting because he was open-minded. After a few more messages, sports made an appearance.

"How supportive was your team when you came out to them because that thought is currently stressing me out," she wrote. While many people accuse transgender people, especially transgender women, of transitioning with the explicit aim of succeeding in sports, Lia did not ask me a single question about the NCAA eligibility rules in our first conversation. Instead, she wondered about coming out to people who might not be as supportive, where could she connect with more trans people for friendship, and what transitioning was like. All her questions surrounded interpersonal stressors that, at the core, asked: "Will I still belong?"

We met in person later that year. The same friend she'd first come out to accompanied her and we sat at a table outside a dorm at Penn. A tall, lanky woman, Lia somehow still seemed small. She spoke quietly, taking long pauses between her thoughts, her misery and duress palpable. I knew the feelings all too well.

There is a certain quality to a person who is not able to be themselves—something deeper than depression or discontentedness, it is the experience of withdrawing oneself from the world, and perhaps most painfully, from oneself.

During that first in-person conversation we continued to focus on coming out and her relationships with her loved ones. Her parents struggled with this newly presented identity and were clearly worried about Lia, who'd just begun her second year at Penn and was struggling deeply. Swimming seemed to be last on the list of priorities, and she frequently considered quitting. She was often unable to attend practice due to the depression and gender dysphoria she was experiencing at the time.

This was a whole "year of knowing I was trans, not transitioning, still swimming, competing, and presenting as a man," she said when she recalled that time. "It put a lot of strain on my ability to swim." And yet, the same season (2018–2019), Lia was somehow able to achieve some of her highest ranking in the men's category. Despite her success in the pool, Lia's mental health continued to deteriorate, and she decided she'd begin her transition once the season ended. Without coming out to either

her coach or teammates, she began hormones—testosterone suppression and estrogen supplements—in May 2019.

When I asked her about that moment, she reflected.

"When I started hormones, there was not a thought about sports or athletics in my mind," she paused and wiped the edge of her eye. "I was trying not to die at that point," she said. "I was doing what I needed to do to live—and that was transitioning, that was HRT, that was trans health-care, and that was the choice I felt I had."

The many who claim that trans women are truly "just men who want to win sports" denigrate trans women's motivation in sport, asserting that their transitions are simply a means to a win in the women's category. In truth, Lia began her transition with no clear plan to compete. She wasn't sure if she'd continue swimming at all, she just knew she needed to transition to stay alive.

In August of that year, with a few months of hormone therapy, Lia was feeling much better. She decided she would consider swimming and began with coming out on the pool deck. After practice one day, she was surprised to be met with overwhelming support from her coach, Mike Schnur (he/him); her assistant coaches; and her teammates. And despite the whirlwind that was the first year on hormones, and continuing to swim on the men's team while she completed her required year of testos-terone suppression, Lia found herself enjoying swimming like she hadn't in years. She was able to acquire a uniform exemption, wearing a wom-en's swimsuit not only in practice but also in competition.

"The biggest thing I've noticed is how much more invested I am in swimming than I was previously. I feel fully engaged with the sport, in the water; I could train and race much better because I was much hap-pier," Lia said.

In the fall of 2021, after a year swimming on the men's team while on testosterone suppressants and estrogen supplements, and then another year of the pandemic, totaling over two years of HRT, Lia began on the women's team. Her subsequent performance and success in the women's category brought an onslaught of attacks like never seen before. Though Lia and I had long discussed the likelihood for this type of backlash, she couldn't have been prepared for what followed after the Zippy Invitational meet when the news broke and protests began.

"It was something I'd expected, to some extent. I knew it would be there. But just the scale of it really shocked me. [...] It was a lot to deal with initially."

Lia has weathered an immense barrage of hatred while somehow still managing to compete at one of the highest levels of competitive swimming. Most of the comments, DMs, and other negative responses to Lia's participation are void of meaning, credibility, and care. But I'd like to address some basic facts that merit further discussion.

Lia Is an Excellent Swimmer

Many accusations insinuate Lia's success in the pool results exclusively from her gender assigned at birth—male. Some even claim that she is taking what other girls have "worked their entire lives for."

This dismisses several truths: (1) Lia has also worked her whole life to be good at swimming. Lia began swimming at five years old and has thousands of practice hours. (2) Lia is not a great athlete because she was assigned male at birth. Lia is a great athlete because she has worked hard for seventeen years to be great at something she loves.

The belief that all folks assigned male at birth are automatically better at sports than those assigned female at birth is rooted in the sexist belief that "boys" are, by default, better at sports than "girls," which is false.

Although arguments commonly rest upon the idea that *all* trans women are somehow biologically inadmissible into the women's category due to "biological sex," the reality is that trans women have competed in the NCAA before Lia Thomas. Not only can most folks not name these women, but these women were also not subjected to the hatred and vitriol that Lia was. Why? Because they didn't succeed at the same level Lia did. Transgender woman Natalie Fahey (she/her) also swam in the women's category—a few years before Lia did—for Southern Illinois University. But, unlike Lia, she broke no records and won no competitions, so there was no media firestorm.

Lia Has Not "Dominated" in the Women's Category

Lia won the 500 freestyle at the NCAA's D1 Women's Swimming and Diving Championships in 2022, becoming the first known transgender athlete to win an NCAA D1 championship title. Lia performed well, and certainly swam exciting races, but the many reports and accusations that have claimed Lia "dominated" and "destroyed" women's sports are inaccurate and manipulative.

Twenty-seven records were broken at the NCAA D1 Championships in 2022.[32] Lia did not break *a single one*. Her winning time in the 500-yard freestyle was not an American, U.S. Open, NCAA, meet, or even pool record. Lia's winning time of 4:33.24 was *not* in the country's top fifty all-time fastest swims and would not have won the same meet six out of the nine years prior. Seven American records were set at the same championship meet, five by University of Virginia's Kate Douglass (she/her). Actually, eighteen of the total twenty-seven records that weekend were broken by Kate Douglass. Of course, no one accused Kate Douglass, a cis woman, of unfair performance or domination.[33]

You'll notice that I've explained quite a few stats to prove to you that Lia did not "dominate," and while all these facts are true, needing to present them is sad. Lia should be allowed to be a great athlete, too. Cis athletes rarely have to qualify their success by saying, "Oh, they're not *that* good." Most people don't look at swimming great Katie Ledecky (she/her) and say, "Well, she *only* won by twenty-six seconds, yeah, that's still fair." (Please do recognize that Katie *has, in fact*, won a national competition by twenty-six seconds before, a margin that is nearly unheard of in elite swimming where many races are won by mere fractions of a second.)

We should not have to prove the fairness of Lia's inclusion by arguing that she's *not* good. Trans women should be allowed to succeed and be celebrated for their success, too.

Lia Did Not Go from a Nobody to a Somebody

A graphic—or meme—depicting Lia before and after her transition, with the text "462nd" and "1st" beneath each respective photo, was widely circulated for a majority of the season. Most obviously, the graphic was aimed at furthering the narrative that Lia's participation in women's sports was unfair.

This was one of many claims that hinged on the argument that Lia was "never in the category of standout athlete" before she transitioned.[34]

In early February 2022, shortly before Lia was seeded to compete at NCAA Championships, sixteen of her teammates anonymously signed a letter condemning the NCAA's allowance of trans women in the women's category.

"Biologically," the letter reads, "Lia holds an unfair advantage over competition in the women's category, as evidenced by her rankings that have bounced from number 462 as a male to number one as a female."[35]

Facts aside for a moment, here I'm going to ask you to please pause to think about Lia, as a person.

As a competitive swimmer for most of my life, I've woken up before the sun has most mornings—either driving on dark highways to practice before school, or walking across the bridge from Cambridge to Allston when I competed at Harvard. Every morning, we'd dive half-awake into a chilly pool where we would swim as a team for two hours, before stumbling to breakfast together and then beginning our days as students. We'd repeat this most afternoons, returning for a second grueling practice, sometimes coupled with strength training.

And we did this all together. We pushed through the physical exhaustion, pain, and fear of the next practice together. I knew my teammates would also be there. I knew they were also hurting and tired. And I knew I would cheer them on during the last set, and I knew they'd do the same for me.

Swimming was worked into every part of every day of my life for a very long time—and for Lia, too. Imagine waking up one morning to find that sixteen of your teammates do not want you to compete. That sixteen of your teammates have gone behind your back to publish an open letter to the entire world sharing this opinion. Imagine the heartache, the pain, the isolation. Imagine not knowing who wanted you there anymore and who didn't. Imagine somehow still walking onto the pool deck that day for practice and hopping in, anyway. Imagine being Lia, just for a moment.

Beyond the cruelty inherent in this letter, the 462nd to first-place ranking comparison used as "proof" that Lia maintained some sort of biological advantage over cis women athletes is fallible at best.

There are countless problems with this alleged "logic."

First, simply: this is not "evidence." Many have contrasted the supposed rankings as "evidence" that Lia was not a standout athlete before and now is, and therefore her inclusion is "unfair." But true evidence is peer-reviewed research with a substantial sample population and methodological integrity, neither of which this claim contains.

The letter fails to provide said "evidence" as to how exactly Lia has an unfair advantage except to claim that she is fast. Essentially, this says: "When cis women are fast, it's okay; when trans women are fast, it's unfair." So, this is not about fairness. This is transphobia incarnate.

Second, factually: neither I nor my teammates could find this 462nd ranking anywhere.

And lastly, most importantly: the statement that Lia was not a standout athlete prior to competing on the women's team is an outright lie intended to deceive you. Lia's highest ranking *before* transitioning was *eleventh in the nation*. Yes, eleventh, when she was swimming against men. She was also ranked twelfth in the 1,000-yard freestyle in 2018 and 2019. Lia ranked thirty-eighth in the 1,650-yard freestyle in 2019, missing qualifying for NCAA Championships by a tenth of a second.[36]

It is far from abnormal or unlikely for an athlete to go from being ranked eleventh to first in the span of a few years. Most (if not all) athletes who succeed at a high level did not begin immediately winning everything. Instead, most improved over the years they competed. If a cis woman went from a lower ranking to first, no one would call this unfair.

Powerful Individuals Have Manipulated the Public

Prior to Laurel Hubbard's Olympic debut, a reporter from the BBC asked me, "Donald Trump Jr. has spoken out against transgender women in sports, what do you have to say about that?"

I took a deep breath to prevent myself from saying what actually ran through my brain: *What the fuck do I care what Donald Trump Jr. has to say about anything, much less about sports specifically?! Was he even an athlete, for crying out loud?*

But because I was live on a major news broadcast, I kept my composure and instead said calmly, "Frankly, Donald Trump Jr., as far as I know, is not a sports expert, sports physiologist, biologist, endocrinologist, or any kind of trans expert, so while he is entitled to his opinion, I would not include it as important or relevant to this issue. If anything, his comments are transphobic, misinformed, harmful, and an irresponsible abuse of power."

Over my career, I've been asked numerous times about my opinion or response to some celebrity, politician, or otherwise public figure's statements about transgender people or athletes—and I always give them a variation of the same answer I gave the BBC.

In Lia's case, one of her loudest opponents was the woman who penned the previously mentioned open letter to the NCAA on behalf of sixteen of Lia's anonymous teammates, Nancy Hogshead-Makar (she/her).

As an Olympic champion and as a civil rights lawyer, I can assure you that there is nothing fair about transgender woman Lia Thomas competing for the University of Pennsylvania in NCAA swimming.

Hogshead-Makar's attempt to qualify herself as an expert is manipulative and wrong. Though being an Olympic champion and a civil rights lawyer both require intensive commitment and are impressive accomplishments, neither qualifies a person to be an expert in discerning the fairness of a transgender woman competing in women's sports. Neither being an Olympic champion nor being a civil rights lawyer are the same thing as being a biologist, a physiologist, an endocrinologist, or an expert in sports physiology. Claiming so is akin to saying, "Because I'm a world-renowned surgeon, I am also clearly qualified to be a lawyer."

This attempt to trick an audience into considering oneself an expert has unfortunately become a common, abusive tactic among those in power. Hogshead-Makar is neither unique nor the first to practice this technique—though she has seemingly mastered it, alongside many others such as governors Ron DeSantis and Greg Abbott.

Lia Is Not a Symbol That Trans Women Will or Have "Dominated" Women's Sport

Most people can't name more than five trans women who have won international or even national athletic competitions. If you can name more than Lia Thomas, that is impressive. There are fewer than a couple dozen in recorded history. Trans women are *not* "dominating" women's sports. Cis women dominate women's sports.

There Will Always Be Great Outlier Athletes Who Seem Impossible to Beat!

Headlines such as, "Michael Phelps Dominates Beijing Olympics," "Olympic Swimmer Katie Ledecky Blows Competition Out of the Water," "This Is What Makes LeBron James a 'Freak Athlete' According to His NBA Coach," grab our attention, but rarely do they raise concern.

Michael Phelps, Shaquille O'Neal (he/him), LeBron James (he/him), Katie Ledecky, and many of the other greats have unique physical characteristics that allowed them advantages in their sport, but no one considered these advantages grounds for disqualification. Some even exclaim in awe that the advantages are unfair. But no one says, "Michael Phelps's arms are too long, he should shorten them to level the playing field," or, "Phelps's lungs are too large, he should be given a handicap so that it's a fair competition." No, they allow him his biological advantages and praise him for being an amazing "freak of nature." However, as soon as the "freak of nature" athlete appears in the women's category—and especially if they somehow do not represent a seemingly acceptable definition of womanhood—their achievements are deemed unfair.

Madison Kenyon (she/her), a nineteen-year-old cisgender runner from Idaho State University, who supported the anti-trans sports ban in Idaho, told NPR, "To step on the field and have it not be fair and to get beat by someone who has advantages that you'll never have, no matter how hard you train—it's so frustrating."[37]

This concept of a "level playing field" is elusive at best. Not only do privilege and oppression make impossible the existence of truly level playing fields, but the belief that one might never triumph over another athlete is far from unique or specific to competing against trans women. Most people in the swim community joke that racing against Katie Ledecky is a race for second place. She has largely been seen as unbeatable—and she has dozens of national and international titles to support her invincibility. But, accusing trans women of being unbeatable just because they're trans is not founded in evidence or fact, and is just transphobic.

Stop Punishing Trans Women for Toxic Cis Men

Once I've whittled away at the transphobic "arguments" that folks use against Lia's or other trans women's participation in sports, some people eventually come down to this:

I understand trans women aren't a threat, an audience member will say. *I get that we should let them play. But if we do,* boys *are going to just pretend to be girls* . . . Men *are going to pretend to be women in order to win!*

My first response usually is to hold back my own laughter at the prospect. This is not how toxic masculinity works! No boy or man who is attempting to boost his ego by becoming a sports champion is going to think that will happen through winning women's sports. Have you seen how trans women in women's sports are treated? Does that look like the glory an insecure man would seek?

Beyond this oversight, the "boys will pretend to be girls" argument also ignores the lengthy and intensive process required by most athletic organizations for a trans woman to compete. You cannot just waltz onto a women's team in most elite-level sports; you've just had a crash course in the many rules and regulations—usually entailing years of hormone therapy—that are often required. Not to mention that skill and training are required to succeed at any sport, regardless of gendered category.

And, even if a man were to pretend to be a woman in order to win, trans women would still not be to blame. If you are afraid of a cis man pretending to be a woman in order to win women's sports, you are afraid of toxic cis men, not trans women!

"Well, so what should we do about those boys who are going to pretend? We can't have them harming girls and women like that!" someone once responded to me as we talked about this.

"Yes, boys and men shouldn't harm women—but the solution is not to exclude trans women (who, again, are not boys or men!). The solution is to teach boys to be better men; to teach men to be better men."

❦ ❦ ❦

TRANS ATHLETES DO not transition to play sports, we transition to live—and happen to also play sports. Trans athletes do not threaten the integrity of sports, women's or otherwise. When we understand that excluding trans women hurts all women, polices the entire women's category, and ignores the true threats to women's sports, we can unify in our fight against the true enemy: patriarchy.

CHAPTER 18

Toxic Masculinity from the Lens of a Transgender Man

M Y FIRST YEAR AT HARVARD WAS, BY FAR, THE MOST DIFFI-cult. I felt anxious during every social event, especially those with my teammates. I'd just barely begun living as what others recognized as a man in the world. In many ways, I felt new and alone. I had never been asked to socialize with dozens of college-aged men—boys, really—and now I was spending almost all my waking hours with a team of forty of them. I felt like I'd missed valuable time learning social practices.

On top of this, I was frequently misgendered by my teammates during my first semester on the men's team. No one misgendered me in class or anywhere else at school—and I tried to give my teammates time. Unlike my classmates, they had known me before I'd transitioned. They'd read about me and seen photos of me. I knew that affected how people saw me. Still, at the pool, being called "she" felt like a burning neon sign, screaming, YOU DO NOT BELONG HERE.

Growing up, I never quite fit in with any groups of kids. I'd gotten used to that and learned to feel at peace. But in college, I was finally me. And on Harvard Men's Swim and Dive, no less! What a journey it'd been to get there. I was so proud, and for the first time in my life, I desperately wanted to belong.

227

In late August, before the start of my first year at Harvard, we were gathered for team bonding at a teammate's house. While at lunch, guys stood up, making jokes. It began silly and fun. Some were funny—most I didn't understand.

At some point, one guy made a very misogynistic joke and everything inside me cringed. Even worse was that he was one of the few who hadn't misgendered me yet and had made a concerted effort to make me feel welcome and cared for. *Should I just laugh and move on? Is that what being a man here will mean?*

I knew there would have been no way I'd have let a joke like his pass by when I was presenting as a woman. I would have easily yelled at him right then and there, in front of everyone.

But surrounded by my hooting and cheering teammates, and with an unfamiliar yearning to fit in, I was overwhelmed with the urge to join them and laugh, too.

It's okay, Schuyler, come on. It's not that bad, you know he didn't mean it. It's just a joke! I tried to convince myself. I knew that laughing was a step to being one of them. To be seen as man enough. To be seen as a man, at all.

But I couldn't do it. I stood up and walked out. There was no cell service where we were. I wandered until my phone would complete a call.

"Please come pick me up, Mom," I said through tears into the phone. "I can't be here . . . I can't be one of them. It's too hard."

Although she tried to convince me to try for a few more days, years later she confessed that she was already in the car, key in the ignition and ready to drive to get me. But my dad had calmed her down, encouraging me to make a decision the following day. The call disconnected due to poor service and I sat on the curb with my head in my hands.

What was I going to do?

A few minutes later, the boy who'd made the joke emerged and approached me.

"Hey, what's wrong? Why did you leave?" he asked, genuinely concerned and deeply clueless.

I debated lying. *What if he just calls me a pussy or a little bitch? Should I tell him what I feel?* But already feeling excluded and different, I figured there wasn't much to lose.

"I didn't like that joke you told—" I started.

"Oh, you didn't understand, let me explain—" he interrupted. I waved him off.

"No, no, I get it, don't worry." I paused, gathering my thoughts. He waited, looking a bit confused but also patient. He sat down next to me and tilted his head. I took a deep breath. "I get it, and I know it was supposed to be funny but... it's very misogynistic and a bit rape-culture-y."

"Oh," he said, considering. "I don't get it."

"Listen, what would you do if one of the guys said that about your mom?" For effect, I repeated the joke to him, replacing the subject with his mother instead of the anonymous woman.

"I mean, I'd be pissed," he answered immediately.

"Okay, what about if someone said it about your sister? Or girlfriend?" I pushed.

"I mean I'd be furious and I'd probably..." He trailed off. "Oh." He joined me in staring at the concrete.

"Right." I was relieved and a bit surprised that my tactic was working. He remained calm, so I did, too. Emboldened, I continued. "Why does a woman have to be your mother, sister, or girlfriend to be respected?"

"You're right..." he mused. "Yeah, okay... Okay."

"I spent my entire adolescence being taunted by boys like you," I ventured. "All the boys on my swim team made gross comments about my body and what they'd want to do with it."

"I'm sorry," he said, listening.

"These days, most women I know have experienced some form of sexual assault by men. And it all starts from small 'just jokes' like what you told today. It tells the younger guys that's okay. And that's a slippery slope... Does that make sense?"

"Yeah," he answered, nodding. I was still taken aback by his lack of defensiveness. I had not expected ease in this conversation.

"But gosh, Schuyler, you gotta understand . . ." he started. "We didn't all grow up like you. We didn't all grow up . . . being treated like a girl, like you did, so we don't understand like you." This made sense. I hadn't considered this.

"I understand that," I nodded. "But women make up some fifty-two percent of the population. I think you all should start considering their perspectives!"

As you probably know, I did *not* end up quitting the team that day.

Instead, accompanied by my teammate, I walked back to where the rest of the guys were and resumed participating in the weekend. Of course, it wasn't all smooth sailing from then on. Sadly, I would face many similar moments in the coming years on the team and in the world among other men—being read as one of them. I've lost count of how many times men have said disgusting things to me about women, expecting me to laugh, agree, or even contribute. And each time, I have the opportunity to choose: Shall I do what is expected of me—potentially bringing me a sense of belonging while simultaneously perpetuating a system of toxic masculinity—or do I resist, risking acceptance?

All this is to say: before I transitioned, I was the object of misogyny. Now, I am expected to be an accomplice to it. This has been an illuminating, difficult, and privileged experience in a variety of ways—and this chapter will attempt to explain some of them.

Before we dive in, here are a few key terms:

Patriarchy: A form of social organization that empowers men over women and others who are not men, placing men in positions of power everywhere—at home, at work, and in society at large. Think: We've never had a woman president. Women did not gain the right to vote until 1920. Women are paid less than men.[1] Women are underrepresented in decision-making roles. Women do at least 2.5 times more unpaid labor than men do.[2] The list goes on.

Misogyny: In short: the hatred of women. With nuance: the inter- and intrapersonal, structural, and systemic oppression and disenfranchisement of women and others who exhibit any kind of femmehood or are not cis straight men. Misogyny is the primary tool of patriarchy.

Sexism: Prejudice toward or discrimination against a person based on their sex or gender, most often women and femmes.

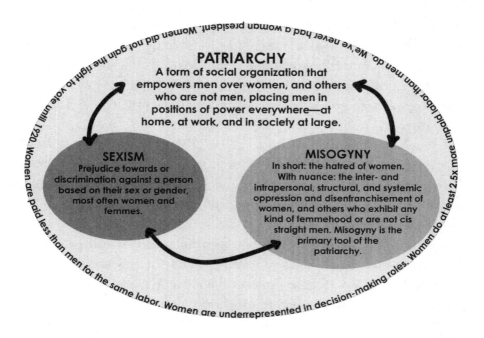

WHAT IS TOXIC MASCULINITY?

As I wrote this section, I struggled with whether or not to begin with *masculinity* or *toxic masculinity*. As you are reading this, it's clear I decided to go with the latter, and here's why.

Although I dislike defining things by what they are not, in this case, masculinity itself is often defined—or, at the very least, stereotyped—by what it is not, by what it lacks, by what it cannot provide.

This stereotype of masculinity is not actually masculinity itself but rather a shell of it, which is most commonly referred to as *toxic masculinity*. In a 2019 *New York Times* article, Maya Salam (she/her) reported that researchers define toxic masculinity as "a set of behaviors and beliefs that include the following: suppressing emotions or masking distress, maintaining an appearance of hardness, [and] violence as an indicator of power."[3] Perhaps contrary to the belief by those who are reactive to this term, toxic masculinity does *not* mean all men are toxic. Toxic masculinity is something that harms men first—and with that pain, repression, and loneliness, men harm others.

Toxic masculinity embodies multiple guises, mostly selling itself as the ticket to fitting in. And, in my experience, I've observed something surprising: engaging in toxic masculinity is not about impressing or courting women but rather is about impressing and fitting in with other men.

I have often commented that my life has felt like a gender studies class. Never quite fitting in anywhere gave me the privilege of watching from the outside in. When I was a kid, the boys who'd previously been my friends suddenly ditched me, as well as other girls, when they realized that their friendships with us were harmful to their social status among the other boys. I listened as they said degrading things and laughed at horrible jokes around other boys but had been previously very kind and protective of me and others.

Sadly, I saw these behaviors continue throughout my college years. I observed as guys would wait and watch for each other's reactions to their jokes, their oversteps, their comments about women—the insecurity and yearning for approval from other men was painfully obvious to me. My suspicions were affirmed twofold: First, I started to find that I felt pressured to engage in what I knew were toxic behaviors, and I witnessed firsthand how doing so could have earned my entry into the mix. Second, as I grew closer with other men in college, I learned that my experience was not unique. Many of my friends who are also men have reported sharing similar feelings.

It is no coincidence that men are far less likely than women to access any kind of mental health resources, including therapy and medication;[4] that men account for 90 percent of domestic violence;[5] and that the demographic most likely to die of suicide are middle-aged white men. While suicide is the twelfth leading cause of death for the U.S. population as a whole, it is the seventh leading cause for men. In 2020, men were nearly four times more likely to die by suicide than women.[6,7]

It might be hard to understand how exactly toxic masculinity can incite the grave consequences that it does, so let's imagine an example.

Johnny is a six-year-old cisgender boy. He's sweet and kind and loves to play with his older sister. They have fun together making up stories with her Barbies. But when he cries, his dad yells, "Stop crying like a girl! Man up." Johnny hides in his sister's room, who gives him a hug but doesn't know what else to do.

His mom tells him that he can play with his sister now, but when he gets older, he's going to have to start to play like a boy, especially with other boys. Johnny tells his mom he doesn't want to. "You will," his mom replies, patting him on the back. "Don't cry. Go, go do your homework."

When Johnny is eight, he is made fun of at school for liking "girly toys." The boys at school call him a fag and laugh at him. By ten, Johnny has stopped hanging out with his sister. He misses her but he is sick of feeling like he doesn't belong anywhere.

By twelve, Johnny refuses to associate himself with boys who seem more feminine for fear of being seen as gay or called a fag. Instead, he's begun to bully them, too. Remembering what his dad has told him, he picks on the boys who are smaller than he is and calls them sissies. He tries his best not to cry.

Sometimes, he gets frustrated because he has difficulty doing his homework. He fights back tears and his dad gruffly reminds him regularly he needs to "be a man." He frequently makes jokes about the "pussies" at work who he thinks aren't man enough. "Real men don't cry at work," he tells Johnny. Johnny takes note.

At thirteen, Johnny watches comedians who make fun of queer and trans people. He laughs when the other boys laugh, and they laugh when he laughs. No one wants to be left out of the joke. No one wants to be labeled not man enough.

At his first football practice when he's fifteen, Johnny takes a hard hit. He doesn't cry. When they're in the car on the way home, his dad grips his shoulder firmly. "You took it like a real man," he says, nodding. Johnny feels proud and loved.

At seventeen, his first girlfriend breaks up with him and he is absolutely heartbroken. His dad speaks a few obscenities about the girl and then ends his diatribe with a gruff, "Don't be so soft. There are more girls."

*At nineteen, Johnny is drunk with his friends at a college party
and a man who is well-known on campus for being openly gay flirts
with him. Johnny punches him in the face. His friends cheer for him,
laughing at the other man.*

At twenty-one . . .

- *Johnny realizes he is gay. Distraught and unable to accept himself, he
takes his own life and dies alone in his college dorm; or,*
- *He takes a girl home from a bar with the intent to have sex. Upon
finding out she is transgender, he beats her senseless and she dies; or,*
- *Johnny and his friend brutally attack and murder a man for supposedly flirting with them.*

Johnny could also do something less extreme:

- *Forever fearful of being "not man enough," Johnny lives much of his
life stuffing his feelings down. During college that means spending most of his time in the gym or at bars, instead of making lasting
friendships. In his adulthood, he struggles to maintain a romantic
relationship; women always tell him he's not "emotionally available."
He doesn't communicate his pain when his mother dies, though the
grief feels unbearable and he goes to her funeral alone. Instead of
being vulnerable with his friends, he drinks heavily by himself. When
he does marry and has kids, he passes the shame of his own emotions
and authenticity to his sons, as well. And so the cycle continues.*

Toxic masculinity begins with a deep and inherently human yearning to belong and can end up stripping us of our humanity. As I see it,
the most insidious, prevalent, and thereby dangerous toxic masculinity is
not solely the violence, murder, or rape, but also the shame and isolation
smaller behaviors inspire.

"Man up," "Grow a pair," "Be a man," "Boys don't cry," "Grow up,"
"Stop acting like a girl," "Don't be a pussy." These are the seeds for violence and destruction, beginning first with young boys and infecting
everyone else.

So am I arguing that cis white straight men are an oppressed group in society? No, not exactly.

Free-speech radicalists, as they call themselves, like aforementioned Canadian psychologist and media personality Jordan Peterson, have argued that society is stupid and "alienating young men," as he told the BBC. "We're telling them that they're patriarchal oppressors and denizens of rape culture. It's awful. It's so destructive. It's so unnecessary. And it's so sad."[8] Although I am sure extremists exist who claim cis white straight men are the sole problem, in reality, Peterson's assertions are incomprehensive.

Demanding accountability from men is not awful or destructive; it is absolutely necessary. But, the problem is not cis men; it's patriarchy, misogyny, and transphobia. The problem is not straight men; it's homophobia. The problem is not white men; it's white supremacy. Understanding these distinctions is crucial to dismantling the systems.

TOXIC MASCULINITY AND TRANS MASCULINITY

As a transgender man, I have been both a victim of misogyny and toxic masculinity, as well as someone who is now expected to—and sometimes demanded to—be an active participant in perpetuating these systems of oppression. As a result, I, along with other trans masculine folks, have a unique perspective from which we can inspire others to challenge patriarchy and toxic masculinity. We are positioned in a way that lends us power. Although I fought hard to be heard when I was presenting as a woman, I often failed to garner respect from other men. This is not uncommon; men are far more likely to listen to other men—which returns us to my earlier assertion that the performance of toxic masculinity is for other men, in seeking approval, admiration, acceptance, and even love from other men.

I have decided to step into that and use the privilege I have of being read as male—and my voice therefore deemed valuable—to gather other men on this journey toward gentle masculinity and more wholesome humanity. And I encourage other men to do the same.

I regularly receive comments from other men that read, "You can't just say you're a man," or, "You're not a real man," or, "You can't just get surgery, that will never change who you are!" And while other facts of ignorance influence these statements, what I recognize most is insecurity.

The roots of these statements run far deeper than simply not believing in my manhood—if that was the only reason, I struggle to understand why they would be so angered. If the only problem is that I am not man enough for them, so what? This does not pose a true problem or threat to another person unless they have attachments to a specific type of manhood. Which they do. In truth, I expect that my manhood is disturbing not because other men don't approve of it but rather because it begs of them the necessity to define manhood altogether. And most cis individuals have not been asked to explain the validity of their gender beyond the appearance of their genitals at birth, while trans individuals, by definition, must. Though not formal, the truth of transness can be an invitation to question one's gender, and thereby question facets of the reality a person has accepted as fact.

This invitation is unfortunately often rejected. It is frightening—and far easier to denigrate the trans person than it is to step into the questions. Doing so first requires the faith that a person is more than their gendered experience of the world. It then demands undoing all the harmful behavior that we have learned to survive, and we can begin doing so through rejecting toxic masculinity.

(SOME SUGGESTIONS FOR) HOW TO REJECT TOXIC MASCULINITY

Let All Boys and Men Express Their Emotions

Teach your sons and other young men in your life that they're allowed to show their feelings, and encourage the expression of your boyfriends', husbands', brothers', and other male friends' emotions. Notice if you feel disdain for men who express emotions usually forbidden to them: grief, pain, fear, softness. Attempt to put this disdain down for a moment and invite those feelings in. Remind yourself and others that all humans should experience the full range of their emotions. If you're someone who dates men, spend some time considering what traits you find attractive in men. If "being my rock" or "is always calm" or "doesn't get too emotional" make the list, consider that many of these typically involve the with-holding of emotions. As with supposed "genital preference," preferences in masculinity can also reflect systems of oppression (in this case, toxic masculinity), and it can be worthwhile to consider unpacking these.

Let Boys and Men Wear Whatever They Want, Including Articles of Clothing That People Might Consider Feminine

Clothing is just clothing—really, it is all just fabric sewn together one way or another, dyed with this color or that. Stop judging people for what they wear. Consider how fashion shifts over time and cultures. Don't forget that symbols of high status for men in the 1700s were pow-dered long-haired wigs, makeup, and heeled shoes. More recently, men's skirts are having a moment, modeled by Brad Pitt (he/him), Jared Leto (he/him), Harry Styles (he/him), and—not to bring up my own mea culpa again—Lil Nas X. If you think your son is going to be bullied for wearing a dress, teach him how to stand up for himself. Don't add to the bullying.

Stop Unnecessarily Gendering Things

Blue is just a color. Sports are for all genders. Barbies can be liked by any-one. Trucks and cars and machines are for kids who like trucks and cars and machines. Makeup is just face paint!

Reject Those Insidiously Harmful Phrases That Perpetuate Toxic Masculinity

Delete "man up," "just grow a pair," "you've got balls," "don't be such a girl," "you're such a pussy," and any other such similarly demeaning phrases from your vocabulary. Encourage others to do the same; don't sit idle while your friends or family use this language.

If You Are a Man, Tell the Men You Love That You Love Them

Share your affection. Share your feelings. Most of us yearn for this and it is only toxic masculinity that allows us to rob ourselves and others of these deep connections.

Reject Ideologies Like "Boys Will Be Boys"

Boys will be what we teach them to be. Teach them to be better.

For some, this list might seem simple. For others, facets of it may feel impossible.

My best friend Kevin (he/him), who is a cis straight man, has always been open to listening to me. Historically, he has always adjusted his behavior if I've shared that something made me uncomfortable—and I've tried to do the same for him. We have built a beautiful friendship on this trust. And even still, I am sometimes nervous to tell him when something upsets me.

In 2020, Kevin was quarantining with me at the beginning of the pandemic. For whatever reason, the words *bitch* and *pussy* had recently entered his daily vocabulary. These weren't directed at me, women, or anyone he or I cared for—they were usually directed at people who weren't kind to me, actually. Still, they didn't feel right.

"Look at this comment," I offered him my phone.

"'I bet all your teammates hate you, fa—'" he stopped before he finished reading the comment aloud.

"They've sent me like twenty comments like this," I said, annoyed.

"That's so dumb," he said. "They are just insecure! What a little bitch!" Even though he was clearly trying to cheer me up, I cringed at his use of the word *bitch*.

"Yeah," I said, not sure if I should address my discomfort in that moment. *Come on, Schuyler, he's just trying to support you. Not everyone uses the right words all the time, give him a break*, I tried to justify. *But it's like the tenth time this week he's said something like that. I should really say something. He'll understand*, I argued back with myself. *But what if he thinks I'm just being too much? What if he thinks* I'm *a bitch or a pussy because I can't handle hearing those words?*

I knew I'd say something eventually—but in all honesty, it took me a lot longer than I'd like to admit.

A few days later, we were sitting on the couch, about to watch a movie together.

"Hey, man," I started, my hands sweating already. He looked at me, a bowl full of Sour Patch Kids in his lap. (I made him use the bowl so as not to spread sugar everywhere.)

"Yeah?" he replied, putting a blue one in his mouth.

"You've been saying *bitch* and *pussy* a lot recently and—"

"Ugh, you're right, I know," he said before I could finish. "I shouldn't. I'll be more careful."

I exhaled, relieved. *That was easy.* And although not all interactions will be as smooth as mine with Kevin, I share this to welcome you if you also feel that challenging your friends is difficult, and to remind you that the response might not be as frightening as you fear.

Going against the dominant behaviors society insists will make you feel included is daunting, yes. And still, I encourage you to go forth. I have found a lot more people willing to challenge the status quo once they see someone else do it. We are less alone that way.

WHAT IS MASCULINITY? WHAT IS MAN ENOUGH?

What remains when we strip away the toxicity from masculinity?

I am not sure if I have an answer to this question. In discussions with friends, both trans and cis, it seems that many of the ways that we know how to describe and define masculinity and femininity reduce both to gender stereotypes. Masculinity is solid and calm; masculinity is opening doors for women, deep voices, and muscular bodies. Femininity is delicate and dainty, quiet and docile; aesthetic and beautiful; soft and warm and curvy.

But the further I attempt to reduce defining either of these, the more similar and, eventually, identical the definitions become.

The *Merriam-Webster* dictionary describes *masculine* as "considered to be characteristic of men," "marked by or having qualities, features, etc. traditionally associated with men," and "of, relating to, or being a man or boy." *Feminine* is defined in the same manner but of women. There are implications to this simple definition: if I am a man, anything I do is masculine; and, masculinity and femininity are purely social concepts that are evaluated based on societal gender roles.

Here's another way to say this: masculinity and femininity can hold different meanings for different people. In many ways, I think describing myself as both masculine and feminine has been a way to communicate my *Schuyleridad,* as my high school Spanish literature teacher put it, in ways that social conventions understand.

When we see "masculinity" and "femininity" as imprecise labels rather than as absolutes that define who we are, I think we can make a lot more space for ourselves and others.

WHAT IS MALE PRIVILEGE?

Before I began my gender-affirmation process, I was living in Boston with my uncle and his family. One afternoon, he dropped me off at my therapy appointment and asked me when I'd need a ride back.

"Don't worry about it," I'd replied. "I'll just walk home." He'd looked at his watch and nodded to himself.

"Okay, sounds good. But if it ends up being dark when you're on your way, don't walk home. Call me, I'll come pick you up. It can be a little bit dangerous for a young woman to walk alone in this area."

I had agreed. I didn't think much of it—I'd been told this countless times before.

Fast forward several months. It was December of my first year at Harvard. We were nearing the semester's end and it had been months since a stranger had misgendered me; in public, I was always perceived as male.

"Let's meet in Central," my uncle texted. "Aim to leave at eleven thirty, okay? By the H Mart."

"Great, see you soon," I replied.

That was 11:30 *p.m.*—the same uncle had proposed a midnight bike ride in Boston to a famous twenty-four-hour bakery. The concern and caution from several months prior was gone—and validly so. I was no longer seen as a woman by the public. And so, I was no longer in the same danger.

This was startling to me, especially at first. In the beginning months of being perceived as a man, I remember walking down the street and hearing the catcalls of men around me. When I'd turn around to ensure my safety or to give the man a dirty look as I usually tried to do, I'd find that there was a woman behind me. She was being catcalled, not me. A mixture of relief and guilt flooded me every time this occurred—relief at my own safety and guilt that while I am safe, she is not.

Safety in public is a primary facet of male privilege. Since transitioning, I have rarely felt unsafe walking alone or at night—sometimes I even forget that I used to fear doing so; the ability to forget is another symbol of my privilege. Few women can ever walk in similar safety.

Here are some other privileges I've experienced as a result of being perceived as a man:

I am always the first to be asked a question if I am in a group of women.

I feel that I am listened to both more and with more trust in my expertise, professionally and otherwise.

I am always considered the leader when in a group of women. While I can likely attribute some of this to my group interaction style (I am comfortable in leadership roles and often take the lead when needed), I am certain it is more than that. Whenever I've been with a group of women at a restaurant, I am always looked to first when the host asks, "For how many?"

I am handed the check after dinner.

I am consistently called "boss" and "brother" by other men in a way that communicates respect, acceptance, and community. I thoroughly enjoy feeling included—though I think this interaction scheme teeters on the edge of misogyny when women are not received with the same care and compassion.

I am listened to by customer service when my wife is not.

I do not experience catcalling or other forms of inappropriate sexual advances from straight cis men. I do, however, experience them from gay cis men—a reminder that sexuality does not preclude the ability to perpetuate toxic masculinity. And, even still, I feel safer in these spaces than I might if I were a woman because I am often entrusted with my own agency and bodily autonomy in a way that women are not.

My assertiveness is more likely to be received as confidence, rather than "bitchiness," "anger," or even "that time of the month."

I am allowed to be shirtless. Well, mostly. Cisgender privilege—or, rather, lack thereof—is also present here. Some folks will attempt to deny me my shirtlessness because they believe trans men are still women. And while I pay them no mind, it's important to note the nuance here, which is, of course, still a product of misogyny.

Women's answers to the question "What would you do if men didn't exist for a day?" include things like "Take a walk at night," "Apply for a promotion because there would be no men to cut the line short," "Roam around this city without a bra," "Go for a run in the city with my headphones on at night," "I wouldn't spend so much money on pepper sprays," "Freely go to public places without looking over my shoulder," and "Go out without having to worry about sharing my live location with people I know."

Because I have not always benefited from male privilege, I have spent a great deal of time thinking about these answers. This is a conflicting reflection: I feel grateful in a way that I imagine most cis men do not—I notice these privileges constantly, especially in the beginning years when they were new to me. And, I also feel guilty or saddened because these should not be privileges.

If you are also someone who the world generally reads as a man, I encourage you to create a similar list. Reflect on what privileges you have due to your perceived manhood. *What do I have that the women around me don't? What does society allow me to do that women cannot? What do I feel safe doing that women do not?*

PEOPLE SAW MY MANHOOD, AND SOMETHING STILL FELT OFF

For me and other trans masculine folks who are read as men in the world, male privilege is built from another, similar, type of privilege: cishet-passing privilege or cishet-assumed* privilege.

---

* The difference between these two terms is that *passing* implies agency on the end of the trans person, and this is not always an accurate reflection. *Assumed* puts the onus of (incorrectly) gendering someone back on others and not on the single trans individual.

When I first began my journey of gender affirmation, I desired to be read by the world as a man. What I failed to articulate at the time was that this was synonymous with wanting to be perceived as a *cis* man. This distinction is important as conflating the two implies that they are one and the same—which then implies that being a cis man is the only way to be a man. This is false.

I am frequently asked: "Schuyler, I understand you are transgender. But you're also a man. So are you a *transgender* man, or *just* a man?"

My answer has remained consistent over the years:

"I am both. I am transgender *and* I am a man. They are not mutually exclusive identities or labels—being transgender is just an additional adjective."

Still, this duality often goes unseen. When I walk through the world I am not perceived as transgender—my history of having been assigned female at birth is invisible to others most of the time. When I first began transitioning, this is exactly what I'd wanted. This was being me! Right...? Unfortunately, I've learned it's not that simple.

Though I have spent years speaking highly of my experience on the men's team and still stand by what I have said, my time there was also fraught with a deep-seated feeling of otherness. When I got to college, I felt the strong urge to be a part of a team for the first time in my life. I was sick of the previous decade during which I never felt like I'd belonged, where I was always too different—too boy—to ever be one of the girls. At Harvard, I was intent on fitting in; I would be one of the guys, I resolved.

Every time I ran into roadblocks where others struggled to relate to me and I to others, I attempted to ignore my feelings. But my transness was often central to how I experienced so many things—especially on a gendered sports team. I felt unable to share with the other guys; I feared doing so would cost me my belonging. And I wanted so badly for my manhood to be just like theirs.

Stop it, I'd tell myself, *I am man enough! I am a man! That's all I need. There's nothing different between me and them.*

At the time, I thought I was affirming myself. I didn't recognize my own internalized transphobia, and instead thought I was just reminding myself that trans men are men. I believed that I should stop trying to see myself as different from cis men. Not having any other role models to correct or guide me through this process, I didn't realize how painful this supposed affirmation was. I was hurting myself—attacking my own trans magnificence and the beauty of being transgender.

Later came the realization that this affirmation was not truly about being man enough—it was really about being *cis* man enough. And again, that distinction is important. In the years since graduating, leaving a toxic relationship with a woman who could not tolerate the implications of my transness, and finally finding myself surrounded by a loving and amazing trans community, I realized that I had been going about finding my own masculinity all wrong.

I am not a cis man. I will never be cis man-enough. Of course, I didn't feel just like the rest of the guys on my team. Of course, my experience in the world is different, my history is different! Of course, attempting to erase my own transness when describing my manhood detracted from both my self-confidence and my own ability to validate—and celebrate—my experience as a transgender man.

I have grown into a deeper appreciation of my identity since having the space to discover my man- and personhood away from the pressures of men's sports and the team environment.

I see my transness as such an integral part of my manhood. I feel that the womanhood I have experienced is inextricably linked to my manhood—I firmly believe that many of the ways in which my mom taught me to be a woman have made me the man I am today. And what a beautifully complex truth that is.

So, as I walk through my life now and people assume I am a cisgender man, I feel a part of me is erased. In an instant, all my transness is gone—my eighteen years walking the world as what people thought was a woman, the hardships I endured, my gender-affirmation journey, my rich history as a complicated human—that all disappears in that moment.

I have spent a large part of my life fighting to be seen as who I am, and I used to think that meant being seen as a man. But now I've arrived here. I'm seen as a man—well, as a cis man. And while this affords me safety, that safety comes at the cost of losing large parts of who I am.

This erasure has proven disturbing and distressing. Recognition brought anger, which took time to morph into grief and acceptance.

Early in my college years, my floormates and I were sitting in my dorm room discussing our Life Sciences 1A homework.

"Well, apparently she can't join us because she's having her period," Rae (she/her) said, annoyed.

"Oh, well, that does make sense, no?" I said, trying to soften Rae's annoyance that Aiyanna (she/her) had bailed last minute. "Getting your period sucks, I know—" I continued.

"What do you mean?" Rae interrupted me. "What do *you* know?"

I had frozen. Confusion quickly shifted into panic. Rae did not know I was trans. She didn't know I'd once menstruated, too.

"Boys always thinking they know what women go through…" Rae muttered.

I had no idea how to proceed. I was very upset that I had accidentally aligned myself with men who mansplain—with the assholes who think they know more about menstruating than those who actually menstruate. But to share that I was not mansplaining, I'd have to share that I was transgender. I was not ready to do that.

"Shoot, I'm sorry, you're right," I said quietly, bowing my head. "My bad, I'm sorry." I repeated.

We moved on and when I eventually did share that I am trans, we looked back on that moment in laughter.

But that moment was pivotal for me.

I'd previously found community with other women—especially those who were also queer or additionally marginalized in some way. I was seen as approachable, as a teammate in fighting patriarchy. I was seen as one of them. Though I revel in the privilege of being seen as myself—as a man—now, I also feel the loss of this community and camaraderie. Sometimes, I'm even perceived as a threat, lumped in with cis men who have perpetrated so much harm against others (and themselves).

Patriarchy not only empowers men over women; it also causes women and other similarly disenfranchised groups to fear cis men. This I'd known in concept, and in practice—but from the other side. Before my transition, *I* had feared cis men. I'd felt unsafe around them. In my high school years, I'd biased my friendships toward women and queer people, finding connection there. But I hadn't imagined what it would be like to be feared once I transitioned. Now, when women, queer folks, or trans folks perceive me as a cis man, they no longer see me as one of them. They see me as a threat. They see me as a tool of patriarchy and even as someone who could perpetuate violence against those disenfranchised by patriarchy.

I think that being seen as toxic or even dangerous irrespective of my actions has been the most uprooting facet of my transition. And I know from talking with other cis-assumed trans masculine individuals that this is a common challenge for us.

The grieving process for this loss and shift in my position in society began first with anger, as I mentioned. *Who are they to think I'm toxic when they don't even know me! I have not benefited from cis male privilege my whole life! I, too, have experienced misogyny and felt unsafe walking the streets alone, how can they think I'm also a threat? How* dare *they consider me a threat!*

Allowing myself the space to feel angry and upset and hurt has been integral to my healing—as well as my ability to reorient: my anger's true direction should be at patriarchy, and not at any singular individual who attaches patriarchal violence to their perception of me as a man.

The anger I felt used to include anger that I should somehow be responsible for holding this erasure and the assumption of my identity. *It's not* my *fault cis men suck, so why am I taking the fall for it?* While I am not responsible for fixing patriarchy on my own, I *am* responsible for understanding how I benefit from it and how I also perpetuate it as someone who society sees as a man.

Sad and disturbing is the reality that a woman might fear for her safety if I, a man, coincidentally walk a few paces behind her at night. I realize now this is not my fault, nor am I at fault for how patriarchy impacts her fear. My absolute responsibility, however, is for understanding how my actions *could* impact her. Regardless of my culpability in this situation, if I do not slow down and adjust my proximity to her, she could be afraid. To mitigate any potential fear, I never walk fewer than ten paces behind a woman at night. I slow down, stop, or cross the street.

Similarly, although the voices of trans men are not often heard and we are also regularly marginalized, I am still mindful of when I speak up or over a woman, especially in a space where my transness has not been shared. If I have not shared that I am trans, I am also careful not to speak about the experiences of women as if I am an authority, despite personal experience walking the world in their shoes.

The list goes on.

Each of these behavioral adjustments requires both the awareness of the impact of patriarchal systems of oppression as well as understanding how my actions could unintentionally align with oppressive behaviors.

Eventually the anger I felt in resisting this demand for my own awareness lessened as I released myself from the blame and moved instead to grief and action. Instead of situating myself in the responsibility for patriarchy itself, I learned that it was more accurate and effective to situate myself in the responsibility of *fighting* patriarchy. This brought grief for what I've lost.

I must also add that this grief does not preclude joy; it never does. Grief and joy can exist together—in fact, I believe they must.

In addition to the joy of feeling at home in my body and being recognized as myself as a man, I grieve that I am no longer assumed to be a teammate by women.

I have, in fact, grieved my womanhood itself. When I've shared this in the past, people (trans and not) accuse of me of wavering: "If you still want to be a woman, you're not trans enough. You're not really trans!" they've said.

Wanting, though, is irrelevant for me. I don't *want* to be a man or woman. I just *am* a man—who was thought to be a woman at first. Additionally, my grieving of my womanhood is not an indicator that I wish to return to it. We can miss something and not want it back; we can value something we used to have and not seek to reclaim it.

I spent over eighteen years believing that I would grow up to be a woman, a mother, a sister, a wife. Though I had not imagined my future with extensive detail, I had dreamed of what I'd become. Then, in a relatively short period of time, I discovered this was not going to be my future. And this was both exciting and beautiful—I could truly be me, a man! And grief ensued, as well. The cost was letting go of a future I'd thought I'd been building—though not *wanting*—my whole life.

I worry that you reading this will internalize this grief as negative. This couldn't be further from the truth.

If you're also trans, I hope you can welcome your own grief. In fact, this invitation extends to anyone experiencing any kind of grief. Grief and joy are two sides of the same coin: they are integral to living life to the fullest. To me, grief is the proper recognition of loss—it is my ability to understand myself and how I changed over the years. It is honoring who I've been and who I am always becoming. Committing to including grief in my life means acceptance that growth is, after all, extremely painful. And it is also how I become all I am supposed to be.

BE CIS ON PURPOSE

"I don't care if you're cis," an unattributed quote has floated around the trans community online. "Just do it on purpose."

Gender isn't something that only trans people have. If you're not transgender, you also have a gender, you also have gendered experiences, and my guess is that you've also had your experience and expression *limited* by gender, as well.

Hear what the model, trans advocate, and writer Devin-Norelle offers:

> We could all benefit from [dismantling gender as we know it] because if we weren't so stuck on adhering to the binary and what it looks like and what it means, think about how many cis men might be more open to expressing themselves outside of masculinity. I think about so many men who probably have so much pent-up anger because they can't be themselves, they don't feel safe to be themselves... I think about the fact that they take that anger and go and police other people and harm other people with that anger, not just themselves... So when I say

that we're oppressing trans people, we're really oppressing everybody, not just trans people.

If we could get to this point where gender isn't a thing that we weren't so concerned over, because we dismantled colonialism, we dismantled white supremacy and the gender standards that came with that... How easy it would be for us to wear any article of clothing, any kind of makeup, without feeling like we might put ourselves in danger. We could do so much more. People would be a lot happier if we dismantled gender.

Considering why you are who you are is a crucial endeavor, not only for your own self-development, self-preservation, and joy, but also for your interactions with others.

When I was kid, I held my dad's hand everywhere we went. My brother did as well, at least when we were little. Though I cannot point to when exactly, at some point my brother stopped doing this. I, as someone who was perceived as a girl, did not. I also continued calling my father "Daddy," as I had since I was young. Most other girls I knew did the same, even past their official childhood.

In the first months of my transition when the world began to gender me as male more consistently, I stood in line at a fast-food restaurant with my dad.

I can't remember what exactly I said, but my sentence included referring to my father as "Daddy" aloud. I continued onward, unaware that people had turned their heads and were staring. After a few moments, my dad tugged on my hand and said gently, "You know, your brother stopped calling me that, at least in public, a little while ago."

Confused, I said, "What? Calling you what?"

"Daddy," he said, quietly. "I just wanted you to know. Most boys stop calling their fathers that at some point."

"Oh," I said, my face falling, embarrassed. "Should I—" I began.

"You can call me whatever you'd like," he answered, preempting my question. "I just wanted to tell you. It's up to you."

As I write this nearly eight years later, with greater understanding of how the world perceives men and masculinity, I cringe at myself. I imagine an eighteen-year-old boy holding his father's hand and calling him "Daddy," and I see now how others saw me then.

And I also hurt for all men who feel like they cannot show that softness with those they love. I often miss the times when it felt easy to hold my dad's hand as I walked together with him—but now it feels awkward and, even, scary. Not because my father would resist in any way, but rather because of how society might receive us.

This is not contained to intimate, loving relationships with parents or best friends—this extends to society at large.

Before I transitioned, when people perceived me as a "woman," wearing clothing that society had gendered as "masculine" was easy. I had no issue wearing button-down shirts, men's jeans, even a suit and tie. I never felt that wearing men's clothing or presenting myself in a more masculine fashion caused me unique danger.

Now, as someone who is perceived as a man, playing with clothing gendered as "feminine" or "woman" can feel scary. The few times I have painted my nails after transition, I've been stared at. I know that if I were to wear a dress in public, I would likely experience even more unwanted attention, including potential violence.

I've found that conventional masculinity leaves far less room for much of my humanity, so I've chosen to discard certain rules. Sometimes I still call my father "Daddy," and sometimes I still reach for his hand. I hug him whenever I see him. My phone lights up with "Daddy" and "Mommy" when we call or email among us. I tell all my friends who are men that I love them, and I tell them often. I tell my women friends often, too.

People might critique me for this: "If you wanted to be feminine, why didn't you just stay a woman?" I did not exit the box of womanhood to jump into somebody else's box of manhood. I am here to be myself—I do not subscribe to the dominant society's strict guidelines of what manhood must look like. In fact, I have found great euphoria and connection through discarding those rules and existing just as myself.

I know that this has also encouraged the men around me to step deeper into their own humanity. And this is my intent in sharing these things with you here.

One night my best friend Kevin and I watched the Disney Pixar film *Coco*. In one of the final scenes, I found myself trying to hold back tears. I wondered why—we'd been best friends for years and neither of us have ever been particularly "masculine" in a way that would preclude our emotions. We'd cried in front of each other many times. Still, I found myself afraid of what he'd think. We were just watching a movie, after all. *I shouldn't be so emotional!* I was berating myself. But after a few short moments, I gave up.

"I'm gonna cry!" I said.

He let out a sob, relieved, and said, "Me, too."

We cried and laughed together through the rest of the movie. And then we chatted about masculinity. We both have often felt insecure about showing affection toward other male friends. Throughout most of college, people thought Kevin and I were a couple—presumably not because we spent most of our time together (we knew many guys who did so as well) but rather because they perceived us to be "too" intimate with each other. This intimacy involved hugs, emotional talks, and sharing sweaters and holidays. My parents lovingly refer to him as their third child.

For most of my life, I have been called "too sensitive." Following my transition, I've been told that I am not man enough for a multitude of reasons: I am not tall enough, I don't have a penis, I am too sensitive, I am too emotional, I am too soft, I think too much, I don't watch or care about (men's) sports, and even, I don't play video games.

While these attacks have felt both painful and ridiculous at times, in every single one, I see men giving up pieces of their own humanity. I see men hiding, repressing, and beating on themselves to be what they think other men want them to be.

In this sense, toxic masculinity is made by men, for men, and at the primary expense of men. Masculinity embodied by these limitations is performed by men, for men. It is this insidious nature of toxic masculinity that instigates harm across gender identity, race, sexuality, class, and so much more. The limitations placed upon men are not truly about height, or body parts, or emotions, or sports, or video games, they are about control.

Transgender men fall into this trap, too. I know several trans men who have assumed behaviors aligned with toxic masculinity because of an overwhelming desire to belong and to be seen as "real" men. Like cis people, trans people are not exempt from perpetuating toxicity: we also desire to belong. But while I have empathy for these trans men—the years during which I was expected to join my teammates in toxicity were long and grueling in many ways—I stand fiercely in my assertion that trans men like myself have a unique capacity for enacting change among cis men and therefore society.

Trans men and trans masculine individuals who have found grounding and security in their masculinity are able to show other men something special: the ability to hold masculinity with gentleness and confidence, with flexibility and intention. As a result, and perhaps risking self-grandiosity and arrogance, I believe that cis men have a great deal to learn from trans men who have found this freedom in masculinity, and from there, we can change the world.

Of course, this expands beyond manhood—cis men *and* cis women will benefit from intentionality in their cishood, because through agency, intentionality invites freedom, too.

As Dylan Kapit puts it:

I just want [cis people] to know that [they're] a cis person and [they're] making choices to reinforce their cis identity, the way that I'm a trans person and I'm making choices to reinforce my trans identity, but both of those things are purposeful gender experiences and cis people are not having that conversation.

I think the world would be a better place if cis people thought about their gender more.

CHAPTER 19

Trans, Korean, Mixed-Race, Athlete: Whew, the Intersectionality!

A s I WRITE THIS CHAPTER, I'M SITTING AT THE DINING TABLE in my grandmother's house. The familiar scent of toasted sesame oil and daenjang (Korean fermented miso paste) fill the air while a soft conversation between Halmoni and my great-aunt drift over from the kitchen while they make kimbap for us to eat later.

I grew up five minutes from here, and I can't remember ever not knowing I am Korean. I can't remember ever not understanding that I am mixed-race. Race was one of the most obvious differences between my parents and thus always apparent in my household. My dad is a white man who is originally from the Midwest; my mom is a Korean immigrant who moved to the States in the 1960s.

Throughout my childhood, I was asked if I was "more Korean" or "more white." I learned to stand firmly in my response: I am both. I am Korean. I am American. I am Korean American. Still, I have spent much of my life feeling stuck in between. I was never white enough to be considered with the white kids, and I was always too white to be included by Koreans or other Asians.

As a kid, I remember craving Korean American connection. Although my parents, and my mom especially, tried very hard to make sure I had exposure to other Asians and Koreans (both in my life and in media I consumed), there was still such a dearth of mixed-race people like me. I always felt like the odd one out. Sometimes I was explicitly excluded by other Asians because I wasn't "full" Asian. I never really felt "full" anything.

This state of identity limbo compounded when I later discovered my queer and trans identities. I feared my queerness further removed me from being welcomed in Asian spaces, but being Asian American stopped me from feeling like I belonged in queer spaces, which were overwhelmingly white. I wasn't enough of anything at all. Belonging fully anywhere was always elusive.

This convergence of marginalized identities can be referred to as *intersectionality*, a term coined by American lawyer and professor Kimberlé Crenshaw (she/her) in 1989. Crenshaw, a leading critical race theory scholar, first used *intersectionality* to discuss the intersections of race and sex, specifically regarding discrimination that Black women are subjected to. Black women exist at the intersection of misogyny and anti-Blackness, and these systems of oppression compound to create what Black queer feminist Moya Bailey (she/her) termed *misogynoir*.[1] On the contrary, white women experience misogyny but not anti-Blackness, and Black men experience anti-Blackness but not misogyny. Black women experience both, and this intersection is significant.

Intersectionality refers to unique dynamics of oppression that result from experiencing multiple marginalized identities, describing overlapping oppressions. It's important to recognize that intersectionality in this context does not simply discuss multiple identities coexisting in one person but rather the *resulting oppression* that can come from the existence of multiple identities in that person. Being white and trans is not intersectionality. Being disabled and trans is. Being Black and trans and a woman is. Being Asian and trans, like me, is.

Intersectionality considers oppression across all identity groups: gender identity, gender expression, gender assigned at birth, sexuality, race, religion, socioeconomic background, ability, age, citizenship and immigration status, and more.

Intersectionality for me has shifted over my life. Before I discovered my transness, I presented myself as a woman, and identified as queer. These both intersected with each other, as well as with my Koreanness and mixed-race-ness. In that perceived womanhood, I was consistently exoticized and sexualized for being mixed-race and Asian American. I was frequently told by strangers, friends, parents of friends, and even teachers that "mixed kids are the most beautiful/sexy/pretty" or that "mixed babies are the most attractive."

Several of my male high school swim teammates discussed in detail what they found attractive about my body while in the locker room—so much so that my brother ceased to shower after practice because of his disgust and discomfort over the boys' endless objectification of me. One teammate pursued me relentlessly.

"He has a thing for Asian girls," another teammate told me. I later learned that he dated Asian women almost exclusively. This, combined with the oversexualization of lesbians, was overwhelming at times. When I told one of my guy friends that I liked girls, his first response was, "Oh, that's hot."

No one prepared me for the shift that occurred after I transitioned. As someone who is now read as an Asian *man*, I experience exactly the opposite of this treatment.

Instead of being oversexualized, exoticized, and fetishized as an Asian *woman*, I am now often forgotten, erased, and seen as extremely undesirable as an Asian *man*. Numerous sources and studies corroborate my personal experience, showing that Asian women (along with white men) are among the most desired categories on dating apps, while Asian men, along with Black women, are by far the least. For *Pacific Standard*, Ravi Mangla (he/him) wrote, "Asian men face the steepest climb." The studies show that the only groups not discriminated against based on category are Asian women and white men.[2,3]

These findings have been consistent on gay dating apps, as well, such as Grindr, where incognito tags like "no rice" or "no curry" are often written, intended to dissuade Asians from communicating any interest.[4]

I can use my own experience as a clear example:

A few months before I got top surgery, a friend and I were hanging out at her house. While I did not understand the role race would play in my future dating life, I was uniquely aware that I would no longer be desired as a woman. This was exciting but the prospect also included grief. I wanted to say goodbye to that part of me.

Somehow, we found ourselves swiping on Tinder, laughing about the ridiculous first lines we'd received. Though I'd recently changed my gender marker to M to reflect my gender identity, that night I impulsively changed it back to F.

"I probably will never be seen like this again," I told my friend. "I'll give it one last go."

So together, we curated my profile with photos of me in exclusively "feminine" presentations. Then I swiped right on every single profile. Within an hour, I had hundreds of matches and dozens of messages. Of course, most of the messages were not particularly pleasant, and many evoked something about my race, as well. Not taking any of it seriously, the process was mostly funny for us at the time, and at the end of the evening, I deleted the profile.

A few years later, after consistently being read as a man, I conducted the same pseudo experiment—uploading all my best photos and swiping right on every profile. I received markedly fewer matches and even fewer messages or engagement, especially from women.

In a less experimental effort, I also tried varying disclosure of my transness—I wanted to see what made me feel comfortable. This made it clear that including my transness (either visually by shirtless photos that exposed my mastectomy scar, or explicitly through naming it in my bio) would reduce matches even further.

In our (Western) society, both Asian men and trans men are seen as less masculine, as less men, as smaller, weaker, meeker. Neither group is displayed often in the media, and when they do appear, at least historically, they're represented as reduced stereotypes.

In my experience as an Asian trans man, I've found that some of the most extreme anti-Asian and anti-trans sentiments target women I've dated, degrading their choice of a man like me. I imagine this stems from insecurity pertaining to an alleged unfairness—that someone they perceive to be less manly is dating someone they've judged to be attractive and desirable.

Still, this intersectional oppression has taken a toll on me. One woman explained why dating me was hard for her: "It's not only that you're trans, you're also Asian, and short, and small, and it's just..." She never finished articulating, but that, in a nutshell, is intersectional oppression.

Yes, I am not only trans, but also mixed-race, Asian American, queer, an immigrant's child, a North Korean's grandchild, an athlete in a world that despises trans athletes, a man who's experienced an eating disorder, the list goes on. Each of these identities plays into the oppression I experience, and thus, the resiliency I have been forced to develop and hold.

I, along with most other trans people like me, am often lauded for my ability to ignore the hatred, to stand courageous throughout, and to still be ourselves.

"You're so brave," I've been told on countless occasions.

I want to remind you that, especially for those of us with intersecting identities, this resilience is not a choice. It may be brave, but it is also mandatory for us to be able to continue forward with our sanity intact and lasting capacity for joy.

This chapter cannot adequately review every identity that, intersecting with transness, increases oppression. This is an incomprehensive list that attempts to provide you with the scaffolding to consider the complexity within our community. If you're also trans, it's an opportunity to examine your own identities and privileges.

RACE

In May 2019, Black trans woman Muhlaysia Booker (she/her) was beaten in broad daylight. The community was deeply affected. I, along with many other activists, made posts about her to raise awareness and crowdfund to help her pay her hospital bills. Despite the horrors that she'd endured, the community seemed hopeful that Muhlaysia was receiving some sort of support and recognition while she was still alive.

A week later, Muhlaysia was murdered by gunshot in Dallas. Three other Black trans women's lives were also taken that weekend.

The years 2020 and 2021 saw record numbers of anti-trans murders, largely of trans women of color at the hands of cisgender men. Black trans women exist at the intersections of three massive systems of oppression: misogyny, anti-Blackness and racism, and transphobia. This intersecting oppression is referred to as *transmisogynoir* and was first coined by the writer Trudy (she/her).[5]

In "The Anatomy of Transmisogynoir," an op-ed for *Harper's Bazaar*, Ashlee Marie Preston reveals how Black trans women are ignored or actively excluded by Black cishet communities because transness is so often seen as a function of whiteness. Black trans women are not included by white trans women because of their Blackness. Black trans women are not included by many cis women because of their transness. Lastly, despite the fact that Black trans women like Marsha P. Johnson (she/her)* and Miss Major Griffin-Gracy (she/her) were crucial figures in the 1969 Stonewall Riots, much of the white, cis, gay, and queer community forgets and fails to pay homage to Black trans women.

"All Black trans women truly have is one another, because we've been exiled from every sector of society," Ashlee writes.[6]

When I asked Ashlee to share the labels she uses to describe herself, she said, "I'm a fat, Black, trans woman." She grinned. I smiled back. Each of these describe a facet of her identity that is both political and powerful, she explained. "The objective of oppression [is] to shatter your ability to dream, to aspire, to envision...it's meant to erase you. To essentially abolish you into the margins. And so, there is something powerful about being fat, Black, trans—and unapologetic," she said.[7]

Ashlee recounted to me her journey: She'd come out in 2004 as trans. Instead of support, she was fired from her job and thrown into financial insecurity. Over the next several years, she was forced to engage in survival sex work, experiencing multiple near-death encounters, and relying on drugs to cope. Unfortunately, this experience is not uncommon, especially among Black trans women—and, Ashlee pointed out, undocumented Black trans women who are even more invisible.

---

* Though the word *transgender* was not widely used in Marsha's lifetime, she usually referred to herself with she/her pronouns in addition to calling herself gay, a transvestite, or a queen.

Many of the Black trans women I have had the privilege to meet and befriend during my career are beacons of courage and models of the most resilient and special kind of strength in self-love. I'm certain that this strength is a direct result of learning to survive—and somehow thrive—despite the oppression. *Some* women like Ashlee find their way through.

"I have survived a lot of traumas that should have broken me," she said, "should have hardened me, made me indifferent..." Somehow, she sat in front of me, glowing and radiant. "Lots of people ask me, 'How did you come out of that?'" she continued. "I didn't lose my ability to love, to forgive, to have compassion, to see beyond a person's behavior or their circumstances, and see the individual behind it all."[8]

In the summer of 2021, I spoke at the Brooklyn Liberation March for Black trans youth in New York City. The march was largely organized and led by trans women of color. I found myself surrounded by amazing community activists whose work I'd long admired: Raquel Willis (she/her), Joela Rivera (she/her), Ianne Fields Stewart (they/she), Junior Mintt (she/her), and of course, Black trans activist, costume designer, and storyteller Qween Jean (she/her).

Tall and stunning in a beautiful white dress with a matching head-dress, Qween led the crowd as we chanted through the streets.

"BLACK TRANS—" she called, and we all replied, "POWER," over and over.

Qween sang her words for the entire time we were out there. My wife and I wondered at how she was able to continue—her voice strong and clear for hours.

"WHAT DO WE DO WHEN WE'RE UNDER ATTACK?"
"STAND UP, FIGHT BACK!"

I found myself holding back tears for a majority of the event. Though we were gathered because of the devastating intersecting oppression Black trans youth experience, unrestrained, unrelenting joy flowed from the crowd. The seemingly unwavering empowerment was infectious—and beyond powerful.

In this moment, joy and pain wove together so tightly in my chest that I was unable to distinguish between the two. It was impossible not to think of all that had brought us here—not only the violence that necessitated the protest itself, but also the resilience and legacy of our trans ancestors that laid the groundwork for us to exist here today.

Qween Jean, who also founded Black Trans Liberation, an organization that aims to empower and resource the trans community,[9] reminded me of famous photos of Marsha P. Johnson—their wide smiles and Black trans joy unwavering in the face of such devastating oppression. Both women seem to fight with joy as their primary tool. Marsha P. Johnson was a Black trans woman and self-identified drag queen (the term *transgender* was not used until after her death), who, along with other queer and trans women of color like Sylvia Rivera (she/her), protested during the Stonewall Riots, lauded as what galvanized the gay rights movement.

As I marched alongside Qween Jean and more trans youth of color than I'd ever been privileged to be in community with, I wept. How painfully beautiful and empowered we are—and always have been. How painful it is we are still fighting this fight. How horrible it is that Black trans folks are still left out of mainstream activism not only due to transness but also due to Blackness. How incredible it is that they rise up, anyway—just like Marsha P. Johnson.

In 2020, shortly after the murder of George Floyd (he/him), I posted a photo of myself holding a whiteboard that read, THE FIRST PRIDE WAS A RIOT. The post went on to clarify: a police riot. Indeed, the Stonewall Riots, which Marsha was a part of, were protests and sometimes destructive riots against police raids and police brutality at gay and queer bars like the Stonewall Inn.

A coworker shared his reception of my post:

"I struggled with this one, to be honest," he confessed to me. He is a white gay cis man. "I really don't understand why they need to be rioting." *They* referred to the Black Lives Matter protesters—of which I would absolutely consider myself a part.

"You wouldn't have any of the rights you do without queer and trans women of color, rioting, who began this movement in the first place," I said.

GENDER IDENTITY

You might have noticed that a majority of anti-trans rhetoric focuses on trans women—often completely ignoring trans men altogether. This creates differing dynamics for each: trans feminine folks are overly visible and heavily sexualized, and, as a result, are subject to disproportionate rates of violence. Trans masculine individuals, on the other hand, are often forgotten or erased from the narrative altogether.

Legislative attacks almost exclusively focus on punishing trans femininity—trans women in sports, trans women in bathrooms, cis men or trans women performing drag, and so on. As previously discussed, none of these efforts are truly based in protecting women or children, but rather in misogyny.

While many trans masculine folks like myself transition into male privilege, trans feminine folks often transition out of it, and into being not only the objects of misogyny, but also targets of transphobia. In childhood, they'll bully trans women for "being a girl," but when she finally comes out and claims her womanhood, they'll bully her for being trans. It often feels there is no winning.

As we walked back to our hotel from the Brooklyn Liberation March, trans flags adorned across our bodies and my person-sized sign reading TRANS ATHLETES BELONG IN SPORTS, we were stopped by a car.

"Yo, let me read your sign," came a voice from a blacked-out window that rolled slowly down. I turned to let him read, still high off the joy from the march.

"Oh, hell no," he said. A slew of transphobia that I don't care to repeat fell out of his mouth. I grabbed my wife's hand and began walking quickly away.

"If you're a man, be a man, you can't be a woman!" he yelled after us. "I'll beat your ass!"

This interaction occurred in broad daylight at a busy intersection in liberal Brooklyn, New York. Not in an alleyway, not under the cover of privacy or night, not in the South, or in a particularly conservative part of the state. And we were lucky he'd not chosen to come after us. There had been three men in that car—who knows what could have happened.

"He thought you were trans and that I was defending you," I explained to my wife once I'd had a moment to digest what had happened. As is common due to the aforementioned visibility of trans women and erasure of trans men, he likely assumed that the femme-presenting person between us (my wife) was trans, instead of me.

After the shakes subsided and we were safely inside, we marveled at how so many trans women and trans femmes, especially those of color, encounter this every time they are in public. And yet somehow, they were able to gather together as they had at the march, dancing, singing, and celebrating our fight.

Something beautiful comes of this complex marginalization, that is certain. But it should not have to. I am hopeful for the day when womanhood and transhood are beautiful not in radical defiance to patriarchy but simply in their own right.

DISABILITY

Recent research suggests that the transgender population exhibits higher rates of disability compared to our cisgender counterparts.[10] This is associated with the fact that compared to cisgender folks, trans people have worse health outcomes and decreased healthcare use. Trans people also suffer from "minority stress," which refers to the distress that marginalized populations experience due to systemic and interpersonal discrimination.

Due to ableism, disabled folks are more likely to experience housing insecurity, medical debt, food insecurity, verbal harassment, and violence. Nearly 25 percent of unhoused folks are disabled; disabled adults are two times more likely to experience poverty; and disabled adults are three times more likely to experience sexual assault.[11-14]

Given that trans folks are also more likely to experience all of these, it follows that the intersection of being trans *and* being disabled can result in even more harm.

For example, the validity of autistic trans folks' trans identities is further doubted by society, and even by medical and mental health professionals, due to their autism. Though many self-advocates—autistic folks who advocate for themselves, as opposed to parent advocates of autistic children—do not consider autism a disorder, but rather evidence of neurodiversity, autism is often deeply pathologized. As a result, autistic trans folks often experience compounded and complex discrimination.

Dylan Kapit reminds us, "Autistic people are very capable of knowing that they are trans, and autistic people's trans identities need to be taken just as seriously as non-autistic people's trans identities. Being trans and autistic is a beautiful thing, but sometimes having two very stigmatized identities at the same time is really difficult."

Some disabled folks draw parallels between their journeys through disability and through transness. When I spoke with Chella Man (he/they), a deaf transgender genderqueer model, artist, and friend, he shared how becoming deaf helped him create the space and framework for discovering his transness:

Both [being disabled and being queer] are very somatic experiences. [...] It's understanding somatically how you're feeling in your body, what your body is capable of and what it's incapable of. [...] Both of my parents are doctors, so I had access to a very medicalized view of my body from a very early age. So, although I didn't have the terminology to articulate my queerness, I was given some level of terminology to explain what I was feeling through my disability. However, it was in a very medicalized way. [...] I was told my body was broken. And that it was becoming more broken as time progressed, which I do not agree with or believe now.

I think I was gaining a lot of really beautiful things that I wasn't able to fully understand and hold close to me at the time. But from a very early age, I struggled with the phrase "losing my hearing" because I don't think it was a loss. As that was happening, I was forced to notice and be conscious of the ways my body was changing—and being in my body more just accentuated the feeling of who I was. Since day one I've always known who I am and in our modern world that is being trans, right? But I just knew the ways I wanted to look, and I knew the ways I wanted to feel, ideally, and what I wanted to be capable of, how I wanted to connect with people.

So being deaf forced/encouraged me to really step into my form more deeply.

When Chella explained this to me, I understood his experience through my own lens as a mixed-race person. Being both Korean and white in a world that constantly asks not *who* but "*what* are you" demanded I ask myself the same. I grappled with this question regarding my race long before I applied the same question to gender, helping me develop a blueprint for self-exploration beyond the tools that were provided to me.

Of course, far more disabilities exist beyond deafness and autism than I can adequately address in this section. I have offered these two examples as thought starters. Physical or cognitive, visible or not, disabilities can cause trans people to experience even more discrimination than we already do just for being transgender. Taking this diversity into consideration when understanding the trans population is key.

MENTAL HEALTH

Due to the long history of pathologization of our transness by healthcare professionals, mental illness can often pose a difficult overlapping struggle. Too many times I have listened to my friends' experiences with providers who invalidate or dismiss their gender identities due to the presence of other mental illnesses such as depression, borderline personality disorder, anxiety, or something else. I, too, was subject to this.

You're not trans, you just have an eating disorder and hate your body.

You're not really trans, you just have borderline personality disorder and don't have a sense of self.

You're not really trans, you're just depressed.

It is true that the trans community exhibits a higher prevalence of mental illness than the general population. But anti-trans rhetoric misses the explanation: trans people do not suffer from mental illness because we are trans, we suffer from mental illness because the world is transphobic.

Because I cannot comprehensively explore the varying ways that different mental illnesses intersect with transness in this chapter, we will focus on one as an example: eating disorders.

Most eating disorder treatment revolves around women—specifically, white, straight, cis women. If you picture *anorexia*, I'll guess that a thin, white girl is what comes to mind. However, studies show that trans folks experience eating disorders and eating disorder behaviors at higher rates than their cisgender peers.[15,16] Despite trans people experiencing eating disorders at rates markedly higher than any other demographic, treatment is not made for us. Finding trans-competent care is next to impossible.

So, in addition to experiencing the hardships and risk of death from an eating disorder, trans individuals with eating disorders struggle to find treatment that will accept them, as well. Once there, they also struggle to have their identities and experiences validated—gender identity often tossed aside as another symptom of the illness.

Understanding transness and, perhaps more importantly, the impact of transphobia on an individual is vital to being able to properly care for a patient of any kind, but especially in mental health. Adjustments that account for gender include large-scale shifts like trans competency training, which I have provided for numerous mental health and eating disorder associations, as well as more minute, but still incredibly important, shifts in language.

For example, while many people will use the words *dysphoria* and *dysmorphia* interchangeably, gender dysphoria is *not* the same as body dysmorphia.

Body dysmorphia is an extreme fixation on specific parts of one's body, usually one or more perceived flaws in appearance. Though widely assumed to appear commonly in those struggling with eating disorders, body dysmorphia most often appears in individuals with body dysmorphic disorder. The *DSM-5-TR* explicitly states, "Body dysmorphic disorder must be differentiated from an eating disorder."[17] People with eating disorders can also experience body dysmorphia, but most often the distress these individuals experience is considered body image disruptions or distortions.

"Body dysmorphic disorder should not be diagnosed if the preoccupation is limited to discomfort with or a desire to be rid of one's primary and/or secondary sex characteristics," the *DSM* reads. This is gender dysphoria.

Unlike gender dysphoria, neither body image distortions nor body dysmorphia are rooted in incongruence of identity but rather in trauma, resulting in disruptions of self-worth and self-image, and a perception of lack of control.

The distinction between body dysmorphia or distortions and gender dysphoria is critical because they can have very different treatment considerations: treatment for gender dysphoria allows and supports physical alterations if desired, while treatment for body dysmorphia does not.

Dysmorphia and body distortions can be weaponized against trans people—claiming that we are just experiencing cognitive distortions and are in need of cognitive reframing tools, or "psychological adjustments" as suggested by David Cauldwell in the 1950s. But being trans is not a mental illness or a cognitive distortion. Treating gender dysphoria through gender-affirming medical care has been shown to be lifesaving, life-giving, an overwhelmingly significant portion of the time.

Trans individuals with eating disorders are often lumped into the same bucket as cisgender individuals, and while eating disorders can present in very similar ways, strategies that manage underlying psychological pain can vary from individual to individual, especially when gender and gender experience are involved.

SEXUALITY

"Stop saying you're queer," she told me after we'd been dating a few months.

"Why?" I'd asked, surprised. She knew I was trans. *What was wrong with being queer?*

"Ew, because you're not. You're just a regular guy who happens to be trans. You date women. You're straight. You're not like those other people."

I hadn't known how to reply. Besides the obvious transphobia, homophobia and queerphobia also creeped in. She went on to tell me how gross it was to imagine me with another man.

While especially painful and scary coming from a romantic partner, these comments were far from unusual.

If you wanted to date men, why not just stay a woman?

How can you be trans and gay?

In addition to weathering transphobia, many trans people who do not identify as straight also face queer- and homophobia. These attacks weave together our gender and our sexuality, somehow attempting to invalidate both of them. This type of queerphobia is different from what a cis gay person might experience where their gender is not likely to be called into question.

I have long feared that showing more femininity—regardless of its tie to my sexuality—would incur attacks on my gender itself. As someone who has fought to be seen as myself, a man, I was not eager to have this discounted due to perceptions of my sexuality.

Admittedly, I have adjusted how I've presented in moments so as not to appear "gay"—not because I fear being seen as gay, but because I fear that gayness attributed to me will result in being seen as "woman."

In college and even the year following, I found myself terrified at the prospect of my teammates finding out that I'd been intimate with men. I felt so relieved that I tended toward dating women; I couldn't bear the idea of adding yet another identity—another reason to discount my gender and me—to my plate.

These days, I share my history and authenticity with far more pride, yet still a touch of hesitance. I understand when people perceive me as "only" trans, I'm seen as a *straight* trans man. As a "regular" trans man. I am all too aware of the privilege and access this brings me—of how other men are more likely to engage with me and trust me if they perceive me to be straight. This is called *palatability*. As a straight man, I am palatable to them. I am worth their respect and their time. Suffice it to say that I should be all these things regardless of my queerness.

In all honesty, I'm not sure if I've learned how to accept all parts of my gender and sexuality. But then again, I'm not sure I ever will. I am fairly certain this will be an ever-evolving journey. An everlasting quest for radical acceptance in a world that wants me to be neither trans nor queer—or mixed-race or Asian, for that matter. And while there is exhaustion and pain in this, there is also great joy. I do not wish to rid myself of my intersections. I wish to hold them sacred.

⁂

RACE, DISABILITY, MENTAL health, and sexuality are far from comprehensive of the many identities that intersect with transness. And while combining each of these can drastically worsen the discrimination a trans person weathers in this world, they also create unique lenses through which we experience the world. The strongest interpersonal bonds I've formed have been with others who either understand or have firsthand experience with the dynamics that result from my intersections. I know the same is true for many other folks with complex identities.

The exercise of looking beyond one identity—be it transness or Blackness or Asianness or disability or queerness—is an exercise in peering into humanity. What else do we find when we consider ourselves to be more than a single label? What else do we find when we consider the diversity of experience within a single label? How can we use this to bolster and empower our own fight? How can we use it to bolster and empower our own radical joy?

CHAPTER 20

Internalized Transphobia and Its Antidote: Radical Trans Joy

I WAS ON A HIGH—I'D JUST FINISHED GIVING A SPEECH TO THE biggest audience I'd ever stood in front of. Over two thousand students had leaped to their feet to give me a standing ovation at the National Association of Independent Schools' Annual Conference. Though I'd already spent more than an hour onstage, I spent almost two hours with the lines of kids who'd gathered to take photos with me. One by one, they excitedly walked up the steps to stand next to me. Their joy in meeting me was overwhelming and touching. I never quite understood what it meant to have your cheeks hurt from laughter or smiling until then—by the thirtieth kid or so, my face muscles ached.

Toward the end of the line, a kid with colorful hair walked slowly to me. They were holding a journal covered in stickers, and wore a "they/them" pronouns pin on their shirt.

"I have a question," they said, nervously.

"Sure thing," I smiled.

"Does it ever get better—" They burst into tears before they could finish the word *better*. I opened my arms, wordlessly asking if they'd like a hug. I wanted to be gentle, but I also knew that if I spoke, I would sob, too.

Unfortunately, their question is not uncommon. Just before writing this book, I received an email that asked the same question: "And lastly, I would like to ask, does it ever get any easier?" wrote a ten-year-old trans boy from a small town in India.

Questions like these create a lump in my throat that I can't always speak through, and the kids and their fear of their own futures take a little piece of me with them.

It *does* get easier. It *does* get better. But it doesn't always get better because *other people* change. It gets better because *we* learn how to deal with it. It doesn't get easier because all parents learn to accept their trans kids or because society stops being transphobic. It gets better because *we* get stronger, *we* build community, *we* find the resources to support ourselves. It gets better because we learn how to be bigger than other people's hatred of us.

This journey is difficult—and sometimes we leave people behind. But ease comes as we realize we do not have to depend on other people's validation or approval. Instead, we find our own communities and spaces. Instead, we learn what trans joy feels like and we harness it.

It gets better—but not because other people accept us; it gets easier because *we* accept us.

But, you might be wondering, *how?* How do we accept ourselves when we live in a world with hundreds of legislative attacks criminalizing and/or banning our healthcare, our privacy, our sports, our ability to express our authenticity, and even use public bathrooms? How do trans people possibly maintain any semblance of our mental health when the world seems to want us gone?

"Reading the news is really hard," says a newer client who I've only seen for a few months. "I know there's logical arguments I can use to respond to the hate, and I've read through your website. We've talked about it before. But it doesn't seem to help—I still feel miserable. How do you stay so positive?"

"I don't," I say, truthfully. He looks surprised. "I'm not positive all the time—and allowing for my grief, pain, anger, sadness—you name it—allows me to make space for the good feelings, too. If I stuff those feelings down, they'll just fester inside and hurt me later."

He nods, mulling this over.

"I just feel like I have this unending well of pain. And anger. I'm so angry. Why do they hate us so much?" His words turn from rage into pain as he begins to cry. I let him, not saying anything.

"It makes me wonder if I *am* just messed up," he admits. "I know better, but I read what they say and . . . How do you stop yourself from believing it?" he asks, distraught.

How do you stop yourself from believing them? This is the crux of it all—and it took me a while to figure it out. I tell him a story about my time at Harvard that I've told only a few people before this book.

⁂

AFTER THE FIRST few months on the men's team, the misgendering had all but come to a halt. While I still didn't quite feel that I belonged, I was starting to glimpse comfort.

One December evening, I walked back from the pool with a guy in my class named Lionel (he/him). He'd been relatively friendly with me—I'd even requested to room with him during our annual training trip that was coming a few weeks later.

"So I guess if you do premed, you'll be the first trans doctor or whatever," he said to me, his voice flat and unamused. It didn't seem like a compliment.

"I guess?" I answered, unsure where he was going.

"I read an article about you. You said you were premed in it." Oh. He was probably referencing the piece I'd done for *The Harvard Crimson* a few weeks earlier. "You also said that you were going to pick people off one at a time?" *What?*

"Huh?" was all I could muster.

"You said you were going to try to beat people. One at a time. The point of this isn't winning and beating people, Schuyler. This is a team." His tone was undeniably condescending now.

I don't remember what I said in response. I was fuming in anger. I remembered what he was likely talking about. The reporter had asked me about how my mental race strategy had shifted from being a winning athlete in the women's category to being in the men's category now. I'd said that I was racing against myself—and hoping to get faster than the next fastest guy, and then go from there. *Nothing's wrong with that! That's how competitive sports work!* I wanted to scream at Lionel.

What did he know about transitioning and "the point of this"?

"You know, you're really not like us," he had continued. "You're always so serious. You need to talk about stupid shit—funny stuff, sports, and girls. When we're around you"—now he was speaking for all the freshmen on the swim team—"we're scared of you getting offended or getting yelled at, so we all feel awkward when you're around."

Yelled at? Talk about serious things? I barely ever say anything around them. I just sit and listen.

"We're all trying really hard. You know, to call you 'he,' and everything. It's just really hard. And yeah, yeah, I know it's hard for you, or whatever," he scoffed. "But don't worry about it. You need to get over it. It's not a big deal."

Unfortunately, by the time he'd finished speaking, we were only about halfway back. I don't remember what I'd said for the remainder of our time together—but I knew I'd have a hard time trusting him after that.

A few months later, the freshmen swimmers gathered in Joseph's (he/him) room to talk about the following year's rooming plans. At Harvard, freshmen create what are called "blocking groups" of up to eight individuals who are sorted into an upperclassman house as a unit. Two blocking groups can link to ensure they are sorted into houses in the same general area. Because every other class on the men's team had blocked together, I'd assumed I would block with my classmates, too. I was excited about the prospect. This was a way I'd continue to foster my belonging on the team.

When I arrived at the room, everyone else was already there.

"There's no space for you in the blocking groups," Lionel announced as soon as I'd sat down. Confused, I surveyed the room. None of the others would make eye contact with me, their heads bowed. I knew what the feeling in my stomach meant.

Someone mumbled about the groups being full because they'd invited some other guys, as well as some girls to block with them.

"Yeah, and we don't really feel like we know you very well," another guy chimed in.

"You've never tried to get to know me," I said, my tone cutting. One of them didn't conceal his shock at my response, his mouth agape.

"I understand what this is," I said, and got up to leave.

Smith (he/him) followed me out, tugging on my arm as I went.

"I'm sorry, Sky," he said, his voice pleading. "That sucked. Do you want to talk?" I didn't, but I nodded anyway.

Back in my room, I held in the tears. Smith confirmed that a majority of the guys were not comfortable with me being in their room or in their suite, or even their blocking group, because I am transgender.

"They think you'll mess up the dynamic or whatever," he explained. "They don't feel comfortable around you. I don't get it. Nothing's wrong with you."

"Thanks, Smith," I said, meaning it. He'd always been nice to me. On the first day we'd met, he'd told me that he'd struggled with depression, too, and that he thought I was brave for sharing about my mental health. He was one of the few guys who'd never misgendered me.

"Listen, I'll block with you if you want. It can just be the two of us," he offered. This felt so kind it almost broke my heart. I knew it wasn't something that would actually make him happy—he was close with many of those guys.

"You don't have to do that, man," I said. "I don't want to take you away from them. Can you tell me what they said about me though?" My curiosity was getting the best of me.

"Some of them think you'll scare their girlfriends away because you're trans. Some of them—yeah, Lionel—straight up doesn't want to live near you because you're trans." He got quieter as he spoke. I'm sure he could see the pain in my face, even though I wasn't crying yet.

"What did Lionel say?" I ventured.

"Aw, Sky, I don't wanna say it," he resisted. "It's fucked-up."

"Please? I really want to know." I did. I wanted to be informed. I'd rather know than wonder.

"Okay. Well. Um," Smith hesitated, looking at me and then settling his gaze on the wooden floor, old and beaten down by years of students living there. He cleared his throat.

"Lionel just doesn't like you, yeah, because you're trans. He thinks you're annoying, and he doesn't believe that you deserve to be a part of the team. He doesn't think you earned your spot here."

That night, I cried harder than I had ever cried before. After Smith left, I'd written out a list of things that I felt, among them: *worthless, not good enough, weird, not part of the team, unliked, strange, freak, an "other,"* and *bad. OUTCAST,* I wrote in big bold letters.

I toggled between feeling tiny and wanting to scream at them—most specifically Lionel. I wondered how I'd show up to practice the next morning, much less make it all four years on the team. *What if I'm a loner forever,* I wrote in my journal. *What if I don't make friends here and I never have a social group. Ugh, I don't want to be seen as weird and queer anymore! I wish I was "normal."*

I felt nauseous as the last line sank into my chest. I'd worked so hard to be proud of myself and my identity and here I was, hoping I could be different. Hoping that the thing I would learn to love most about myself was gone, erased.

Feeling the internalization beginning to take hold, I grabbed the stack of blank paper I kept in my desk drawer. I taped them one by one to the wall next to my bed, creating a poster I could write on. Then, tears still streaming down my face, I began to write:

Their words do not define me.
Their words do not define me.
Their words do not define me.
Their words do not define me.
Their words do not define me.
Their words do not define me.
Their words do not define me.

Over, and over again, until the tears finally stopped.

THOUGH I DIDN'T know it then, this was the beginning of an extremely important practice of active self-validation and self-affirmation that has been lifesaving for me over the years—one that I've honed and taught my clients and support group attendees, as well.

Even though my experience on the men's team improved dramatically after that first year, I have continued to interface with transphobia, and I imagine, as a very openly trans person, that I always will. I receive bigoted, hateful comments every day on social media, the worst of which usually contain some kind of wish for my death—either that I be murdered violently or that I kill myself. "They should bring back the gas chambers for your kind," one commenter wrote a few years ago.

I share these not to create space for the hatred, but rather to illustrate the sheer vile nature of what most trans people must weather.

But somehow, I have still found immense joy, fulfillment, and peace. Somehow, I still stand strong and proud of who I am—most of the time.

So without further ado, here is how.

A FRAMEWORK

Validate My Pain

Before I do any kind of reframing, I spend time with my feelings.

Hold space for the ugliest of feelings. If you need, validate yourself aloud, as you would a friend:

Of course it hurts deeply to be told that I am not man enough—that I am too weird, strange, or other to be included in my teammates' blocking group.

Of course I feel upset and am tripping over future worries of what this will mean.

Of course being excluded feels horrible.

Put Space Between My Truth and Theirs

While other people's words can hurt, they are not always facts. Those boys' opinions of me were not facts and did not have to impact my truth.

If someone attempts to invalidate who I am, it doesn't mean I am invalid. It means a lot about them—their character, their insecurities and fears, their views of the world. It does not mean anything about who I am.

Again, we can validate our own anger and pain. But do not use their words as weapons against yourself.

Decide If I Want to Engage

In the case of Lionel and the other guys, I chose to disengage. I encouraged Smith to block with them, and I found other friends who welcomed me into their group and would provide important support for me throughout college.

Lionel never told me to my face that he didn't believe I belonged there. And while I fantasized about confronting him, I didn't. I realized I was not there to prove to him I was man enough or that I belonged on that team—I wasn't there to prove anything to him. *Why am I here?* I repeatedly asked myself in an effort to re-center. *I'm here to swim.* And so I did.

Coincidentally, Lionel and I specialized in the same stroke. The first year, he beat me in both the 100 and the 200. The second year, I beat him in the 100. And the final two years, I beat him in both. This was my quiet way of reminding myself—and him—I belonged there. And while the victory was sweet, I would have succeeded whether or not I'd swum faster than he did because I would have done what *I* had come to do.

In the face of transphobia or any other bigotry perpetrated against your own identities, you get to decide if you'd like to engage. Give yourself permission to disengage, to not confront, to let them go. Not every battle is yours to fight. Not every battle is worth the win.

I try to choose engaging only when the following criteria are *all* satisfied:

DEPTS:

• Desire: I want to.
• Energy: I have the energy. (Another way to verify this one is to ask: Will engaging be harmful to me?)

- Productivity: I think it is productive—for the recipient *and* for me.
- Time: I have the time.
- Safety: It is physically safe to do so.

Affirm Myself

When the outside voices are too loud or too prevalent as they often are in the world we live in, we have to reinforce our own voices and our own truths. Doing so takes active affirmation. I know, I used to think it was stupid, too. *What, I'm going to write down, "I'm man enough," and one day I'll believe it?* Well actually, yeah.

I encourage writing down affirmations on days you feel good—sometimes it's easier to imagine them when the meaner voices are quieter. Then, keep the list around for tougher times.

Here are a few to get you started:

- I know who I am even if my teammates/coworkers invalidate me.
- I know who I am even if my parents invalidate me.
- I know who I am even if my supervisors/managers invalidate me.
- I am enough, regardless of others' views of me.
- I am allowed to know and am capable of knowing who I am, no matter my age.
- My sexuality is valid. My gender identity is valid.
- I am worthy of love even if my parents/family/peers do not show me this.
- I belong in this world.
- I belong on this team.
- I belong in this role.
- I am resilient. I will get through this.
- I am allowed to grieve.
- Disappointing others does not mean I am a disappointment.
- I am doing enough.
- Their words do not define me.

SPEEDOS AND SCARS

When I was first recovering from top surgery, I posted shirtless photos with pride nearly every day. And nearly every time, I received comments with recommendations about how I could make the scars less red. My scar grew thicker with time—and deeper in color. Now my scar is about three-quarters of an inch in width, and a soft purple-red, depending on how cold I am. Other people, trans and not, assumed that I would want to change this.

"Use vitamin E oil," dozens have recommended. Use this product, use that one.

I ignored it all. I am so proud of my scar. It is my history—my story—written in bold across my chest. I fought hard to get this, and I am not planning on hiding it.

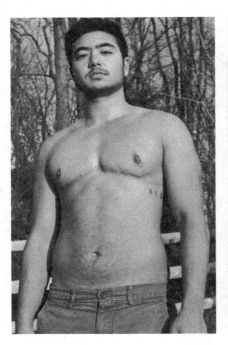 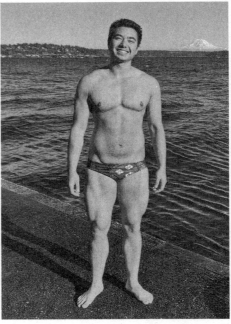

The first time I wore the tiny little triangular swim brief that most people call a "Speedo," I was terrified. I had stood in front of the mirror in my dorm room for hours trying to will myself into thinking it looked good enough. It never quite did and I decided I'd have to do it anyway. So that day, I walked on deck feeling more naked than usual. And I did it. And I never stopped.

Despite the fact that I stopped competing years ago, I still wear my speedo every chance I get—whether or not I'm practicing in the pool or just hanging out at the beach. If I'm honest, the anxiety hasn't fully dissipated and I don't think it ever will. And that's okay. I tug the suit on anyway, sporting not only my beautiful scar, but also my bulgeless briefs.

I feel I am so obviously and openly trans—and there is still a piece of me that feels I should hide this. When I walk, nearly naked, through the men's locker room or on the pool deck or beach, I still worry what some people might think.

"You do?" one of my trans friends asked me when I shared this with him. He was incredulous. "I thought you were able to do it because you just don't care! I thought that you didn't even think about it!"

I was so surprised at his surprise. *Of course I do, look at the world we live in.*

"I am absolutely nervous," I assured him. "I just do it anyway."

And this has remained my motto. I refuse to let someone else's disdain or dislike of my transness stop me from doing something I love so much—in this case, swimming. Over the years, this override has become a practice with which I have learned to find both peace and ease. But neither peace nor ease erase fear and anxiety, and I've found that that is okay.

"I know it sounds kind of weird, but I tell fear and anxiety to come with me," I confessed to my friend. "'Come along for the ride,' I'll say to them. You can't drive the car, but hang out in the back seat. I hear you, I see you, and I'll be okay anyway."

This is how I remind myself that my body is not wrong.

This is how I remind myself that I am no less a man.

This is how I remind myself that their words do not define me.

I do.

PART 4

GENDER AND YOU

CHAPTER 21

Allyship

Y ou're such a fag," the textbook bully on my high school team would jeer at any guy who bothered him. Sometimes, for no reason at all, he would use a stereotypical "Asian" accent with random phrases like "Give me eggroll" or "You want fried rice?" Most of the guys would laugh when he did, some even mimicking his actions.

As a closeted queer kid who is also Asian American, I felt extremely uncomfortable with his remarks—and perhaps, more importantly, the lack of concern from everyone else. *Why was no one saying anything? Why were they all laughing? Why didn't the coach do anything?*

At first, this guy was surprisingly nice to me. I'm not sure why—I assume it was because he perceived me as attractive. (I was presenting as a woman at the time.) But his demeanor quickly changed as I failed to engage with his racist and homophobic behavior. Anytime he'd say anything to me in his mocking "Asian" accent, I would stare back, my face either blank or disappointed.

"Why are you talking like that?" I eventually asked him. Stunned and with nothing to say in response, he just turned around and continued with someone else. I felt alone, especially given that I was new to the team. But I had no tolerance for how he spoke to me or to others. I thought of my grandparents' Korean accents and how my friends sometimes struggled to understand their English. Anger rushed through my veins.

Each time he tried to engage me, he met no welcome.

"Stop talking like that, it's racist," I'd say firmly.

"It's really not funny," I'd reply, my mouth a flat line.

To my satisfaction, the more I resisted him, the more others began to as well. At first, it was among the girls in the girls' locker room.

"He's always been like this, he's so annoying," they'd complain.

"Yeah, he's such a dick."

Quickly, they, too, began to call out his slurs and racism. Within a few months, practically no one was reacting to his "jokes," including the guys.

At this point, he began to target me in particular.

"Oh, you think you're so fast, Schuyler?" he spat at me after we had raced the 200 breaststroke one day. Though at the time I was competing against girls, my coach frequently made the fastest girls race against the boys at practice.

"Well, how come I just beat you by so much, huh?" he taunted. "Nationals cut whatever..." And he turned away.

I was fifteen years old then and someone he saw as a girl. He was eighteen or nineteen and the biggest guy on the team. His pride in his faster speed was ridiculous.

I gave him no response. Surprisingly, a teammate stood up for me, telling him to leave me alone. He ignored her and dove into the pool. About a month later, he left the team.

⬡ ⬡ ⬡

I BEGIN THIS chapter with this memory because it exemplifies the power of standing up. It is not always easy to do so, but if you can, many others will likely join you.

Look at you all here, reading along with me. You have chosen to join me, and I am so grateful.

I firmly believe that allyship is *active* work—it can be tiring, trying, and painful. But your allyship has already begun by reading this book.

And the most impactful allyship will come when you take what you've learned here and translate that into actions in your daily life.

This chapter will further equip you with tangible skills and practices to help you create a framework for your allyship. My hopeful intention is this scaffolding might help this work be less daunting and more effective.

WHAT IS ALLYSHIP?

The word *allyship* entails advocating for, supporting, and/or engaging with work that contributes to the liberation of a marginalized group whose identity you do not share. For example, a cisgender person who fights for trans rights, or a white person who bolsters equity for Black, Indigenous, and other people of color (BIPOC), or a man who fights for women's rights.

Over the years, the social justice movement has adopted other terms, such as *accomplice*, to explain allyship that includes the fight to dismantle systemic oppression. By any term, allyship is not truly allyship if it does not get at the root cause of oppression, if it is not active, loud, and in collaboration with the marginalized people for which it exists. So, for this reason and for simplicity, I will continue using *allyship* to describe these actions.

Allyship develops in two primary arenas that feed into and overlap with each other.

First, internal—where we observe, question, and then shift ourselves to align with allyship.

Second, external—integrating what we've learned into our interactions and creating tangible societal change.

INTERNAL

Beneath our actions lie our belief systems that drive our actions—conscious or not. And while we could simply try to change our actions, it is far more effective to begin with examining the reasons underlying them first.

A famous quote (falsely attributed to Morgan Freeman [he/him]) says, "I hate the word *homophobia*. It's not a phobia. You are not scared. You are an asshole."

While there are certainly assholes out there, and many people—both bigoted and not—do act like assholes, I believe that the *reason* they are assholes *is* because they are afraid. Fear is at the root of transphobia and queerphobia: our queer or transness stirs in them something they are not ready or do not know how to confront. And that is, absolutely, terrifying.

So, people *are* afraid. But what we miss is that they're not afraid of *us*; they're afraid of what we elicit in *them*. They are afraid of the freedom and the realm of possibility our existences suggest, or … demand.

"The moral panic people experience is about themselves: if *you* can choose this … did *I* choose?" Dr. McLean explains what might be running through the minds of cis people.[1] Of course, trans people do not *choose* to be trans. Still, I have witnessed comments like this often, usually in the flavor of *Well if you can just choose to be a man, then what does that mean manhood is? It makes manhood meaningless!*

We see this same argument frequently when discussing marriage equality. "Gay marriage ruins the sanctity of my marriage," straight people have often said. In reality, no one else's marriage can ruin the sanctity of your marriage. Only you can do that.

In the same vein, proclamation of my manhood does not render manhood itself meaningless, nor does it revoke any manhood from another man. But I understand why it feels like it could: *if manhood is not awarded at birth through a penis or other biological, concrete factors, then what is it?*

And this is where the fear sets in.

"It undoes a lot. People watch the world they thought they knew so well fall apart around them," Dr. McLean reflected.[2]

True and grounded allyship must then begin with awareness, wherein we can observe ourselves and our beliefs. Through this, we can recognize that transphobia is not truly about trans people, but rather our own internal bias, fear, and imagined limitations.

"I think that transness is a commitment to the future," says Dr. shawndeez. "And it's a very radical commitment—what becomes possible when we not only entertain this type of life, but are open to new forms of existence and expression?" This is why the first and most important step in allyship is observation of ourselves.

IN OCTOBER 2021, I was honored with the Matthew Shepard Foundation's Spirit of Matthew Award. My dad flew across the country to meet me in Denver, where the black-tie gala took place. Hundreds of people were there, and I was nervous—for my acceptance speech, but more importantly because the pandemic still raged and I was deeply uninterested in catching the virus.

During the cocktail hour prior to the dinner, my dad and I socialized with other attendees. Far more gregarious and experienced at networking than I was, my dad jumped right into the fray. I've always envied his ease in these settings—he seems able to talk to anyone. But as I've grown older and more aware of how my own identities impact how I am received, I've noticed that people's reception of my dad can be a result of his identities, too. As a tall, successful, generally good-looking white man, people defer to him automatically. Space is always made for him. People always listen to him.

As we stood at one of those tiny standing tables people gather around at these fancy events, I grew frustrated with my dad. He frequently interrupted the people we were talking with, his hand motions were not mindful of the space his own body took up as he nearly whacked the man in front of him, and he was standing far too close to his listener, who was wearing a mask—clearly still nervous about COVID exposure like I was.

I tried unsuccessfully to subtly tell him to take a step back. After a few attempts, he stepped aside, annoyed. I followed him outside to chat—or argue, more accurately.

"What are you doing?" he asked, annoyed. "What's the problem?"

"You're standing too close to people and you're going to whack someone with your hands," I said, trying to be calm but failing.

"You always want people to act a certain way, Schuyler! You can't control how everyone acts. You can't have everyone be a robot. I'm not a fucking robot!" he spat. He was furious now, his voice coming out in something that was somehow both whispering and yelling.

In many ways, my dad is the person I've felt most understood by in this world. He's always been my biggest cheerleader and fiercest supporter—but then, in moments like these, he's somehow unable to digest that his privilege could hurt me, or others. He is so blinded by his privilege that understanding feels like it disappears. Witnessing this disconnect is so jarring that I am rarely able to hold in my temper or pain. I usually feel like exploding—and so, outside that gala in 2021, I did.

"You are not queer or trans or a person of color!" I did not whisper-yell. I yell-yelled. "You need to be more mindful!" Though we were alone at that moment, my voice echoed against the concrete pillars, reminding me to quiet.

"We are surrounded by queer and trans people," I adjusted my volume. "You are acting as if you are allowed to take up all the space in the world—physically and verbally. This is not only upsetting to me, it's also embarrassing. This is my life *and* my work. So much of what I teach people is how to understand their privilege! How can my own father not understand his? I, and lots of marginalized people like me—including your wife, who is a Korean woman—have spent our lives being talked down to by white cis men." His expression shifted, his anger falling. He looked like he was about to speak but I wasn't finished.

"I've been made to feel small and worthless because men like you speak over me or don't think my contributions matter. I have felt unimportant because men like you don't consider how their actions impact others and take up space because they think they are entitled to it. Don't be one of these men."

I was short of breath. I wiped the tears from my eyes, fearful their remnants would show on my face during my speech, which was fast approaching. I hoped no one was watching us out here. *The famous transgender educator and advocate who couldn't even have a calm conversation with his own dad.* I was embarrassed by my outburst, even though I knew my emotions were valid.

"Oh," he mumbled. "I didn't understand . . . I didn't understand this was about privilege."

When I began writing this section of this book, I informed my dad that I'd include this story. Though I did not feel the need to ask for his approval or permission, I asked him what he thought. He sent this reply:

For me, our discussions about taking up space have been most impact-ful. Whether that be in conversations, mixed social settings, Zoom calls, parenting roles, subways, and even my posture... The attitude of a white cis man is unannounced, unfettered; it is expected and nur-tured by everyone around them. Cis white men are deferred to, granted preference, spoken to, offered the bill, and, intentionally or not, we step into this as expected most of the time. We take that space from those who should have just as much—or more—right to it. Even in situations where it is clear we should not have preference or prior-ity, the system perpetuates this deferential behavior toward us. It takes conscious and deliberate action to step down and step back and take less space. Most cishet white men reading might gloss over a section that speaks to this—and even this is a behavior we learn as part of our "right." Criticisms of our privilege are sloughed off (per the training of the system) as misplaced or misunderstood. And this allows us to keep going, blinded and perpetuating harm.

As I read his response, tears welled in my eyes. I've yelled louder and with more fury at my father than any other living being on this earth. And while I am not proud of this, it comes from the knowing that I can-not lose him. And that I know he *can* understand. We've had our fair share of arguments and screaming fits and both my wife and my mother always ask me why I keep going. Why don't I just hang up the phone—or leave the room?

"Because I want him to understand. And I know he can."

Although I strongly discourage the yelling, I encourage the invita-tion to observe oneself. My father's misunderstanding of my criticisms is not one-sided—I have many-a-time failed at communicating the core of my discomfort, focusing on what he did instead of how it made me feel. I've learned that telling him more about how his actions impact me breeds a more productive conversation and therefore is a more effec-tive tactic.

But as he insightfully noted in his reflection, observing oneself with honesty requires relinquishing the gender-given birthright to be put first, to be listened to, to be deferred to. It requires observing where those assumptions first took place, why they're there, and what we can do to dismantle them so that others have a bit more space. And, yes, this *does* mean that the white cis man will then have *less* space.

I have repeatedly been asked why these attacks on trans people are culminating *now*—why are there so many anti-trans bills, why is there so much anti-trans rhetoric, why are trans people seen as a threat?

These attacks are here because trans people *are* a threat—but not in the way the current accusations portray. Trans people are not a threat to children, women, or sports. No, trans people are a threat because our very identities disrupt the most basic conventions of Western society: cis white patriarchal power—the system of oppression that has built and controlled this country since its conception. Trans people are a threat because we know ourselves even when those in power say it is impossible for us to exist. Somehow, we exist.

Transness is incredibly powerful—and terrifying to those *in* power. Our truth demands the world to ask themselves what is possible when cis white straight men do not make all the rules and control all other bodies. Because these attacks are not truly "just about fairness," or "just about protecting women," or just about bathrooms, healthcare, or even just about trans people...

No, this is about concentrating power back in the hands of the cis white men who are so afraid of losing it in the first place. The oppressive system they built all those centuries ago has begun eroding as the oppressed have finally been able to stand up for ourselves.

The system that has disenfranchised anyone who is not a cis white straight man *is* threatened. The system views diversity as weakening its stronghold—because it does. In an effort not to crumble, they are scrambling to shore up their power through age-old methods. If we remove the right to vote, Black people cannot organize and will remain disenfranchised. If we ban abortion, poor people, especially BIPOC women, will remain impoverished.[3-7] If we ban LGBTQ+ content in schools, people will struggle to learn about their identities, amassing mental illness instead of celebrating who they are. If we do not focus media on the missing and murdered Indigenous women and children, they will not carry on knowing their culture and history, eventually eliminating them as a threat to the system. The list is endless.

But what those in power fail to realize is that they can never take our knowing away from us. No number of legislative bans will ever stop me from knowing I am transgender. No bans from sports or bathrooms, no removal of my medical care, no attempts to reduce me to a statistic will ever stop me from knowing who I am. And I think this is our innate power that we are just discovering—and that they can never take from us.

This is true for you, too, reader. Nothing can take your identities away from you. Trans people do not exist to steal a cis person's man- or womanhood. You are still you. When we can understand and accept that, we can move forward.

OBSERVE, QUESTION, SHIFT

"Hi!" she said quickly, eager to ask her question. "I am a cisgender ally and I call my trans friends the right pronouns, but if I'm honest with myself, sometimes I'm just calling them the right pronouns but I'm not actually seeing them as themselves—as their real gender. I know this is bad, so how do I start to see people for who they really are instead of how they 'look' to me? Do you have any recommendations for helping undo the gender binary?"

"Oof," I'd begun. "That's a great question. My short answer is a framework: Observe, Question, Shift."

THE FRAMEWORK
Observe

Develop an awareness of our biases and how they function in our lives—most specifically, how they impact our actions.

Here are some questions to ask yourself as you *observe*:

- What gendered biases do I hold? (This is a way to begin to bring consciousness to these biases.)

- What feelings do I have in response to reading this book? Do I feel resistance or anger? What comes up for me?
- How do I gender people? (Or, start by simply noticing that you do gender everyone you meet reflexively.)
- What causes me to gender people one way or another? (Notice what factors contribute to your ultimate conclusion of what someone's gender is.)
- What do I assume about people based on their gender?
- What actions do I partake in that are gendered? Which feel good? Which don't?
- When and how do I notice my own gender?
- What space do I feel entitled to?

These questions should be asked with curiosity, not judgment. The goal is not to punish yourself for your biases, beliefs, or practices. You are only trying to bring awareness to where you are starting from: this is you recording your baseline.

Question

Unpack the observations you've collected to create more space.

Here are some things to ask yourself as you *question*:

- Why did I gender that person that way? Why did I assume what their gender was based on those factors?
- Why did I assume XYZ about that person based on their gender?
- Why do I do XYZ gendered action? (E.g., sit in this way, talk in this way, relate to other people in this way, restrict/control your emotions in this way, etc.)
- Why do I feel XYZ about trans people?
- Why do I feel entitled to the space I feel entitled to?

Shift

Here, we work to undo the actions that stem from the harmful biases we've now learned to notice, and instead do actions that align with our goals of equity, allyship, and inclusion. Translating the internal work of observation and questioning demands willingness to relinquish pieces of how we understand the world—and to invite the curiosity we've cultivated to get to this point.

Remember, this is not a game of shaming yourself or your thoughts. The goal is to invite all of you in, along with your biases, so that you might examine yourself holistically and act in defiance of the bias. Change does not require the absence of bias altogether—it demands radical action in spite of it.

Here are some questions to ask yourself as you *shift*:

- Can I interrupt this process of automatic gendering? What would it look like to entertain the notion that the person I've automatically gendered is *not* the gender I imagined?
- Can I introduce new information and facts that I've been presented and integrate this information?
- What can I glean from someone's presentation other than gender?
- What is important to me about someone I've just met other than gendered assumptions? (E.g., name three things you notice about someone other than their gender.)
- How would I act if I did not gender them in this way? How would I like myself to act?
- What space *should* I be entitled to? Where and how can I make more space for others who do not have the space I do?

BRIDGING FROM INTERNAL TO EXTERNAL

At this point, you've begun to build your allyship from the inside, a wonderful internal endeavor. Next, we'll extend this journey beyond ourselves to cultivate impactful *external* allyship. But, before we do so, let's take a pause to consider a crucial detail.

This book is filled with intimate and private disclosures that not only were difficult for me to write but also took careful consideration for me to share with you. I have provided answers to otherwise inappropriate questions as well as invited you into deeply private parts of my life, all in hopes of allowing you to truly witness me, a small window into transness.

But not every trans person will do this. And they should not have to.

When I am educating, I work diligently not to communicate in anger or frustration because I have found that it does not invite the audience to learn. The decision to assume this disposition is a choice—*my* choice—facilitated by access to a host of privileges that have allowed me the mental space to hold the pain and discomfort, the informational tools to defend myself with science, and the support to grow my own confidence in the face of confrontation.

At the end of nearly every speech, someone approaches me with a variation of this:

"I really enjoyed your presentation. You're so calm and kind. I've seen other people doing this and they yell and get angry . . . and you didn't make it an issue, you just explained it all factually. I love how you invited us to ask all the questions we wanted and how you answered them so graciously. It really helped me learn."

You might have read that and nodded your head in agreement. *What's the problem with that?*

In short—this is not a compliment. It, too, is a microaggression.

"You are so calm while others are not" actually says: "I only respect and value pain when it is presented to me in a way I accept." It demands: "Do not show me the pain that this system—of which I am a part and likely perpetuate—has caused you. Pretend it doesn't exist so that I am more comfortable in your presence."

"I love how you invited us to ask all the questions" also says: "I am glad you do not have any boundaries I have to respect!"

This is called *tone policing*. Tone policing demands that ideas are communicated in a particular way that is palatable to the receiver—usually calm, kind, patient. Tone policing dismisses communication delivered in an angry, frustrated, or otherwise negative manner.[8,9]

I do not deny that using a different tone can be productive. I know few who enjoy being yelled at or spoken to in fury. Yes, most of us learn better when we feel safe and welcomed—and that is why I try my best to regulate my emotions when I am educating. But again, this is *my choice*.

The crucial distinction is validity versus productivity. When someone asks me an inappropriate question, it is absolutely *valid* for me to get upset and answer angrily; it is not always productive. However, even in this dichotomy, it is important to ask: Productive for whom? I see three viable options: productive for the inappropriate question-asker; productive for me, the disrespected trans person; or productive for the greater society / others / purpose of learning. Because I want to educate, I often choose to prioritize the benefit to the question-asker and greater society, instead of myself.

My choices, of course, are not everyone's. It is not every trans person's job to educate you on transness because they are trans. But it *is* my job—in speeches, when consulting, and here in this book. In scenarios wherein I choose to maintain a calm disposition, I have not only *chosen* to do so, I've also likely been *paid* to do so. Recognize that this is likely not the case for other trans folks in your life.

So, know this: If you ask an inappropriate, disrespectful, or uncomfortable question, a trans person's angry response is valid. Do not expect them to offer their pain to you on a silver platter. Your question might have seemed harmless to you, but that trans person might have been asked it more times than they've been gendered correctly. So yes, you need to accept the impact and consequences of your actions that align with systemic oppression and take responsibility for your part in perpetuating it, regardless of intention.

From here we can dive into interacting with others—we've contextualized where you're coming from, and how trans people might be receiving you. Now it's time for you to act.

EXTERNAL: HOW TO BE AN ALLY, INDIVIDUAL TO INDIVIDUAL

Interpersonal interactions are arguably the most widely accessible arena in which we can make societal change because nearly everyone has someone they can talk to and engage with about these issues. Here is your toolbox:

Correct Other People When They Misgender/Deadname Trans People

Calling us by the right name and pronouns is one of the simplest and yet most impactful ways to say, "I see you." This respect should continue into correcting others when appropriate. If someone is misgendered or called the wrong name by others, correct them, even if the person being mis-gendered isn't in the room or you don't know them personally.

As you go about this, please be careful not to out folks. They might use different pronouns in different scenarios. Before you correct any mis-gendering, make sure you're aware of where they use which pronouns because they might not be out in all places.

Do Not Rely on Trans People to Educate You

Again, it is not every trans person's responsibility to educate you on trans-ness. That is your responsibility.

I'm supposed to learn directly from trans people, but I'm not supposed to ask them to educate me? What?!

Yes! Do not ask random trans people to educate you. Ask the trans folks who have already consented to do so, access the resources (like this book) we have already created for you, ask those who do this for a living, and do not forget to compensate us for the labor.

Use Your Privilege to Educate Others

Have conversations with transphobic people. The most important shifts occur when you take what you've learned and go *beyond* your echo cham-bers. Trans people do not have endless energy to educate, and we are in desperate need for our cisgender allies to step in and help.

Use your privilege, whatever that may be, to reach people who would never be here—those who would never buy this book, or go to an inclusion training, or ever want to listen to a trans person at all. Talk to your trans-phobic uncles, aunts, boyfriends, girlfriends, team members, and work-mates. Share what you learn, invite them in, and engage with compassion.

Here are some helpful tools for engagement:

Try to Add Perspective Instead of Aiming to Change It

No one likes entering a conversation in which the other person's sole goal is to convince you that you are wrong because they are right. If your goal is to convince the other person they are wrong, you might be done before you begin. I have learned that shifting my own perspective in these conversations is useful. When someone tells me that trans athletes should not participate in sports, I enter the conversation not to convince them we should, but rather to share more context that might lead them to consider that they have come to a conclusion with incomplete information. Rather than, *I was wrong*, I hope they think, *Oh, I hadn't considered that additional detail—doing so widens my perspective and might change my conclusion.*

When All Else Fails, Ask Them with Genuine Curiosity, "Why Do You Care About This?"

If you are repeatedly running into the same wall with someone, pause and ask them this question.

Several years ago, I was at a public school in Seattle. After my presentation, a middle school student came up to talk to me. He identified himself and then told me that he was very upset by my suggestion to introduce ourselves with our pronouns.

"That's so dumb, nobody does that anywhere!" he said angrily.

"Well," I said gently, "it sounds like you haven't seen it that often, but I actually travel around quite a bit and I know lots of people who do! Whole companies, even!"

He continued to argue with me and after a few more similar retorts from him, I decided to switch directions.

"Hmm. Okay, it sounds like you care a lot about this, Jack. It sounds like pronouns and gender matter a lot to you! I'm curious why? Why does this matter to you?" I asked with genuine curiosity.

"Well," he said, confused by the shift. He thought about it.

"Well, I just... My parents and I are Christians, and my parents, they're very Christian, and it's very important to me." He told me this with pride. "I'm a Christian, too, and I talk about this a lot with my parents! And the Bible says 'no' to trans people!"

At the core of his rejection of pronoun usage was his fear that accepting me and trans people and our pronouns would fuel a disconnection with his parents—a very real and terrifying concept. I empathized with him. In the end, we had a very different conversation about his connection to his parents through religion. I can't report that I changed his views on trans people, but I sure confirmed a truth that is prevalent: rejection of transness is rarely about transness itself but rather something it stirs or threatens in others. Understanding this can help us to reorient the conversation and address the true root of a resistance to trans people.

Understand the Difference Between Validity and Productivity

As we discussed in Chapter 10, angry or otherwise intensely emotional reactions are valid responses in the face of difficult statements from others. However, answering with that anger might not be the most productive method of conversing with another person.

If you can, and especially if you're an ally, regulate your emotions to communicate calmly so your listener might learn. If you feel frustrated, instead of yelling or screaming or demeaning, try naming your feelings: "This is a tough conversation—you might hear frustration in my voice because what you've said is difficult for me to hear. But I really want to talk through it together," or, "I hear what you're saying, and I understand your feelings. I'm a bit upset by what you've shared but I'd love to keep trying to understand each other if you're open to it."

A friend has said, "I try to engage in conversations with others in a way that will make it most likely for them to want to continue engaging with me." This is spot-on. But in practice, this can be very difficult to achieve. Sometimes it is impossible—and in that event, it may be worthwhile to take a step back instead of potentially creating a fissure that might be hard to reconcile later.

Call In, Instead of Call Out

One of my personal guiding principles is *conversation over confrontation*. I try to call the other person *in* to the conversation instead of calling them out. Calling in entails refraining from character-centered feedback ("you *are* horrible") and emphasizing action-centered feedback ("you *did* something horrible"). Calling in is often more private and aims to give the other an opportunity to learn and shift, while calling out is more public and aims to chastise or shame.

Speak from your experienced truths using I-statements instead of making assertions based on assumptions about the other person, their motives, or their background that could potentially be incorrect. Calling out usually includes attacking jargon, attitudes, and tones—all of which can be fueled by valid emotions, but usually only encourage the other person to engage their defenses, not their minds or hearts.

Understand that doing this requires privileges—sometimes of not being transgender, thereby distancing you from the pain itself; sometimes of emotional groundedness, of the ability to articulate yourself and your ideas; of energy to engage; of the ability to suppress and manage certain emotions as you discuss.

Remember this is a practice you are working to develop. Keep trying.

Know When to Disengage

Sadly, some people embrace transphobia and will not listen to reason, logic, facts, or experts. Most of the time, engagement with these individuals is a waste of time. Committing to allyship does not mean working tirelessly and at your own expense with every person, all the time. Be mindful of your environment, and exit, especially if anything threatens your safety or well-being.

"There will always be people who don't get it," Kevin Tyrrell (he/him), my Harvard swim coach, told me. "Don't spend your energy on them." Though simple, this proved to be one of the most useful pieces of advice he ever gave me.

Let's say I have one hundred units of energy. I could spend all one hundred units on one person who is never going to budge—who doesn't care what I have to say, who doesn't listen, and who doesn't want to listen. Or I could distribute the one hundred units among one hundred people who are willing to listen and learn, and actually create change. Be economical with your energy when you can.

Accept Rejection

Along your journey, I'm sure you will ask someone a question they do not want to answer. Perhaps a result of that person's available energy, or inappropriate content in your question—whatever the reason, accept their rejection. You may even apologize if you notice you've overstepped or offended.

I strongly discourage you from defending your asking a potentially inappropriate question with, "I'm just curious." As I've repeated in this book, curiosity does not necessitate an answer, nor does it excuse an inappropriate question or entitle a person to an answer. If you're truly "just curious," then be curious! Don't demand an answer.

Resisting a trans person's rejection of your question places the burden of education on them, which is inappropriate and unkind. If someone invites you to ask questions, do so respectfully, but if their consent changes, receive that information and adjust your actions accordingly.

Set Boundaries

If you are attempting to converse with someone who is exhibiting hatefulness or bigoted behavior and is clearly not listening, failing to indicate any intent to learn, or causing you to worry about your safety, set boundaries. Boundaries can be physical (leaving the room), they can be technological (blocking, deleting, unfriending), and they can be contextual (refusing to discuss certain topics).

Integrate Feedback Without Defensiveness

You are bound to make mistakes and others are bound to have something to say about that. Regardless of how calmly they respond to you, do your best to hear the feedback itself. This is something I've practiced as someone who interacts with an enormous amount of feedback online. You might wonder why I don't call it "criticism" or "attacks." I call it *feedback* with intention: this is an effort not to judge or to police how others share how they feel with me.

Feedback can tell me lots of different things. A message like "You're such a fag, I hope u die" (a real message I've received, unfortunately numerous times) gives me the feedback that my content is reaching people who likely do not follow me and are not very supportive of my community. Another that reads, "Stupid tranny, this is anti-Black as fuck" (also a real comment—from when I posted about Lil Nas X), gives me the feedback that what I posted hurt someone and perpetuated anti-Blackness.

My point is: Sometimes people will say mean things when they are upset or angry, and I try my best to let these go so that I may hear the important feedback in their statements. I try my best to delete all the noise—the phrases, words, slurs, or statements that one might consider hateful or attacking—that cloud the central message. I ask myself, *What is the core of what they are trying to communicate with me?* and then I try to address that.

By not internalizing these comments intended as attacks, I've been able to reduce the amount of tone policing I perpetuate against others and integrate meaningful feedback so that I may better myself and my actions. I encourage you to use a similar method to reduce the likelihood you will tone police trans people when you've offended, hurt, or upset them, and thus improve your allyship.

I've also honed another method that helps me disengage ego as I've received feedback: the separation of self and work—of what you do, and who you are. If we integrate feedback we receive onto the sphere of work, instead of self, we are far more likely to improve action and maintain our mental well-being.

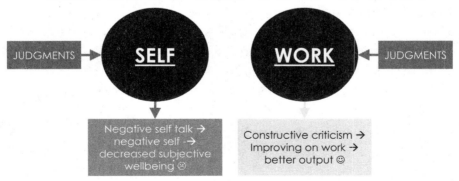

SEPARATE SELF AND WORK

JUDGMENTS → **SELF**   **WORK** ← JUDGMENTS

Negative self talk → negative self → decreased subjective wellbeing ☹

Constructive criticism → Improving on work → better output ☺

MOVING BEYOND INTERPERSONAL SUPPORT AND SHOWING
ALLYSHIP IN A GROUP

In the summer of 2022, I spent a few days with a dozen trans kid athletes from around the country. The youngest was seven, the oldest was eighteen. Most were nine to twelve years old. The event was titled Let Kids Play, and it lived up to its name—at least for the three days it lasted. The kids spent most of that time playing with each other, and I listened to the glorious noise of children screaming with delight as they ran around together.

But most of those kids went home to states like Texas and Florida where they could no longer continue to play sports—where they were bullied by their classmates, where they weren't allowed to hold their transness publicly, much less with pride.

During the last afternoon, I sat with a group of them crowded around me. I read them a chapter from my novel, *Obie Is Man Enough*, which is about a transgender athlete in middle school. And then I let them ask me questions.

What do I do when I get bullied for being transgender at school?

What do I do when my teachers tell other kids that I'm transgender and they make fun of me?

Will I ever be able to play sports like you did?

These questions broke my heart. I didn't have answers. Because despite the fact that everyone at the event called the kids the right pronouns and names, didn't ask them invasive questions, and the kids got to just be kids for a few days, they still were returning home to legislative and systemic nightmares. Which is to say that no amount of interpersonal kindness can give a kid access to sports or healthcare or their autonomy when the government installs barriers.

And this is where you come in.

Making change requires moving beyond interpersonal relationships to the group (meso) and systemic (macro) levels. Everything builds from those interpersonal connections.

Here are a few scenarios to outline how we can make changes at these levels.

A FRAT MEMBER COMES OUT AS TRANS

"I am the president of a fraternity alumni group—so we've got people ranging from eighteen to . . . ninety years old, really. One of our members recently came out as trans and I want to be supportive, but I'm not sure how to help her. We have a reunion upcoming. What would you suggest? How can I help her, especially when there might—definitely—be some, well, other opinions."

"This is a fantastic question," I began. "I'll answer with an anecdote about my coach, who is not the president of a frat—although he was, once—but I'll admit that a men's sports team is not all that dissimilar from a frat!" The question-asker chuckled. I could see several muted Zoom faces laugh.

"The first thing I always recommend when someone wants to support someone else's journey of presenting themselves anew is *ask*. Ask them what they need—ask them what they want. Ask them what would be most helpful.

"When my coach and I began telling the swim team that I am trans, we had no model to use. Kevin asked me how I wanted to do so, and I chose writing an email. He sent my note to the whole team. When it was time for me to actually join, he began asking me about physical accommodations—which locker room was I more comfortable using and did I feel safe around campus being openly trans? I chose the men's locker room and although I felt safe, Kevin gave me his phone number and encouraged me to call him if anything happened.

"With the member in your frat, make sure you consider safety, especially given that trans women are more likely to experience physical violence. If the event is in person, let her know that you understand safety could be a concern and ask if you can provide any support. My first year, Kevin contacted other coaches whose teams we competed against to ensure my safety at their pools—this can be done in a myriad of situations, but you should always check to make sure that the trans individual is okay with it because you will likely have to out them in order to do this.

"Lastly, we tackled interpersonal interactions on the team—what did I want to do if (when) someone said or did something transphobic? Did I want him to intervene, or would I handle it? Usually, I chose to handle it, given that most of these moments did not happen at practice. But he continued to model his acceptance of me through calling me my correct pronouns and never treating me any differently on the pool deck.

"Each of these steps—individual, interpersonal/team, and beyond—can be translated into your fraternity, or for any other audience members"—I motioned to everyone in the Zoom room—"to any other group dynamics such as at a workplace, school, or other organization."

Here is a quick breakdown:

Individual Considerations

- What physical accommodations does the individual need or want to use? (Bathrooms, locker rooms, changing rooms, etc.)
- What method of coming out or dispersing information is most productive? (Email, in person in a group setting, in person individual by individual, via a recorded video, etc.)
- Who should do the coming out? (The trans individual or another person on behalf of individual—the latter is often productive at a school.)

Team Considerations

- How should we navigate questions people have? (Who should answer them, what resources should we provide, what questions is the trans person comfortable answering, etc.)
- How should we navigate transphobia that the individual will likely interface with?

Systemic Considerations

- What would happen if some governing body revokes a basic right that impacts this trans person's ability to be present in a given scenario?
- How will the group support and show compassion to the individual in an event of systemic transphobia?

- How can we advocate for trans people to have more rights?
- How can we use our privileges to raise the volume in the fight for trans rights?

ADVOCATING FOR A TRANS CHILD'S PRONOUNS

"My child is trans and I love and support him. My husband and I call him the name he asked for and we call him his correct pronouns. But what do I do when other adults are misgendering him? How do I advocate for him at school and with other parents?"

Individual Considerations

- Does the child want other people to call him he/him pronouns? This might sound like a silly question, but some kids are not ready for their pronouns to be public, and that's okay. Go at their pace and ensure that this is something they're ready for.
- What kind of support does the child want when he is misgendered?
  » Does he want to correct others himself?
  » Does he want to do nothing? Remember this is valid, too.
  » Does he want you and others around him to correct people when they misgender him? If so, here are a few methods of doing so at increasing severity of misgendering:
    ○ Interrupt and interject the correct pronoun each time misgendering occurs. *"He," "him," "you mean 'his.'"*
    ○ If a specific person continues to misgender him, pull them aside and have a conversation. *Why are you struggling to gender my child correctly? Do you need to practice?* Here, you could also explain the pain misgendering causes, inviting them to understand the impact of their actions.
    ○ If someone still refuses to gender your child correctly, consider next steps: distancing from, leaving, removing this person from being able to harm your child.
- What emotions arise for the child as you converse about this? Making space for the trans child's feelings throughout these conversations is key.

Group Considerations

- What would the child prefer to have others know about his pronouns?
  - » Does he want a parent to inform each of his teachers?
  - » Does he want to tell his peers and teachers himself about his pronouns?
- How will you protect your child?
  - » If you choose to repeatedly bring your child into a space where his trans identity is not affirmed and where he is rejected and harmed (verbally or physically) then you are communicating to him he is not worth protecting. This is a harsh and painful reality for many trans people whose parents prioritize their social relationships and standing over the well-being of their trans child.
  - » Consider removing or distancing from the people in your life who harm your child.
  - » Communicate validation to your child instead of attempting to dismiss transphobic actions of family members or other problematic loved ones. Too many parents will dismiss transphobic grandparents or other relatives with comments such as, "Oh, but grandma/grandpa loves you." Perhaps they do, or maybe they don't, but I encourage you to foster love that is more than a feeling. Cultivate love that protects.
- How will you care for yourself if you need to distance yourself from people you love?
  - » It is okay to grieve, but it is not okay to blame your child for this grief. Lean on your friends, partners, therapists, and other adults, but do not put your child in a place to hold your pain about their journey. That is for you to hold.

Systemic Considerations

- If legislative bans exist that affect your child's ability to be safe and included at school (to use the bathrooms that align with their gender identity, retain privacy regarding their transness, play sports with their peers), fight these. If you can, vote. Organize PTA meetings. Advocate for your child's rights at their school, sport, or other arena.

These considerations apply to more than just parents. Anyone can foster love that protects. Though I rarely felt a sense of belonging at school and in other social settings, a few teachers made sure the classroom was a place I wasn't bullied. At a time when so many had something to say about my clothing, my hair, my gender, Lida (she/her), my seventh-grade science teacher, let me be me. I felt welcomed as my quirky, cargo-shorts-wearing, nerdy self. She never once asked me to prove my gender as other teachers had. She never made a big deal about my pronouns. My memories of her classroom have barely faded: I remember most everything she taught us. Today, Lida and I are friends and she is one of my biggest supporters.

So many children do not have the privilege of supportive parents and teachers as I did. Having at least one supportive adult in a trans child's life can reduce the likelihood of suicide by 40 percent.[10] Be that supportive adult. It might save a child's life.

SUPPORTING A TRANS COLLEAGUE

"A colleague of mine recently disclosed that they are transgender. They haven't told our manager yet and I want to make sure that I will be a support whenever I can. They told me they want to come out soon. What would you suggest in order to support them best?"

Individual Considerations

- How does the colleague prefer to come out? Via email or in person? In a group/mass communication style or one at a time? Can you help disseminate information if they would like that help?
- Does your colleague want support surrounding coming out to your manager? (E.g., you could attend the meeting itself, you could give them a pep-talk beforehand, or you could eat lunch together after to debrief.)

Group Considerations

- After the colleague has come out, ask if they would like you to help correct people when misgendering or deadnaming occurs, and if they say yes, correct others who misgender or deadname the colleague.
- Offer support to your colleague if conflict arises through helping bring incidents of transphobia to your manager or supporting your colleague when they do, speaking up in the face of transphobic jokes, advocating for gender-neutral bathrooms, including pronouns in email signatures or on name tags, etc.

Systemic Considerations

- Ensure company antidiscrimination policies include gender identity and gender expression and maintain these regardless of any state or federal laws that remove protections.
- Encourage the company to release statements in support of the trans community.
- Encourage the company to donate money to trans grassroots organizations.

⁂

As I WRITE these suggestions, I hope that they feel somewhat obvious. Maybe you even thought, *This is how I should support anyone going through a big change.* Yes! In many ways, supporting a trans person at work, in school, or in a social group requires considering the trans person a human with autonomy and emotions that deserve to be protected. Which is to say: I have deep faith you have the skills to support a trans person even if you do not think you do. Let your heart lead—your compassion and empathy will foster greater allyship than any step-by-step suggestions could.

To my trans readers, if you cannot find the support you need from your parents or primary caretakers, find others who will. There *are* other people who will accept you exactly as you are. It might take some time to find them, but I promise they're there.

CHAPTER 22

Love Transcends

Y MOTHER AND I DROVE IN HER OLD SILVER PRIUS TO MY
grandmother's house. It was only about five minutes away from
the home in which I'd grown up, but the drive along the thickly forested
road felt like it took forever. I watched the trees whip by as I held the letter I'd typed. I tried not to damage the paper with my extremely sweaty
hands. It was probably the tenth version I'd tried. It had taken me weeks
to write, and still more weeks to gather the courage to decide I'd read it
out loud.

It was mid-June of the year I would begin at Harvard. Although I'd
come out in a grand Facebook post to my peers online, I still had to tell
my grandparents. The last on the list, they were the people I most feared
telling—especially Halmoni. My grandmother had spent my childhood
gifting me frilly dresses and blouses, pink T-shirts and makeup, none of
which I'd ever felt fit me. She lamented that I was, according to her, so
pretty but didn't flaunt it—why not?

I saw my grandmother as a devoutly Catholic woman, who'd immi-
grated to the United States from Korea in the late 1960s. To me, she
was stuck in her ways. I'd never heard her talk about gayness, much less
transness, and I only supposed that she'd reject it.

A year earlier, we'd been driving in her car—one that somehow smells exactly like her house. She had been quiet for a while before she asked me a question.

"Schuyler, I saw something on FaceTime," she started.

"FaceTime?"

"Yeah, FaceTime, on the computer." She nodded.

"Face*book*, you mean?" Easy to confuse, I guess.

"Ah, yes. Yes. I saw something—rainbow one." She paused, thinking. It was clear she'd been trying to figure out how to ask me this question, probably for the whole car ride.

"A rainbow?" I wasn't sure what she was talking about. *Did I accidentally post something about being gay?* I was beginning to panic.

"Yes, rainbow something. Title . . . Gay something?"

"Mm," I said, curtly. It was all I could manage. I was racking my brains—I never posted about my sexuality. *What could this be? Did someone else post something on my wall?*

"What is that?"

"I don't know, Halmoni," I said, pulling out my phone, the green bumper case around the edges was worn. I scrolled through my Facebook wall until I found what she was referencing.

"Oh," I said, relieved. "It's just a repost. From another account. My friend sent it to me. She's gay," I said. "I thought it was funny," I offered as Halmoni's face soured. She didn't say much else.

Though all my close friends (outside of swimming) and my nuclear family knew that I had identified as lesbian, I'd never told my grandmother. I figured that one day, I would likely marry a woman—and I'd tell her then. But in the meantime, what was the point?

Coming out as transgender was a different story. Not only would my appearance change fairly drastically, but I knew that my story had the potential to be widely publicized. I had already been approached for multiple interviews. But when I came out on Facebook to my peers, I wasn't ready to come out to Halmoni. Not wanting a repeat of her questioning, I blocked her. I did not want her to find out from the internet.

My mother and I talked extensively about coming out and what it would look like—what could happen and what was likely. We were fairly pessimistic.

"I'm not sure what Halmoni is going to say," Mom confessed. "I know she'll blame me—not all the blame will land on you, at least?" This was supposed to be comforting. It was not.

My mom let me take the lead—on timing, on how I shared, and on what I shared. She ensured she would be there with me. But I could see how nervous she was, too.

By the time I'd prepared my letter and decided I'd do it, I wasn't feeling particularly hopeful. I had resolved that I would tell Halmoni because I loved and respected her. This was the right thing to do, regardless of how she'd react.

When the forever-five-minute-drive was over, we sat around the kitchen table—my grandfather, my grandmother, my great-aunt, my mom, and myself.

"Schuyler-neun keun mal-eul eesohyoh," *Schuyler has something big to tell you,* my mom announced.

I wondered if they noticed how I shook as I sat down. I wondered if this would be the last time I ever sat at this table. I wondered if I'd ever be welcome in this home again.

I read the letter, my voice somehow stronger than I expected it to be. When I finished, I waited, my words hanging in the air.

My grandfather began a slow clap. *Clap, clap, clap.* Each rang out quietly.

"So, you come out of closet now," he said in his Korean accent, his voice hoarse with age. "Congratulations." He broke the word into syllables slowly. *Kohn-grah-doo-lay-shuns.* He smiled.

Stunned, I smiled awkwardly. *What? How did Harabuhji know that this was called "coming out"? Some days, it felt like he didn't speak much English at all but he knew this very colloquial phrase?*

My great-aunt sat silently. She reached out and squeezed my hand—as if to wish me good luck with my grandmother. Unlike how I had worried about Halmoni or Harabuhji's reactions, I'd never worried about my keun imo's reaction, not even for a second. My great-aunt stood up to refill everyone's tea, knowing her love had been communicated.

My gaze shifted to Halmoni. Her face showed an unreadable expression.

"Okay. Now I have two grandsons from your mother. That's fine." She said this so matter-of-factly, as if I'd just informed her what we were having for lunch.

Dumbfounded, I said nothing. I heard my mother begin to cry.

Halmoni raised her pointer finger in the air.

"But." My relief faltered. This was more along the lines of what I'd been expecting—where was the disappointment?

"In Korean culture," she continued, "daughters take care of their parents. Your mother has been such a good daughter to me. She takes such good care of me."

My mom was sobbing now. It is also not typical in Korean culture to offer praise, especially not to your daughters. I had never before heard Halmoni speak about my mom in reverence. I'd never heard her give my mother any compliments.

"She lives nearby so she can take care of me. She makes sure I am okay. She is a good daughter. The best daughter." Halmoni continued, her expression stern. I hadn't heard my mom cry like that. I reached out and held her hand as she tried to compose herself. She wiped her eyes and nose with a napkin because, for some unknown reason, my grandparents never keep tissues out in the open. Instead, they're stuffed in the back of the pantry closet. I squeezed her hand as Halmoni continued.

"So, you can be boy, son, brother." She paused and thought. "You can be a doctor now!" she exclaimed with excitement. I laughed. *Gender roles, Halmoni! I could have done that as a woman, too.* (Don't worry, we've talked about that one since.)

"You can be a man, but your mother has no more daughters, now, Schuyler. It is still your responsibility to take care of your mother like she takes care of me. Take care of your parents." I nodded furiously, tears now in my eyes, too.

"Of course, Halmoni," I promised.

A few years later, I tattooed my grandmother's words in her hand-writing beneath my mastectomy scar, next to my heart. 부모효도. *Boo-moh-hyoh-doh.* Take care of your parents.

The tattoo is a tribute to my history, my culture, my grandmother, and the people from which I come. It is a tribute to all the strong womanhood that birthed me. It is a tribute to the daughterhood I was assigned, never truly identified with, but the duties of which I abso-lutely will fulfill.

When I got the tattoo, I sent Halmoni a photo of it. She replied, thanking me for taking the "eternal vow" to care for my parents.

Somehow, remarkably, Halmoni has been the most supportive family member I've had. She switched pronouns and gendered epithets over-night, despite the fact that her native tongue doesn't even have gendered pronouns. She almost immediately began calling me handsome, as well as her "superman."

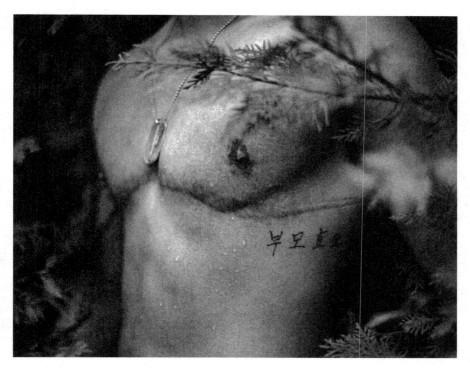

"Oh, our handsome man returns from college," she'd say upon the end of the semester. "You are superman!"

She took on the task of sharing my identity with her very large Korean family back in Korea—she is one of seven and my grandfather is one of six.

When they next returned to Korea to visit our extended family and my parents, brother, and I accompanied them, I was nervous.

"What will they say about me being...me?" I asked Halmoni.

"Nothing!" she said, indignantly.

"What do you mean? What if someone...says something mean?"

"They won't," she said, certain. "But if they do, I yell at them." She nodded at me. She wasn't joking.

The trip passed without struggle.

Halmoni even asked me if I wanted Harabuhji to give me a new Korean name. We were sitting at their kitchen table one day and I'd asked if my Korean name was gendered.

"Yes," Halmoni had said after a few moments. "I think so." Harabuhji had nodded in agreement.

"Girl's name," he said.

"But a boy can have. If you want." Halmoni said. But Harabuhji was already standing up, getting a pen. "Harabuhji can give you new name. You want?"

In our Korean family, my grandfather names the children. My grandfather had given me the name Miwon, 미원, meaning "foundation of beauty." The first character, 미, is also the first character of the word for America, 미국, which means "beautiful country." Harabuhji had given me this name because I was the first child of my Korean family to be born in the United States—I am the American foundation. My first character 미 is also the second character of my mother's Korean name, 여미, which means "beautiful dawn" because she was born early in the morning.

"No," I answered Halmoni. "I love my name. I don't care if it is a girl's name. It's about where I come from. I want to keep it." Halmoni smiled and Harabuhji put his pen down.

I wear my scar—my history, my story—and my tattoo with great pride. Both are a promise to myself that I will never forget where or who I come from; not my assigned gender, nor my Korean culture, not my parents or my grandparents, not my own personal history nor my body as it was and always is and will be—because these make me who I am, and I refuse to forget who I am.

These days, I see the oldsters as often as I can. They are ties to my history and my culture, and they are evidence of a love that transcends any boundaries. My grandparents and great-aunt had every excuse I can think of to reject me: language, religion, age, generation, and culture. But they chose instead to lead with love.

If my Korean Catholic immigrant grandparents can do this, anyone can. Does that mean anyone will? Unfortunately, sometimes tragically, of course not: it is still a privilege that I was received with open hearts by my family.

Welcoming acceptance and unconditional love should never be a privilege in one's own family: kindness costs nothing and should be something commonly expected and freely given.

I am fighting for that day—I hope you will fight with me.

Until then, my family near and far serves as proof of this possibility—as examples of the kind of love we all deserve, and the kind of love we can all provide to others. Love can transcend all barriers if we let it.

CHAPTER 23

As You Embark, Take Me with You

DEAR READER,
I hope you've enjoyed this journey with me. I'm so grateful you decided to pick up this book, and even more grateful you made it this far.

Now the hard work of allyship truly begins as you close these pages to enter back into the real world and integrate what you've learned into your daily lives and actions.

I hope this book can help you be an ally to the people who have not read this book—and probably never will. Those are the people who need shifting the most. Use this to support and diffuse those difficult conversations. Extend the care and compassion you have hopefully garnered for trans people through reading this to yourself as well.

Thank you, again, for your willingness to connect, learn, and educate yourself and others.

I hope through inviting you into my humanity, you've also been invited into your own.

Here it sits, waiting for you.

❖ ❖ ❖

AND TO MY fellow transgender readers:

Being transgender is one of my life's greatest joys.

I mean that.

I hold tightly to all that this gender roller coaster has taught me.

I throw away the expectations the world had of me with glee—and grief.

"This is me," I whisper. *"This is me!"* I shout into the air.

I taste my tears in my enormous smile.

And no one can ever take this from me.

No one can ever take your identity away from you.

So no matter where you are or who knows who you are, I hope you breathe in deep the power that your transness holds.

How magical it is to hold these multitudes.

AFAB: abbreviation for *assigned female at birth*, pronounced "ay-fab."

Agender: someone who does not experience having a gender.

Ally: someone who fights for a marginalized identity group but who does not share that identity, e.g., someone who is not transgender, but who supports and fights for the trans community.

AMAB: abbreviation for *assigned male at birth*, pronounced "ay-mab."

Biological sex: often shortened to just *sex*, this technically refers to the anatomical, physiological, and biological makeup of one's reproductive organs and secondary sex characteristics, usually categorized into a noncomprehensive binary of either "male" or "female." Colloquially, *biological sex* is most often used to refer either to one's external genitalia or to a person's gender assigned at birth.

Body dysmorphia: according to the *DSM-5-TR*, preoccupation with one or more perceived defects or flaws in physical appearance that are not observable or appear slight to others. *Not* the same thing as gender dysphoria.

Bottom surgery: gender-affirmation surgery to reconstruct genitalia. This is sometimes called "gender/sex reassignment surgery" or "genital reassignment surgery" or, even more infrequently, "sex change," but these are antiquated and/or inaccurate terms. Reconstruction of genitalia does not "reassign" gender identity or truly change someone's gender; surgery is an affirmation of one's gender identity that has *always been there.*

Cis man: a man assigned male at birth.

Cis woman: a woman assigned female at birth.

Cisgender: an adjective that describes someone who is not transgender—someone whose gender identity matches the gender they were assigned at birth.

Cishet: a compound adjective, combining abbreviated versions of *cisgender* and *heterosexual*, and describes people who are neither transgender nor queer.

Cisheteronormative: describing a societal/world view that assumes everyone is both cisgender and straight.

Cisnormative: describing a societal/world view that assumes everyone is cisgender and/or conforms to cisgender expectations of body.

Cissexism: a system of beliefs that assumes gender is defined by genitals, that only two genders exist, and that everyone is therefore cisgender. This is systemic transphobia. Cissexism also purports (whether unconsciously or consciously) that cisgender bodies and gender identities are more legitimate and natural than those of trans people, that being trans is inherently inferior to being cis. Cissexism is the control center from which transphobia is enacted.

Enby: an abbreviation for *non-binary*—the phonetic pronunciation of the letters N and B.

Femme: a noun referring to or an adjective describing a person who aligns and/or identifies themselves with femininity and/or womanhood. An umbrella term with ever-evolving and individualized uses, *femme* can be used to describe people who are perceived as women by societal gender standards.

FTM: *female-to-male*, a label trans folks assigned female at birth, mainly trans men, might use for themselves. I refrain from using *FTM* because it implies I was once female, which is inaccurate. I recommend using *trans man* or *assigned female at birth* instead of *FTM* unless an individual uses it for themselves.

Gender affirmation: an umbrella term that some use instead of or in addition to *transition* and is more likely to be accurate and inclusive, in that it encompasses exactly what it is: a vague and therefore individualized process of affirming one's gender—an identity that existed before any affirmation processes began.

Gender-affirming care: social, psychological, behavioral, and/or medical interventions that support and affirm a person's gender identity.

Gender-affirming surgery: surgery that seeks to affirm one's gender identity.

Gender assigned at birth: sometimes abbreviated to AGAB, this refers to the sex printed on someone's birth certificate at birth, which is usually deduced from the appearance of the newborn's external genitalia.

Gender binary: often regarded as a Euro-colonial construction of gender, the concept that there are only two distinct genders of male and female, and that gender itself is determined by sex, specifically genitals at birth.

Gender dysphoria: the distress or discomfort that can arise from the incongruence between gender assigned at birth and gender identity. Often shortened to *dysphoria*.

Gender expression: this refers to how folks present their gender, including how we talk, how we act, how we look. Gender expression is bound into gender roles by social construction and it can change based on epoch, culture, geographic location, and other socially influenced factors.

Gender identity: a person's knowledge and understanding of their own gender.

Gender nonconforming: describes people whose gender identity and/or gender expression does not align with societal standards or expectations of gender.

Genderfluid *or* **Genderqueer:** describing someone whose gender is not fixed and shifts over time or depending on a situation.

Heteronormative: describing a societal/world view that assumes everyone is straight and is/should be in straight relationships.

HRT/GAHT: acronyms that stand for *hormone replacement therapy* or *gender-affirming hormone therapy*. The administration of a cross hormone—one that is not produced at high concentrations during an individual's natal puberty—for gender-affirmation purposes.

Intersectionality: a term coined by American lawyer and professor Kimberlé Crenshaw in 1989, originally used to discuss the intersections of race and sex, specifically regarding discrimination that Black women are subjected to. Intersectionality refers to unique dynamics of oppression that result from experiencing multiple marginalized identities.

LGBTQ+: an acronym that represents the queer and trans community. The letters stand for lesbian, gay, bisexual, transgender, and queer, with the + representing other marginalized gender and sexual identities not enumerated in the acronym.

Also common:

LGBTQI+: includes intersex.

LGBTQIA+: includes both intersex and asexual spectrum identities.

LGBTQ2S+: includes 2S for two spirit.

Microaggression: according to the *Merriam-Webster* dictionary, a microaggression is "a comment or action that subtly and often unconsciously or unintentionally expresses a prejudiced attitude toward a member of a marginalized group (such as a racial minority)." In the words of my best friend Kevin, if you are talking about a marginalized group and you say something you don't think is offensive but it still offends someone from that group, it's a microaggression.

Misogynoir: a term coined by Black queer feminist Moya Bailey to describe the compounded discrimination that Black women experience, existing at the intersection of misogyny and anti-Blackness.

Misogyny: in short: the hatred of women. With nuance: the inter- and intrapersonal, structural, and systemic oppression and disenfranchisement of women and others who exhibit any kind of femmehood or are not a cis straight man.

MTF: *male-to-female*, a label trans folks assigned male at birth, mainly trans women, might use for themselves. I recommend using *trans woman* or *assigned male at birth* instead of *MTF* unless an individual uses it for themselves.

Natal puberty: puberty that ensues without medical intervention—e.g., for someone assigned female at birth, this would usually entail estrogen-driven puberty; for someone assigned male at birth, this would usually entail testosterone-driven puberty.

Non-binary: an umbrella term that describes individuals whose gender does not fit current (Euro-colonial) social constructions of "man" or "woman."

Patriarchy: a form of social organization that empowers men over women, and others who are not men, placing men in positions of power everywhere—at home, at work, and in society at large.

Queer: an umbrella term that can encompass a variety of marginalized sexual and gender identities. Queerness can describe sexuality, gender, or a combination of both. *Queer* is most commonly used to describe someone who is not cisgender, not straight, or neither cisgender nor straight.

Sexism: prejudice toward or discrimination against a person based on their sex or gender, most often women and femmes.

Sexuality: the classification of one's romantic, sexual, or emotional attraction toward others (e.g., gay, straight, bisexual, pansexual, queer, asexual, etc.).

TERF: an acronym standing for "Trans Exclusionary Radical 'Feminist'" that describes supposed feminists who reject that trans women are women.

Trans feminine: an umbrella term that can refer to a person assigned male at birth who does not identify as a boy or man.

Trans man: a man assigned female at birth.

Trans masculine: an umbrella term that can refer to a person assigned female at birth who does not identify as a girl or woman.

Trans woman: a woman assigned male at birth.

Transgender: an adjective that describes someone whose gender identity differs from the gender they were assigned at birth. Do *not* use "transgendered" (implies that something happened to someone to make them trans, which is false), "a transgender" (reduces someone to a label, which is unkind), or "the transgenders" (same as previous).

Transition: any steps a person takes to affirm their gender identity, which could or could not include surgery, hormone therapy, pronoun changes, wardrobe or name changes, and haircuts.

Transmisogynoir: a term coined by Trudy to describe the compounded discrimination that Black trans women experience, existing at the intersection of transphobia, misogyny, and anti-Blackness.

Transphobia: the dislike of, prejudice against, or discrimination toward transgender people based on their transgender identity.

Transsexual: an outdated term that describes transgender individuals and has been used in a variety of ways, mostly to describe a trans person who has chosen to undergo medical transition, namely surgery. Because it is often considered pejorative, do not use *transsexual* to describe someone unless they use it to describe themselves.

Top surgery: chest reconstruction surgery—a breast reduction, mastectomy, or a breast augmentation, though the term *top surgery* is less common in the trans feminine community where *breast augmentation* or simply *BA* is more often used.

Toxic masculinity: a group of beliefs, behaviors, and expectations of men that require them to suppress emotions, mask distress, maintain a stoic or hardened external disposition, and use violence or aggression as indicators of power.

TRANS TERMINOLOGY QUICK SHEET

INSTEAD OF THIS...	TRY THIS...
✗ He is a transgender ✗ He is transgender<u>ed</u> "Transgender" is an adjective. Using it as a noun or verb is not only grammatically incorrect but also a) dehumanizing, or b) implies something has happened to make us trans, which is false.	✓ He is <u>transgender</u> ✓ He is a transgender <u>man</u>
✗ He <u>transgendered</u> last year	✓ He <u>transitioned</u> last year
✗ He <u>changed genders</u> I didn't change my gender. I changed my presentation. I've always been myself—a boy, a man. I just haven't always had the words or resources or confidence to explain that.	✓ He <u>transitioned</u> ✓ He <u>affirmed his gender</u>
✗ He was <u>born a girl</u> ✗ When he <u>was a girl</u> ✗ Before he <u>became a boy</u> These imply I was once a girl. But I was never truly a girl. Though I may have "looked like" or presented as a girl, I have always been me; a boy, a man. Even when I couldn't explain that. For me, this extends to "FTM" as well. When relevant, I prefer to say I was "assigned female at birth, and identify as male," instead.	✓ He was <u>assigned female</u> at birth ✓ When he <u>presented as</u> a woman OR When he was <u>perceived as</u> a woman The difference between these two is that the former implies the trans person intended to present as a woman, whereas in the latter, it's just about others' perception. ✓ Before he <u>transitioned</u>
✗ Being trans means you're gay	✓ Gender identity and sexual orientation are not the same
✗ Did you get the surgery?	✓ Don't ask about surgeries and/or private parts unless a person explicitly invites that conversation!

ACKNOWLEDGMENTS

I have poured every part of myself into this book. Every person I've met, every opportunity I've been privileged to have, and every heartbreak I've grieved has shaped my writing here. I am all that I have experienced and all that I have loved and all who have loved me—and so is this book.

A comprehensive list of acknowledgements is impossible; instead, here are a few.

My team at Hachette Go—Sharon Kunz, Michael Barrs, Ashley Kiedrowski, Abimael Ayala-Oquendo, Mary Ann Naples, Michelle Aielli, Terri Sirma, Sean Moreau, Logan Hill, Erica Lawrence, Kay Mariea, Robie Grant, Linda Mark, Bart Dawson, and, of course, Renee Sedliar, my editor, whose direction was more than editing—driven by compassion and care for the work that made *He/She/They* what you have read here.

My team at Penguin Life UK—Martina O'Sullivan and Susannah Bennett—who joyously brought this to the UK, Australia, and New Zealand.

My team at Fortier; my agents Susan Canavan, who has always believed in the power of this book, and Scott Waxman, who knew I'd write this long before I did and has supported my career before its conception.

Those I interviewed, who added invaluable insights, depth, and humanity to this book.

Ellen Oh, whose encouragement and faith sparked the writing of the proposal. (And my writing career itself!)

The YES! Institute of Miami, where I first received education about gender identity, transness, and the complexity of biological sex.

Josephine, who saved my life and in whose therapy sessions I first found myself and my manhood.

My teachers Lida and Clay, my coaches Steph, Kevin, Ron, and Peter, my therapist Deb, and my other mentors who have guided me over the years.

Michael, who has been the gentle older brother I never had.

Saren, in whose company I feel a safety I never even knew to look for.

Kevin, my best friend and teammate, who is one of the primary reasons I was able to get through my college years with joy and laughter and peace.

Every teammate I've ever had.

Every friend who has loved me.

Emma, without whom I'm not sure I'd have survived high school, and who was the first person to ever hear me utter the words, "I think I am transgender."

Kayden, Ely, Dylan, Taylor, Saren, Hansa, Kris, and others, who were sounding boards when I got stuck writing.

Every trans person who showed me that my life was possible, particularly our transcestors, especially the Black trans individuals who paved the way, who broke in before they opened the doors to us, who made certain we had a place here.

Each social media follower and supporter—and social media itself, the first place I ever asked for my pronouns, the first place I announced, "I am transgender."

My clients and support group attendees who teach me about the beautiful diversity our community holds, who continuously remind me of the power of softness, of empowering from within, of trans and queer joy.

The trans children I've met whose unfettered thirst for life as their true selves sparkle through transphobia and bigotry.

To my eight-year-old self, who knew who he was with clarity and ease, and who survived all that life brought us so that I may be who I am today.

My brother, who was my first best friend and confidante, who always pushes me to think beyond myself and my own echo chamber.

My mother- and father-in-law, whose warmth, love, and ease of acceptance I only ever dreamed of having one day.

My father's parents, whose home and hearts were filled with art, who loved without needing to always understand.

My Halmoni, Harabuhji, and my Kumja—my immigrant Catholic grandparents—who could have used every excuse to reject me but chose instead to lead with love, who are examples that all of us can and should follow.

My parents, who have ensured that I have never, ever felt alone. My dad, who still laughs during my speeches even though he's heard my words hundreds of times; whose gentle masculinity has invited me into my own; who has always taught me to be myself. My mom, whose love is fiercer than that of anyone else I know; whose strong womanhood has taught me to be a better man; who edits my writing with the most careful eye; who is the reason I am equipped to write at all.

And, of course, my wife, Sarah, who held me as I sobbed from exhaustion and frustration writing this book. Sarah, who listened intently as I read her sections and eventually the entire manuscript over and over. Sarah, who brought me homemade, lovingly curated snack plates and easy-to-eat dinners when I refused to leave my desk as I wrote for days on end. Sarah, whose patience, love, and companionship I do not ever wish to live without.

And you, dear readers, for picking up this book and diving in heart first.

REFERENCES

"1 in 6 People Globally Affected by Infertility." World Health Organization, April 4, 2023. https://www.who.int/news/item/04-04-2023-1-in-6-people-globally-affected-by -infertility#:~:text=Around%2017.5%25%20of%20the%20adult,care%20for%20 those%20in%20need.

"1.2 Million LGBTQ Adults in the US Identify as Nonbinary." Williams Institute, June 22, 2021. https://williamsinstitute.law.ucla.edu/press/lgbtq-nonbinary-press-release/.

"2015 Word of the Year Is Singular 'They.'" American Dialect Society, January 8, 2016. https://americandialect.org/2015-word-of-the-year-is-singular-they.

"AACAP Statement Responding to Efforts to Ban Evidence-Based Care for Transgen-der and Gender Diverse." American Academy of Child and Adolescent Psychi-atry, November 8, 2019. https://www.aacap.org/AACAP/Latest_News/AACAP _Statement_Responding_to_Efforts-to_ban_Evidence-Based_Care_for_Transgender _and_Gender_Diverse.aspx.

Academic Dictionaries and Encyclopedias. "David Oliver Cauldwell." Accessed March 12, 2023. https://en-academic.com/dic.nsf/enwiki/11600702.

"Accepting Adults Reduce Suicide Attempts Among LGBTQ Youth." The Trevor Proj-ect, June 27, 2019. https://www.thetrevorproject.org/research-briefs/accepting -adults-reduce-suicide-attempts-among-lgbtq-youth/.

"Access to Health Services." Healthy People 2030. Accessed March 16, 2023. https://health.gov/healthypeople/priority-areas/social-determinants-health /literature-summaries/access-health-services#cit11.

Achille, Christal, Tenille Taggart, Nicholas R. Eaton, Jennifer Osipoff, Kimberly Tafuri, Andrew Lane, and Thomas A. Wilson. "Longitudinal Impact of Gender-Affirming Endocrine Intervention on the Mental Health and Well-Being of Transgender Youths: Preliminary Results." *International Journal of Pediatric Endocrinology* 2020, no. 1 (December 2020): 8. https://doi.org/10.1186/s13633-020-00078-2.

Adderly, Mila Jam. Interview, October 27, 2022.

Agence France-Presse. "A Spate of Drownings: Classes Help Black Americans Learn to Swim." VOA, October 22, 2022. https://www.voanews.com/a/a-spate-of-drownings -classes-help-black-americans-learn-to-swim-/6801549.html.

Ahmad, Syed W., Gianfranco Molfetto, David Montoya, and Ariday Camero. "Is Oral Testosterone the New Frontier of Testosterone Replacement Therapy?" *Cureus* 14, no. 8 (August 2022): e27796. https://doi.org/10.7759/cureus.27796.

Ahmed, Ayesha. "Quick Facts About Sexual Assault in America." *PlanStreet* (blog), May 25, 2022. https://www.planstreetinc.com/quick-facts-about-sexual-assault-in-america/.

Alfonseca, Kiara. "Why Abortion Restrictions Disproportionately Impact People of Color." *ABC News*, June 24, 2022. https://abcnews.go.com/Health/abortion-restrictions-disproportionately-impact-people-color/story?id=84467809.

American Psychiatric Association. *Diagnostic and Statistical Manual of Mental Disorders: DSM-5*. 5th ed. Washington, DC: American Psychiatric Association, 2013.

American Psychiatric Association. *Diagnostic and Statistical Manual of Mental Disorders: DSM-5-TR*. 5th ed., text rev. Washington, DC: American Psychiatric Association Publishing, 2022.

Aragão, Carolina. "Gender Pay Gap in U.S. Hasn't Changed Much in Two Decades." Pew Research Center. Accessed March 16, 2023. https://www.pewresearch.org/fact-tank/2023/03/01/gender-pay-gap-facts/.

Artiga, Samantha, and Latoya Hill. "Health Coverage by Race and Ethnicity, 2010–2021." *KFF*, December 20, 2022. https://www.kff.org/racial-equity-and-health-policy/issue-brief/health-coverage-by-race-and-ethnicity/.

Asarch, Steven. "A Social-Media Trend Has People Identifying as 'Super Straight.' The Transophobic Campaign Was Meant to Divide LGBTQ People." *Insider*, March 8, 2021. https://www.insider.com/super-straight-flag-meaning-tiktok-superstraight-ss-movement-origin-2021-3.

Aschenbrenner, Diane S. "First Oral Testosterone Product Now Available." *The American Journal of Nursing* 119, no. 8 (August 2019): 22. https://doi.org/10.1097/01.NAJ.0000577424.31609.23.

Austin, Ashley, Shelley L. Craig, Sandra D'Souza, and Lauren B. McInroy. "Suicidality Among Transgender Youth: Elucidating the Role of Interpersonal Risk Factors." *Journal of Interpersonal Violence* 37, nos. 5–6 (March 2022): NP2696–2718. https://doi.org/10.1177/0886260520915554.

Bainbridge, Carol. "What Is a Social Construct? Why Every Part of Society Is a Social Construct." Verywell Mind, March 14, 2023. https://www.verywellmind.com/definition-of-social-construct-1448922.

Barnes, Katie. "How Two Transgender Athletes Are Fighting to Compete in the Sports They Love." ESPN.com, May 29, 2018. https://www.espn.com/espn/story/_/id/33460938/how-two-transgender-athletes-fighting-compete-sports-love.

Baxter, Kevin. "The First U.S. Boxer to Fight as a Woman, and Then as a Man." *Los Angeles Times*, August 4, 2017. https://www.latimes.com/sports/boxing/la-sp-pat-manuel-20170804-htmlstory.html.

Beauchamp, Zack. "Jordan Peterson, the Obscure Canadian Psychologist Turned Right-Wing Celebrity, Explained." *Vox*, May 21, 2018. https://www.vox.com/world/2018/3/26/17144166/jordan-peterson-12-rules-for-life.

Beers, Lee Savio. "American Academy of Pediatrics Speaks Out Against Bills Harming Transgender Youth." American Academy of Pediatrics. Accessed March 16, 2023.

https://www.aap.org/en/news-room/news-releases/aap/2021/american-academy-of-pediatrics-speaks-out-against-bills-harming-transgender-youth/.

Berman, Sarah. "2022 NCAA Division I Women's Swimming and Diving Championships Records Roundup." SwimSwam, March 20, 2022. https://swimswam.com/2022-womens-ncaa-division-i-swimming-and-diving-championships-records-roundup/.

"Black Americans Are Systematically Under-Treated for Pain. Why?" Frank Batten School of Leadership and Public Policy, University of Virginia, June 30, 2020. https://batten.virginia.edu/about/news/black-americans-are-systematically-under-treated-pain-why.

"Black Trans Liberation." Black Trans Liberation. Accessed March 16, 2023. https://www.blacktransliberation.com.

"Black Trans Women and Black Trans Femmes: Leading & Living Fiercely." Transgender Law Center. Accessed March 16, 2023. https://transgenderlawcenter.org/black-trans-women-black-trans-femmes-leading-living-fiercely.

Block, Melissa. "Idaho's Transgender Sports Ban Faces a Major Legal Hurdle." NPR, May 3, 2021. https://www.npr.org/2021/05/03/991987280/idahos-transgender-sports-ban-faces-a-major-legal-hurdle.

Boerner, Heather. "What the Science on Gender-Affirming Care for Transgender Kids Really Shows." *Scientific American*, May 12, 2022. https://www.scientificamerican.com/article/what-the-science-on-gender-affirming-care-for-transgender-kids-really-shows/.

Bose, Nandita. "Roe v Wade Ruling Disproportionately Hurts Black Women, Experts Say." Reuters, June 27, 2022. https://www.reuters.com/world/us/roe-v-wade-ruling-disproportionately-hurts-black-women-experts-say-2022-06-27/.

Boskey, Elizabeth. Interview, March 10, 2023.

Bowlby, John. *Attachment and Loss*. Basic Books, 1969.

"Breast Augmentation." UCSF Gender Affirming Health Program. Accessed March 16, 2023. https://transcare.ucsf.edu/breast-augmentation.

Bridges, Khiara M. "Implicit Bias and Racial Disparities in Health Care." *Human Rights Magazine*. Accessed March 16, 2023. https://www.americanbar.org/groups/crsj/publications/human_rights_magazine_home/the-state-of-healthcare-in-the-united-states/racial-disparities-in-health-care/.

Brummitt, Chris. "Serena Williams Says 'Williams Brothers' Comment Was Case of Bullying." *The Independent*, October 19, 2014. https://www.independent.co.uk/sport/tennis/serena-williams-says-williams-brothers-comment-was-case-of-bullying-sexist-and-racist-9804563.html.

Carmichael, Polly, Gary Butler, Una Masic, Tim J. Cole, Bianca L. De Stavola, Sarah Davidson, Elin M. Skageberg, Sophie Khadr, and Russell M. Viner. "Short-Term Outcomes of Pubertal Suppression in a Selected Cohort of 12 to 15 Year Old Young People with Persistent Gender Dysphoria in the UK." Edited by Geilson Lima Santana. *PLoS One* 16, no. 2 (February 2, 2021): e0243894. https://doi.org/10.1371/journal.pone.0243894.

Chan, Sewell, "Marsha P. Johnson," *New York Times Overlooked*, March 8, 2018, https://www.nytimes.com/interactive/2018/obituaries/overlooked-marsha-p-johnson.html.

Cheung, Kylie. "Simone Biles Should Be Praised, Not Punished for Achieving a Feat That Was Deemed Impossible." *Salon*, May 26, 2021. https://www.salon .com/2021/05/26/simone-biles-yurchenko-double-pike-gymnastics-scoring/.

"Child Abuse in the U.S.—Perpetrators by Race/Ethnicity 2020." Statista. Accessed March 16, 2023. https://www.statista.com/statistics/418475/number-of-perpetrators -in-child-abuse-cases-in-the-us-by-race-ethnicity/.

"Children and Teens: Statistics." RAINN. Accessed March 14, 2023. https://www.rainn .org/statistics/children-and-teens.

Clements, KC. "What Does It Mean to Be Cissexist?" Healthline, June 1, 2021. https: //www.healthline.com/health/transgender/cissexist.

"Closing Gender Pay Gaps Is More Important than Ever." UN News, September 18, 2022. https://news.un.org/en/story/2022/09/1126901.

Commissioner, Office of the. "FDA Approves New Oral Testosterone Capsule for Treatment of Men with Certain Forms of Hypogonadism." FDA, March 24, 2020. https://www.fda.gov/news-events/press-announcements/fda-approves-new -oral-testosterone-capsule-treatment-men-certain-forms-hypogonadism.

"Cosmetic Surgery in Teens: Information for Parents." HealthyChildren.org. Accessed March 14, 2023. https://www.healthychildren.org/English/ages-stages/gradeschool /puberty/Pages/Cosmetic-Surgery-in-Teens-Information-for-Parents.aspx.

Costa, Rosalia, Michael Dunsford, Elin Skagerberg, Victoria Holt, Polly Carmichael, and Marco Colizzi. "Psychological Support, Puberty Suppression, and Psychosocial Functioning in Adolescents with Gender Dysphoria." *The Journal of Sexual Medicine* 12, no. 11 (November 2015): 2206–2214. https://doi.org/10.1111/jsm.13034.

Dammeyer, Jesper, and Madeleine Chapman. "A National Survey on Violence and Discrimination Among People with Disabilities." *BMC Public Health* 18, no. 1 (March 15, 2018): 355. https://doi.org/10.1186/s12889-018-5277-0.

Daniels, Morg. "Ancient Mesopotamian Transgender and Non-Binary Identities." Academus Education, June 30, 2021. https://www.academuseducation.co.uk/post /ancient-mesopotamian-transgender-and-non-binary-identities.

De Bellefonds, Colleen. "Why Michael Phelps Has the Perfect Body for Swimming." Biography, May 14, 2020. https://www.biography.com/athletes/michael -phelp-perfect-body-swimming.

de Vries, Annelou L. C., Jenifer K. McGuire, Thomas D. Steensma, Eva C. F. Wagenaar, Theo A. H. Doreleijers, and Peggy T. Cohen-Kettenis. "Young Adult Psychological Outcome After Puberty Suppression and Gender Reassignment." *Pediatrics* 134, no. 4 (October 1, 2014): 696–704. https://doi.org/10.1542/peds.2013-2958.

de Vries, Annelou L. C., Thomas D. Steensma, Theo A. H. Doreleijers, and Peggy T. Cohen-Kettenis. "Puberty Suppression in Adolescents with Gender Identity Disorder: A Prospective Follow-Up Study." *The Journal of Sexual Medicine* 8, no. 8 (August 2011): 2276–2283. https://doi.org/10.1111/j.1743-6109.2010.01943.x.

Dehlendorf, Christine, Lisa H. Harris, and Tracy A. Weitz. "Disparities in Abortion Rates: A Public Health Approach." *American Journal of Public Health* 103, no. 10 (October 2013): 1772–1779. https://doi.org/10.2105/AJPH.2013.301339.

Denny, Kara N., Katie Loth, Marla E. Eisenberg, and Dianne Neumark-Sztainer. "Intuitive Eating in Young Adults. Who Is Doing It, and How Is It Related to Disordered

Eating Behaviors?" *Appetite* 60, no. 1 (January 1, 2013): 13–19. https://doi .org/10.1016/j.appet.2012.09.029.

Deran, Elle. Interview, October 13, 2022.

Diamond, Adele. "Executive Functions." *Annual Review of Psychology* 64, no. 1 (January 3, 2013): 135–168. https://doi.org/10.1146/annurev-psych-113011-143750.

Diamondstein, Megan. "The Disproportionate Harm of Abortion Bans: Spotlight on Dobbs v. Jackson Women's Health." Center for Reproductive Rights, November 29, 2021. https://reproductiverights.org/supreme-court-case-mississippi-abortion-ban -disproportionate-harm/.

Diemer, Elizabeth W., Julia D. Grant, Melissa A. Munn-Chernoff, David A. Patterson, and Alexis E. Duncan. "Gender Identity, Sexual Orientation, and Eating-Related Pathology in a National Sample of College Students." *Journal of Adolescent Health* 57, no. 2 (August 2015): 144–149. https://doi.org/10.1016/j.jadohealth.2015.03.003.

"Discriminatory Policies Threaten Care for Transgender, Gender Diverse Individuals." Endocrine Society, December 16, 2020. https://www.endocrine.org/news -and-advocacy/news-room/2020/discriminatory-policies-threaten-care-for -transgender-gender-diverse-individuals.

"Doctors Agree: Gender-Affirming Care Is Life-Saving Care." American Civil Liberties Union, April 1, 2021. https://www.aclu.org/news/lgbtq-rights/doctors-agree -gender-affirming-care-is-life-saving-care.

Druke, Galen. "Native American 'Two-Spirit People' Serve Unique Roles Within Their Communities." Wisconsin Public Radio, June 27, 2014. https://www.wpr.org/native -american-two-spirit-people-serve-unique-roles-within-their-communities.

"Eating Disorders Among LGBTQ Youth." The Trevor Project, February 17, 2022. https://www.thetrevorproject.org/research-briefs/eating-disorders-among -lgbtq-youth-feb-2022/.

Ehrensaft, Diane, Shawn V. Giammattei, Kelly Storck, Amy C. Tishelman, and Colt St. Amand. "Prepubertal Social Gender Transitions: What We Know; What We Can Learn—A View from a Gender Affirmative Lens." *International Journal of Transgenderism* 19, no. 2 (April 3, 2018): 251–268. https://doi.org/10.1080/155327 39.2017.1414649.

"Endocrine Society Alarmed at Criminalization of Transgender Medicine." Endocrine Society, February 23, 2022. https://www.endocrine.org/news-and-advocacy /news-room/2022/endocrine-society-alarmed-at-criminalization-of-transgender -medicine.

Ennis, Dawn. "NCAA Champion CeCé Telfer Says 'I Have No Benefit' by Being Trans." Outsports, June 3, 2019. https://www.outsports.com/2019/6/3/18649927 /ncaa-track-champion-cece-telfer-transgender-athlete-fpu-trans-testosterone.

"Fatal Violence Against the Transgender and Gender Non-Conforming Community in 2021." Human Rights Campaign. Accessed March 14, 2023. https://www.hrc .org/resources/fatal-violence-against-the-transgender-and-gender-non-conforming -community-in-2021.

Feder, Jill. "Why Are Persons with Disabilities 3 Times More Likely to Experience Sexual Assault?" Accessibility.com, June 14, 2022. https://www.accessibility.com /blog/disability-and-sexual-assault.

Ferguson, Heather J., Victoria E. A. Brunsdon, and Elisabeth E. F. Bradford. "The Developmental Trajectories of Executive Function from Adolescence to Old Age." *Scientific Reports* 11, no. 1 (January 14, 2021). https://doi.org/10.1038/s41598-020-80866-1.

Fitzsimons, Tim. "Trans Teens Face Higher Sexual Assault Risk When Schools Restrict Bathrooms, Study Finds." *NBC News*, May 6, 2019. https://www.nbcnews.com/feature/nbc-out/trans-teens-face-higher-sexual-assault-risk-when-schools-restrict-n1002601.

"Frontline Physicians Oppose Legislation That Interferes in or Criminalizes Patient Care." American Psychiatric Association, April 2, 2021. https://www.psychiatry.org:443/news-room/news-releases/frontline-physicians-oppose-legislation-that-inter.

"Gender Affecting Domestic Violence." Counseling Services, Valparaiso University. Accessed March 16, 2023. https://www.valpo.edu/counseling-services/gender-affecting-domestic-violence/.

"Gender Dysphoria Diagnosis." American Psychiatric Association. https://www.psychiatry.org/psychiatrists/cultural-competency/education/transgender-and-gender-nonconforming-patients/gender-dysphoria-diagnosis.

"Gender Incongruence and Transgender Health in the ICD." World Health Organization. Accessed March 14, 2023. https://www.who.int/standards/classifications/frequently-asked-questions/gender-incongruence-and-transgender-health-in-the-icd.

Grannis, Connor, Scott F. Leibowitz, Shane Gahn, Leena Nahata, Michele Morningstar, Whitney I. Mattson, Diane Chen, John F. Strang, and Eric E. Nelson. "Testosterone Treatment, Internalizing Symptoms, and Body Image Dissatisfaction in Transgender Boys." *Psychoneuroendocrinology* 132 (October 2021): 105358. https://doi.org/10.1016/j.psyneuen.2021.105358.

Grant, Jaime M., Lisa A. Mottet, Justin Tanis, Jody L. Herman, Jack Harrison, and Mara Keisling. "National Transgender Discrimination Survey Report on Health and Health Care." National Center for Transgender Equality and the National Gay and Lesbian Task Force, October 2010. https://cancer-network.org/wp-content/uploads/2017/02/National_Transgender_Discrimination_Survey_Report_on_health_and_health_care.pdf

Green, Amy E., Jonah P. DeChants, Myeshia N. Price, and Carrie K. Davis. "Association of Gender-Affirming Hormone Therapy with Depression, Thoughts of Suicide, and Attempted Suicide Among Transgender and Nonbinary Youth." *Journal of Adolescent Health* 70, no. 4 (April 2022): 643–649. https://doi.org/10.1016/j.jadohealth.2021.10.036.

Grierson, Jamie. "Most Child Sexual Abuse Gangs Made Up of White Men, Home Office Report Says." *The Guardian*, December 15, 2020. https://www.theguardian.com/politics/2020/dec/15/child-sexual-abuse-gangs-white-men-home-office-report.

Handelsman, David J., Angelica L. Hirschberg, and Stephane Bermon. "Circulating Testosterone as the Hormonal Basis of Sex Differences in Athletic Performance." *Endocrine Reviews* 39, no. 5 (October 2018): 803–829. https://doi.org/10.1210/er.2018-00020.

Hasenbush, Amira, Andrew R. Flores, and Jody L. Herman. "Gender Identity Nondiscrimination Laws in Public Accommodations: A Review of Evidence Regarding

Safety and Privacy in Public Restrooms, Locker Rooms, and Changing Rooms." *Sexuality Research and Social Policy* 16, no. 1 (March 1, 2019): 70–83. https://doi.org/10.1007/s13178-018-0335-z.

Heid, Markham. "The 7th Most-Common Killer of Men—and How You Can Avoid It." *Men's Health*, June 13, 2016. https://www.menshealth.com/health/a19522651/7th-leading-cause-of-death/.

Hesse, Monica. "We Celebrated Michael Phelps's Genetic Differences. Why Punish Caster Semenya for Hers?" *The Washington Post*, May 3, 2019. https://www.washingtonpost.com/lifestyle/style/we-celebrated-michael-phelpss-genetic-differences-why-punish-caster-semenya-for-hers/2019/05/02/93d08c8c-6c2b-11e9-be3a-33217240a539_story.html.

Hisle-Gorman, Elizabeth, Natasha A. Schvey, Terry A. Adirim, Anna K. Rayne, Apryl Susi, Timothy A. Roberts, and David A. Klein. "Mental Healthcare Utilization of Transgender Youth Before and After Affirming Treatment." *The Journal of Sexual Medicine* 18, no. 8 (August 2021): 1444–1454. https://doi.org/10.1016/j.jsxm.2021.05.014.

Hoffman, Joanna. "Athlete Ally & Chris Mosier Respond to NCAA New Trans Inclusion Policy." Athlete Ally, January 20, 2022. https://www.athleteally.org/athlete-ally-mosier-respond-ncaa-new-trans-policy/.

Hoffman, Kelly M., Sophie Trawalter, Jordan R. Axt, and M. Norman Oliver. "Racial Bias in Pain Assessment and Treatment Recommendations, and False Beliefs About Biological Differences Between Blacks and Whites." *Proceedings of the National Academy of Sciences of the United States of America* 113, no. 16 (April 19, 2016): 4296–4301. https://doi.org/10.1073/pnas.1516047113.

"How Common Is Infertility?" NIH Eunice Kennedy Shriver National Institute of Child Health and Human Development. Accessed March 14, 2023. https://www.nichd.nih.gov/health/topics/infertility/conditioninfo/common.

ICT Staff. "PBS Documentary Explores Navajo Belief in Four Genders." *ICT News*, September 13, 2018. https://ictnews.org/archive/pbs-documentary-explores-navajo-belief-in-four-genders.

Imani, Blair (@blairimani). "#SmarterInSeconds: Tone Policing." TikTok, October 10, 2022. https://www.tiktok.com/@blairimani/video/7155978031603944750?lang=en.

IMDb. s.v. *Irrefutable Proof That Serena Williams Is a Man* (2014). Accessed March 16, 2023. https://www.imdb.com/title/tt5282834/.

"IOC Framework on Fairness, Inclusion and Non-Discrimination on the Basis of Gender Identity and Sex Variations." International Olympic Committee, n.d. https://stillmed.olympics.com/media/Documents/Beyond-the-Games/Human-Rights/IOC-Framework-Fairness-Inclusion-Non-discrimination-2021.pdf.

Italie, Leanne. "Merriam-Webster Declares 'They' Its 2019 Word of the Year." AP News, December 10, 2019. https://apnews.com/article/0b88fde3eeb023355fc2be0f8955a0b5.

Jackson, Hallie, and Courtney Kube. "Trump's Controversial Transgender Military Policy Goes into Effect." *NBC News*, April 12, 2019. https://www.nbcnews.com/feature/nbc-out/trump-s-controversial-transgender-military-policy-goes-effect-n993826.

Jaffee, Kim D., Deirdre A. Shires, and Daphna Stroumsa. "Discrimination and Delayed Health Care Among Transgender Women and Men: Implications for Improving Medical Education and Health Care Delivery." *Medical Care* 54, no. 11 (November 2016): 1010–1016. https://doi.org/10.1097/MLR.0000000000000583.

James, S. E., J. L. Herman, S. Rankin, M. Keisling, L. Mottet, and M. Anafi. *The Report of the 2015 U.S. Transgender Survey.* Washington, DC: National Center for Transgender Equality, 2016. https://transequality.org/sites/default/files/docs/usts /USTS-Full-Report-Dec17.pdf.

Jones, Stephen C. "Subcutaneous Estrogen Replacement Therapy." *The Journal of Reproductive Medicine* 49, no. 3 (March 2004): 139–142.

Kaltiala, Riittakerttu, Elias Heino, Marja Työläjärvi, and Laura Suomalainen. "Adolescent Development and Psychosocial Functioning After Starting Cross-Sex Hormones for Gender Dysphoria." *Nordic Journal of Psychiatry* 74, no. 3 (April 2020): 213–219. https://doi.org/10.1080/08039488.2019.1691260.

Kapit, Dylan. Interview, September 16, 2022.

Klink, Daniel, Martine Caris, Annemieke Heijboer, Michael van Trotsenburg, and Joost Rotteveel. "Bone Mass in Young Adulthood Following Gonadotropin-Releasing Hormone Analog Treatment and Cross-Sex Hormone Treatment in Adolescents with Gender Dysphoria." *The Journal of Clinical Endocrinology & Metabolism* 100, no. 2 (February 2015): E270–275. https://doi.org/10.1210/jc.2014-2439.

Kuper, Laura E., Sunita Stewart, Stephanie Preston, May Lau, and Ximena Lopez. "Body Dissatisfaction and Mental Health Outcomes of Youth on Gender-Affirming Hormone Therapy." *Pediatrics* 145, no. 4 (April 2020): e20193006. https://doi.org /10.1542/peds.2019-3006.

Lake, Jaboa, Valerie Novack, and Mia Ives-Rublee. "Recognizing and Addressing Housing Insecurity for Disabled Renters." Center for American Progress, May 27, 2021. https://www.americanprogress.org/article/recognizing-addressing-housing -insecurity-disabled-renters/.

Lee, Janet Y., Courtney Finlayson, Johanna Olson-Kennedy, Robert Garofalo, Yee-Ming Chan, David V. Glidden, and Stephen M. Rosenthal. "Low Bone Mineral Density in Early Pubertal Transgender/Gender Diverse Youth: Findings from the Trans Youth Care Study." *Journal of the Endocrine Society* 4, no. 9 (July 2020): bvaa065. https://doi.org/10.1210/jendso/bvaa065.

Leland, John. "A Spirit of Belonging, Inside and Out." *The New York Times*, October 8, 2006. https://www.nytimes.com/2006/10/08/fashion/08SPIRIT.html?_r=0.

"The Lens of Systemic Oppression." National Equity Project. Accessed March 14, 2023. https://www.nationalequityproject.org/frameworks/lens-of-systemic-oppression.

"LGBTQ Americans Aren't Fully Protected from Discrimination in 29 States." Freedom for All Americans." Accessed March 14, 2023. https://freedomforallamericans .org/states/.

Linehan, Marsha. *Cognitive-Behavioral Treatment of Borderline Personality Disorder.* New York: Guilford Press, 1993.

López de Lara, Diego, Olga Pérez Rodríguez, Isabel Cuellar Flores, José Luis Pedreira Masa, Lucía Campos-Muñoz, Martín Cuesta Hernández, and José Tomás Ramos Amador. "Psychosocial Assessment in Transgender Adolescents." *Anales de Pediatría*

(English Edition) 93, no. 1 (July 2020): 41–48. https://doi.org/10.1016/j.anpede.2020.01.004.

Lopez, German. "Anti-Transgender Bathroom Hysteria, Explained." *Vox*, February 22, 2017. https://www.vox.com/2016/5/5/11592908/transgender-bathroom-laws-rights.

López Torres, Núria. "Intimate Portraits of Mexico's Third-Gender Muxes." *The New York Times*, September 27, 2021. https://www.nytimes.com/2021/09/27/travel/mexico-muxes-third-gender.html.

Macdonald, V., A. Verster, M. Mello, K. Blondeel, A. Amin, N. Luhmann, R. Baggaley, and M. Doherty. "The World Health Organization's Work and Recommendations for Improving the Health of Trans and Gender Diverse People." *Journal of the International AIDS Society* 25, no. S5 (October 2022). Accessed March 16, 2023. https://onlinelibrary.wiley.com/doi/10.1002/jia2.26004.

Maglaty, Jeanne. "When Did Girls Start Wearing Pink?" *Smithsonian Magazine*, April 7, 2011. https://www.smithsonianmag.com/arts-culture/when-did-girls-start-wearing-pink-1370097/.

Mangla, Ravi. "The Race Dynamics of Online Dating: Why Are Asian Men Less 'Eligible'?" *Pacific Standard*, June 14, 2017. https://psmag.com/social-justice/why-are-asian-men-less-eligible-on-tinder.

"A Map of Gender-Diverse Cultures." PBS, August 11, 2015. https://www.pbs.org/independentlens/content/two-spirits_map-html/.

"Mapping Attacks on LGBTQ Rights in U.S. State Legislatures." American Civil Liberties Union. Accessed June 13, 2023. https://www.aclu.org/legislative-attacks-on-lgbtq-rights.

"March 26, 2021: State Advocacy Update." American Medical Association, March 26, 2021. https://www.ama-assn.org/health-care-advocacy/advocacy-update/march-26-2021-state-advocacy-update.

Marcin, Ashley. "Navigating Puberty: The Tanner Stages." Healthline, February 10, 2023. https://www.healthline.com/health/parenting/stages-of-puberty#tanner-stages.

McLean, Shay-Akil. Interview, September 22, 2022.

Media Matters Staff. "Tucker Carlson Calls Preferred Pronoun Choice 'a War on Nature.'" Media Matters for America, January 21, 2021. https://www.mediamatters.org/fox-news/tucker-carlson-calls-preferred-pronoun-choice-war-nature.

"Medical Organization Statements on Transgender Health Care." TLDEF Trans Health Project. Accessed March 14, 2023. https://transhealthproject.org/resources/medical-organization-statements/.

Merriam-Webster. s.v. "nonbinary *(adj.)*." Accessed March 10, 2023. https://www.merriam-webster.com/dictionary/nonbinary.

Merriam-Webster. s.v. "social construct *(n.)*." Accessed March 1, 2023. https://www.merriam-webster.com/dictionary/social+construct.

Merriam-Webster. s.v. "they *(pronoun)*." Accessed March 12, 2023. https://www.merriam-webster.com/dictionary/they.

"Merriam-Webster: Non-binary Pronoun 'They' Is Word of Year." *BBC News*, December 10, 2019. https://www.bbc.com/news/world-us-canada-50735371.

"Merriam-Webster's Words of the Year 2019." *Merriam-Webster*. Accessed March 12, 2023. https://www.merriam-webster.com/words-at-play/word-of-the-year-2019-they.

Meyerowitz, Joanne. *How Sex Changed: A History of Transsexuality in the United States*. Cambridge, MA: Harvard University Press, 2004.

Migdon, Brooke. "Sixteen Penn Swimmers Say Transgender Athlete Lia Thomas Holds 'Unfair Advantage.'" *The Hill*, February 4, 2022. https://thehill.com/changing-america/respect/diversity-inclusion/592822-sixteen-penn-swimmers-say-transgender-athlete/.

"Milan Garçon (@milangarcon)." Accessed March 12, 2023. https://www.instagram.com/milangarcon/.

Mitchell, Hilary. "The Complex, Divisive History of the Word TERF—and Why It's Not Actually a Slur." *PinkNews*, March 2, 2021. https://www.thepinknews.com/2021/03/02/terf-meaning-jk-rowling-definition-what-is-robert-webb-graham-linehan/.

Moore, Indya. Interview, October 4, 2022.

Mosier, Chris. "Transgender Athletes in the Olympics." Transathlete.com. Accessed March 14, 2023. https://www.transathlete.com/olympics.

Mozes, Alan. "Most Transgender Children Stick with Gender Identity 5 Years Later: Study." HealthDay, May 4, 2022. https://consumer.healthday.com/5-4-most-transgender-children-stick-with-gender-identity-5-years-later-study-2657223343.html.

Muller, Natalie. "Singular 'They' Named Word of the Decade." dw.com, January 4, 2020. https://www.dw.com/en/singular-they-crowned-word-of-the-decade-by-us-linguists/a-51884397.

Murphy, Jessica. "Toronto Professor Jordan Peterson Takes on Gender-Neutral Pronouns," November 4, 2016. https://www.bbc.com/news/world-us-canada-37875695.

"Myths and Facts About Sexual Assault." California Megan's Law Website. Accessed March 14, 2023. https://www.meganslaw.ca.gov/mobile/Education_MythsAndFacts.aspx.

"Nancy Hogshead-Makar Explains Problems with Lia Thomas Situation." *Swimming World News*, December 25, 2021. https://www.swimmingworldmagazine.com/news/nancy-hogshead-makar-explains-problems-with-lia-thomas-situation/.

National History Museum, Los Angeles County. "Beyond Gender: Indigenous Perspectives, Muxe." Accessed March 12, 2023. https://nhm.org/stories/beyond-gender-indigenous-perspectives-muxe.

Ndugga, Nambi, and Samantha Artiga. "Disparities in Health and Health Care: 5 Key Questions and Answers." *KFF*, May 11, 2021. https://www.kff.org/racial-equity-and-health-policy/issue-brief/disparities-in-health-and-health-care-5-key-question-and-answers/.

Oliven, John F. *Sexual Hygiene and Pathology: A Manual for the Physician and the Professions*. 2nd ed., fully rev. and enl. Philadelphia: Lippincott, 1965.

Olson, Kristina R., Lily Durwood, Rachel Horton, Natalie M. Gallagher, and Aaron Devor. "Gender Identity 5 Years After Social Transition." *Pediatrics* 150, no. 2 (August 2022): e2021056082. https://doi.org/10.1542/peds.2021-056082.

Oluo, Ijeoma. *So You Want to Talk About Race*. 1st ed. New York: Seal Press, 2018.

Oxford English Dictionary. s.v. "Korean (*adj.* and *n.*)." Accessed March 16, 2023. https://www.oed.com/view/Entry/104363.

Oxford English Dictionary. s.v. "they (*pron., adj., adv., n.*)." Accessed March 16, 2023. https://www.oed.com/view/Entry/200700.

Panek, Kathryn, and Gabrielle A. Carlson. "Child Psychiatry Opposes AR HB1570." American Civil Liberties Union, March 31, 2021. https://www.aclu.org/letter/child-psychiatry-opposes-ar-hb1570.

Parker Harris, Sarah, Rob Gould, and Courtney Mullin. "Research Brief: Experience of Discrimination and the ADA." ADA National Network. Accessed March 16, 2023. https://adata.org/research_brief/experience-discrimination-and-ada.

"Perpetrators of Sexual Violence: Statistics." RAINN. Accessed March 16, 2023. https://www.rainn.org/statistics/perpetrators-sexual-violence.

Preston, Ashlee Marie. "The Anatomy of Transmisogynoir." *Harper's Bazaar,* September 9, 2020. https://www.harpersbazaar.com/culture/features/a33614214/ashlee-marie-preston-transmisogynoir-essay/.

————. Interview, October 25, 2022.

Pruden, Harlan, and Se-ah-dom Edmo. "Two-Spirit People: Sex, Gender & Sexuality in Historic and Contemporary Native America." National Congress of American Indians. https://www.ncai.org/policy-research-center/initiatives/Pruden-Edmo_TwoSpiritPeople.pdf.

"Pubertal Blockers for Transgender and Gender-Diverse Youth." Mayo Clinic, June 18, 2022. https://www.mayoclinic.org/diseases-conditions/gender-dysphoria/in-depth/pubertal-blockers/art-20459075.

Qian, Yue. "Asian Guys Stereotyped and Excluded in Online Dating." *The Conversation,* February 9, 2020. http://theconversation.com/asian-guys-stereotyped-and-excluded-in-online-dating-130855.

Reback, Cathy J., Kirsty Clark, Ian W. Holloway, and Jesse B. Fletcher. "Health Disparities, Risk Behaviors and Healthcare Utilization Among Transgender Women in Los Angeles County: A Comparison from 1998–1999 to 2015–2016." *AIDS and Behavior* 22, no. 8 (August 2018): 2524–2533. https://doi.org/10.1007/s10461-018-2165-7.

"Renée Richards Documentary Debuts at Tribeca Film Festival." *Tennis Panorama,* April 22, 2011. https://web.archive.org/web/20120403155400/http:/www.tennispanorama.com/archives/9472.

Resneck Jr., Jack. "Everyone Deserves Quality Medical Care Delivered Without Bias." American Medical Association, August 22, 2022. https://www.ama-assn.org/about/leadership/everyone-deserves-quality-medical-care-delivered-without-bias.

Rhodan, Maya. "Why Do We Have Men's and Women's Bathrooms Anyway?" *Time,* May 16, 2016. https://time.com/4337761/history-sex-segregated-bathrooms/.

Riley, John. "School Investigated Athlete's Gender After Her Competitors Complained." *Metro Weekly,* August 19, 2022. https://www.metroweekly.com/2022/08/school-investigated-athletes-gender-after-her-competitors-complained/.

Riley, Wayne J. "Health Disparities: Gaps in Access, Quality and Affordability of Medical Care." *Transactions of the American Clinical and Climatological Association* 123 (2012): 167–174.

Rondinone, Nicholas. "Federal Judge Dismisses Lawsuit Seeking to Bar Trans-gender Athletes from CT Girls Sports." *Connecticut Post*, April 25, 2021. https://www.ctpost.com/news/article/Federal-judge-dismisses-lawsuit-seeking -to-bar-16128048.php.

Russo, Juniper. "Definition of 'Cissexism.'" *The Queer Dictionary*. Accessed March 16, 2023. http://queerdictionary.blogspot.com/2014/09/definition-of-cissexism.html.

Salam, Maya. "What Is Toxic Masculinity?" *The New York Times*, January 22, 2019. https://www.nytimes.com/2019/01/22/us/toxic-masculinity.html.

Schillace, Brandy. "The Forgotten History of the World's First Trans Clinic." *Scientific American*, May 4, 2021. https://www.scientificamerican.com/article/the-forgotten -history-of-the-worlds-first-trans-clinic/.

Schrager, Allison. "No Abortion Means Poor States Will Get Poorer." *Bloomberg*, May 4, 2022. https://www.bloomberg.com/opinion/articles/2022-05-04/roe-v-wade -outlawing-abortion-will-keep-more-women-poor.

Scott, Charlie Amaya. Interview, September 21, 2022.

Seip, Nick. "Why LGBT Youth Homelessness? Why Not All Youth?" True Colors United, April 26, 2016. https://truecolorsunited.org/2016/04/26/why-lgbt-youth/.

Serano, Julia. "Julia's Trans, Gender, Sexuality, and Activism Glossary." juliaserano.com. Accessed March 16, 2023. http://www.juliaserano.com/terminology.html.

"Sexual Assault and the LGBTQ Community." Human Rights Campaign. Accessed March 16, 2023. https://www.hrc.org/resources/sexual-assault-and-the-lgbt-community.

"Sexual Assault: The Numbers." Office of Justice Programs, Office for Victims of Crime. Accessed March 16, 2023. https://ovc.ojp.gov/sites/g/files/xyckuh226/files /pubs/forge/sexual_numbers.html.

"Sexualized Violence Statistics." Supporting Survivors, Cal Poly Humboldt. Accessed March 16, 2023. https://supportingsurvivors.humboldt.edu/statistics.

shawndeez. Interview, October 14, 2022.

Simon, Barbara. "Medical Association Statements Supporting Trans Youth Healthcare and Against Discriminatory Bills." GLAAD, April 19, 2021. https://www.glaad .org/blog/medical-association-statements-supporting-trans-youth-healthcare -and-against-discriminatory.

Singh, Devita. "A Follow-Up Study of Boys with Gender Identity Disorder." PhD thesis, University of Toronto, 2012. 341.

Smith-Johnson, Madeline. "Transgender Adults Have Higher Rates of Disability than Their Cisgender Counterparts." *Health Affairs* 41, no. 10 (October 2022). https:// doi.org/10.1377/hlthaff.2022.00500.

Snipes, B. Hawk. Interview, September 15, 2022.

Sorbara, Julia C., Lyne N. Chiniara, Shelby Thompson, and Mark R. Palmert. "Mental Health and Timing of Gender-Affirming Care." *Pediatrics* 146, no. 4 (October 1, 2020): e20193600. https://doi.org/10.1542/peds.2019-3600.

Stahl, Shane. "Mythbuster: Debunking Anti-Transgender Messages." Freedom for All Americans, March 14, 2021. https://freedomforallamericans.org/mythbuster -debunking-anti-transgender-messages/.

Steensma, Thomas D., Roeline Biemond, Fijgje de Boer, and Peggy T. Cohen-Kettenis. "Desisting and Persisting Gender Dysphoria After Childhood: A Qualitative

Follow-Up Study." *Clinical Child Psychology and Psychiatry* 16, no. 4 (October 2011): 499–516. https://doi.org/10.1177/1359104510378303.

"Suicide Statistics." American Foundation for Suicide Prevention, November 15, 2019. https://afsp.org/suicide-statistics/.

"Super Straight." LGBT+ pride Wiki. Accessed March 14, 2023. https://lgbt-pride .fandom.com/wiki/Super_Straight.

"Sweet 16 Birthday Breast Implants Spark Uproar in Britain," *The Morning Journal*, January 5, 2001. https://www.morningjournal.com/news/sweet-16-birthday -breast-implants-spark-uproar-in-britain/article_1ba78a3c-af99-5660-9058 -cc119fa3ef45.html.

Szilagyi, Moira. "Why We Stand Up for Transgender Children and Teens." AAP Voices. American Academy of Pediatrics, August 10, 2022. https://www.aap.org /en/news-room/aap-voices/why-we-stand-up-for-transgender-children-and-teens/.

Tennison, Crissonna. "Feminism 101: What Is Cissexism?" *FEM*, May 29, 2016. https://femmagazine.com/feminism-101-what-is-cissexism/.

Terlizzi, Emily P., and Benjamin Zablotsky. "Mental Health Treatment Among Adults: United States, 2019." Centers for Disease Control and Prevention, September 2020. https://www.cdc.gov/nchs/products/databriefs/db380.htm.

"Top Times/Event Rank Search." USA Swimming. Accessed March 16, 2023. http: //www.usaswimming.org/times/popular-resources/event-rank-search.

Tordoff, Diana M., Jonathon W. Wanta, Arin Collin, Cesalie Stepney, David J. Inwards-Breland, and Kym Ahrens. "Mental Health Outcomes in Transgender and Nonbinary Youths Receiving Gender-Affirming Care." *JAMA Network Open* 5, no. 2 (February 2022): e220978. https://doi.org/10.1001/jamanetworkopen.2022.0978.

Trans Legislation Tracker. "2023 Anti-Trans Bills: Trans Legislation Tracker." Accessed June 13, 2023. https://translegislation.com.

"Transgender Teens with Restricted Bathroom Access at Higher Risk of Sexual Assault." Harvard T.H. Chan School of Public Health, May 7, 2019. https://www .hsph.harvard.edu/news/hsph-in-the-news/transgender-teens-restricted-bathroom -access-sexual-assault/.

TransHub. "Feminising Hormones." Accessed March 16, 2023. https://www.transhub .org.au/clinicians/feminising-hormones.

Turban, Jack. "The Evidence for Trans Youth Gender-Affirming Medical Care." *Psychology Today*, January 24, 2022. https://www.psychologytoday.com/us/blog /political-minds/202201/the-evidence-trans-youth-gender-affirming-medical -care.

Turban, Jack L., Brett Dolotina, Dana King, and Alex S. Keuroghlian. "Sex Assigned at Birth Ratio Among Transgender and Gender Diverse Adolescents in the United States." *Pediatrics* 150, no. 3 (September 1, 2022): e2022056567. https://doi .org/10.1542/peds.2022-056567.

Turban, Jack L., Dana King, Jeremi M. Carswell, and Alex S. Keuroghlian. "Pubertal Suppression for Transgender Youth and Risk of Suicidal Ideation." *Pediatrics* 145, no. 2 (February 2020): e20191725. https://doi.org/10.1542/peds.2019-1725.

Turban, Jack L., Dana King, Julia Kobe, Sari L. Reisner, and Alex S. Keuroghlian. "Access to Gender-Affirming Hormones During Adolescence and Mental Health

Outcomes Among Transgender Adults." *PLoS One* 17, no. 1 (January 2022): e0261039. https://doi.org/10.1371/journal.pone.0261039.

Turban, Jack L., Dana King, Sari L. Reisner, and Alex S. Keuroghlian. "Psychological Attempts to Change a Person's Gender Identity from Transgender to Cisgender: Estimated Prevalence Across US States, 2015." *American Journal of Public Health* 109, no. 10 (October 2019): 1452–1454. https://doi.org/10.2105/AJPH.2019.305237.

Turban, Jack L., Stephanie S. Loo, Anthony N. Almazan, and Alex S. Keuroghlian. "Factors Leading to 'Detransition' Among Transgender and Gender Diverse People in the United States: A Mixed-Methods Analysis." *LGBT Health* 8, no. 4 (June 1, 2021): 273–280. https://doi.org/10.1089/lgbt.2020.0437.

"Two-Spirit Community." Researching for LGBTQ2S+ Health. Accessed March 14, 2023. https://lgbtqhealth.ca/community/two-spirit.php.

van der Loos, Maria Anna Theodora Catharina, Sabine Elisabeth Hannema, Daniel Tatting Klink, Martin den Heijer, and Chantal Maria Wiepjes. "Continuation of Gender-Affirming Hormones in Transgender People Starting Puberty Suppression in Adolescence: A Cohort Study in the Netherlands." *The Lancet Child & Adolescent Health* 6, no. 12 (December 2022): 869–875. https://doi.org/10.1016/S2352-4642(22)00254-1.

van der Miesen, Anna I. R., Thomas D. Steensma, Annelou L. C. de Vries, Henny Bos, and Arne Popma. "Psychological Functioning in Transgender Adolescents Before and After Gender-Affirmative Care Compared with Cisgender General Population Peers." *Journal of Adolescent Health* 66, no. 6 (June 2020): 699–704. https://doi.org/10.1016/j.jadohealth.2019.12.018.

"Varsity Odds." ScholarshipStats.com, August 31, 2020. https://scholarshipstats.com/varsityodds.

Vasuian, Ana. "Do You Regret Having Cosmetic Surgery?" Medical Accident Group, May 28, 2014. https://www.medicalaccidentgroup.co.uk/news/do-you-regret-having-cosmetic-surgery/.

"Victims of Sexual Violence: Statistics." RAINN. Accessed March 14, 2023. https://www.rainn.org/statistics/victims-sexual-violence.

Webb, Karleigh. "Trans Boxer Patricio Manuel Wins First Match in Four Years, Improves to 2-0." Outsports, March 22, 2023. https://www.outsports.com/trans/2023/3/22/23650980/patricio-manuel-hien-hunyh-boxer-trans-win-long-beach.

Weissmann, Jordan. "So, Let's Talk About Republicans and Sex Crimes." *Slate*, April 9, 2022. https://slate.com/news-and-politics/2022/04/from-hastert-to-gaetz-lets-talk-about-republicans-and-sex-crimes.html.

Wertheim, Jon. "She's a Transgender Pioneer, But Renée Richards Prefers to Stay Out of the Spotlight." *Sports Illustrated*, June 28, 2019. https://www.si.com/tennis/2019/06/28/renee-richards-gender-identity-politics-transgender-where-are-they-now.

West, J., and D. I. Templer. "Child Molestation, Rape, and Ethnicity." *Psychological Reports* 75, no. 3, pt. 1 (December 1994): 1326. https://doi.org/10.2466/pr0.1994.75.3.1326.

"What Does It Mean to Be Transgender?" *Them*, April 25, 2022. https://www.them.us/story/inqueery-transgender.

"What Is Executive Function? And How Does It Relate to Child Development?" Center on the Developing Child, Harvard University. Accessed March 16, 2023. https:// developingchild.harvard.edu/resources/what-is-executive-function-and-how -does-it-relate-to-child-development/.

Wikipedia. s.v. "Fallon Fox." Accessed March 7, 2023. https://en.wikipedia.org/w/index .php?title=Fallon_Fox&oldid=1143444121.

Wikipedia. s.v. "Rape by Deception." Accessed, March 10, 2023. https://en.wikipedia .org/w/index.php?title=Rape_by_deception&oldid=1143895880.

Zeigler, Cyd. "Read the Olympics' New Transgender Guidelines That Will Not Man-date Surgery." Outsports, January 21, 2016. https://www.outsports.com/2016/1/21 /10812404/transgender-ioc-policy-new-olympics.

Zelazo, Philip David, Clancy B. Blair, and Michael T. Willoughby. "Executive Func-tion: Implications for Education." National Center for Education Research, 2016. https://eric.ed.gov/?id=ED570880.

Zuckerman, Diana, "Teenagers and Cosmetic Surgery," Virtual Mentor 7 no. 3 (March 2005): 253–256, https://journalofethics.ama-assn.org/article/teenagers-and-cosmetic -surgery/2005-03.

NOTES

INTRODUCTION

1. "Mapping Attacks on LGBTQ Rights in U.S. State Legislatures," American Civil Liberties Union, accessed June 13, 2023, https://www.aclu.org/legislative-attacks-on-lgbtq-rights.

2. "2023 Anti-trans Bills Tracker," Trans Legislation Tracker, accessed June 13, 2023, https://translegislation.com.

CHAPTER 1

1. Elle Deran, Interview, October 13, 2022.

CHAPTER 2

1. Amy B. Wisniewski "Complete Androgen Insensitivity Syndrome: Long-Term Medical, Surgical, and Psychosexual Outcome." *The Journal of Clinical Endocrinology & Metabolism* 85, no. 8 (August 2000): 2664–2669. https://doi.org/10.1210/jcem.85.8.6742.

2. B. Kulshreshtha, P. Philibert, M. Eunice et al. "Apparent Male Gender Identity in a Patient with Complete Androgen Insensitivity Syndrome." *Arch Sex Behav* 38, 873–875 (2009). https://doi.org/10.1007/s10508-009-9526-2.

CHAPTER 3

1. Shay-Akil McLean, Interview, September 22, 2022.

2. Jamey Jesperson, "Honouring Trans Lives, Historicising Trans Death," *History Workshop*, November 20, 2020, https://www.historyworkshop.org.uk/queer-history/honouring-trans-lives-historicising-trans-death/.

3. McLean, Interview.

4. *Merriam-Webster*, s.v. "social construct (*n.*)," accessed March 1, 2023, https://www.merriam-webster.com/dictionary/social+construct.

5. Carol Bainbridge, "What Is a Social Construct? Why Every Part of Society Is a Social Construct," Verywell Mind, March 14, 2023, https://www.verywellmind.com/definition-of-social-construct-1448922.

6. McLean, Interview.

7. McLean, Interview.

8. Morg Daniels, "Ancient Mesopotamian Transgender and Non-Binary Identities," Academus Education, June 30, 2021, https://www.academuseducation.co.uk/post/ancient-mesopotamian-transgender-and-non-binary-identities.

9. "Two-Spirit Community," Researching for LGBTQ2S+ Health, accessed March 14, 2023, https://lgbtqhealth.ca/community/two-spirit.php.

10. John Leland, "A Spirit of Belonging, Inside and Out," *The New York Times*, October 8, 2006, https://www.nytimes.com/2006/10/08/fashion/08SPIRIT.html?_r=0.

11. Harlan Pruden and Se-ah-dom Edmo, "Two-Spirit People: Sex, Gender & Sexuality in Historic and Contemporary Native America," National Congress of American Indians, https://www.ncai.org/policy-research-center/initiatives/Pruden-Edmo_TwoSpiritPeople.pdf.

12. Indya Moore, Interview, October 4, 2022.

13. "A Map of Gender-Diverse Cultures," PBS, August 11, 2015, https://www.pbs.org/independentlens/content/two-spirits_map-html/.

14. Galen Druke, "Native American 'Two-Spirit People' Serve Unique Roles Within Their Communities," Wisconsin Public Radio, June 27, 2014, https://www.wpr.org/native-american-two-spirit-people-serve-unique-roles-within-their-communities.

15. ICT Staff, "PBS Documentary Explores Navajo Belief in Four Genders," *ICT News*, September 13, 2018, https://ictnews.org/archive/pbs-documentary-explores-navajo-belief-in-four-genders.

16. Núria López Torres, "Intimate Portraits of Mexico's Third-Gender Muxes," *The New York Times*, September 27, 2021, https://www.nytimes.com/2021/09/27/travel/mexico-muxes-third-gender.html.

17. "Beyond Gender: Indigenous Perspectives, Muxe," National History Museum, Los Angeles County, accessed March 12, 2023, https://nhm.org/stories/beyond-gender-indigenous-perspectives-muxe.

18. Pruden and Edmo, "Two-Spirit People."

19. "A Map of Gender-Diverse Cultures."

20. Indya Moore, Interview, October 4, 2022.

21. shawndeez, Interview, October 14, 2022.

22. "1.2 Million LGBTQ Adults in the US Identify as Nonbinary," Williams Institute, June 22, 2021, https://williamsinstitute.law.ucla.edu/press/lgbtq-nonbinary-press-release/.

23. *Merriam-Webster*, s.v. "nonbinary (adj.)," accessed March 10, 2023, https://www.merriam-webster.com/dictionary/nonbinary.

24. *Merriam-Webster*, s.v. "nonbinary."

25. B. Hawk Snipes, Interview, September 15, 2022.

26. Charlie Amáyá Scott, Interview, September 21, 2022.

27. Elle Deran, Interview, October 13, 2022.

28. McLean, Interview.

29. Scott, Interview.

30. Snipes, Interview.

31. Dylan Kapit, Interview, September 16, 2022.

32. Kapit, Interview.

33. Snipes, Interview.

34. Snipes, Interview.

35. Milan Garçon (@milangarcon), Instagram account, accessed March 12, 2023, https://www.instagram.com/milangarcon/.

36. *Oxford English Dictionary*, s.v. "Korean (*adj.* and *n.*)," accessed March 16, 2023, https://www.oed.com/view/Entry/104363.

CHAPTER 4

1. "Feminising Hormones," TransHub, accessed March 16, 2023, https://www.transhub.org.au/clinicians/feminising-hormones.

2. Stephen C. Jones, "Subcutaneous Estrogen Replacement Therapy," *The Journal of Reproductive Medicine* 49, no. 3 (March 2004): 139–142.

3. Syed W. Ahmad et al., "Is Oral Testosterone the New Frontier of Testosterone Replacement Therapy?," *Cureus* 14, no. 8 (August 2022): e27796, https://doi.org/10.7759/cureus.27796.

4. Office of the Commissioner, "FDA Approves New Oral Testosterone Capsule for Treatment of Men with Certain Forms of Hypogonadism," FDA, March 24, 2020, https://www.fda.gov/news-events/press-announcements/fda-approves-new-oral-testosterone-capsule-treatment-men-certain-forms-hypogonadism.

5. Diane S. Aschenbrenner, "First Oral Testosterone Product Now Available," *The American Journal of Nursing* 119, no. 8 (August 2019): 22, https://doi.org/10.1097/01.NAJ.0000577424.31609.23.

6. "Access to Health Services," Healthy People 2030, accessed March 16, 2023, https://health.gov/healthypeople/priority-areas/social-determinants-health/literature-summaries/access-health-services#cit11.

7. Wayne J. Riley, "Health Disparities: Gaps in Access, Quality and Affordability of Medical Care," *Transactions of the American Clinical and Climatological Association* 123 (2012): 167–174.

8. Nambi Ndugga and Samantha Artiga, "Disparities in Health and Health Care: 5 Key Questions and Answers," *KFF*, May 11, 2021, https://www.kff.org/racial-equity-and-health-policy/issue-brief/disparities-in-health-and-health-care-5-key-question-and-answers/.

9. Jaime M. Grant et al., "National Transgender Discrimination Survey Report on Health and Health Care," National Center for Transgender Equality and the National Gay and Lesbian Task Force, October 2010, https://cancer-network.org/wp-content/uploads/2017/02/National_Transgender_Discrimination_Survey_Report_on_health_and_health_care.pdf.

10. Kim D. Jaffee, Deirdre A. Shires, and Daphna Stroumsa, "Discrimination and Delayed Health Care Among Transgender Women and Men: Implications for Improving Medical Education and Health Care Delivery," *Medical Care* 54, no. 11 (November 2016): 1010–1016, https://doi.org/10.1097/MLR.0000000000000583.

11. Kim D. Jaffee, Deirdre A. Shires, and Daphna Stroumsa, "Discrimination and Delayed Health Care."

12. Cathy J. Reback et al., "Health Disparities, Risk Behaviors and Healthcare Utilization Among Transgender Women in Los Angeles County: A Comparison from 1998–1999 to 2015–2016," *AIDS and Behavior* 22, no. 8 (August 2018): 2524–2533, https://doi.org/10.1007/s10461-018-2165-7.

13. "Breast Augmentation," UCSF Gender Affirming Health Program, accessed March 16, 2023, https://transcare.ucsf.edu/breast-augmentation.

CHAPTER 5

1. Media Matters Staff, "Tucker Carlson Calls Preferred Pronoun Choice 'a War on Nature,'" Media Matters for America, January 21, 2021, https://www.mediamatters.org/fox-news/tucker-carlson-calls-preferred-pronoun-choice-war-nature.

2. Jeanne Maglaty, "When Did Girls Start Wearing Pink?," *Smithsonian Magazine*, April 7, 2011, https://www.smithsonianmag.com/arts-culture/when-did-girls-start-wearing-pink-1370097/.

3. S. E. James et al., *The Report of the 2015 U.S. Transgender Survey* (Washington, DC: National Center for Transgender Equality, 2016), https://transequality.org/sites/default/files/docs/usts/USTS-Full-Report-Dec17.pdf.

4. *Merriam-Webster*, s.v. "they (*pronoun*)," accessed March 12, 2023, https://www.merriam-webster.com/dictionary/they.

5. "Merriam-Webster: Non-binary Pronoun 'They' Is Word of Year," *BBC News*, December 10, 2019, https://www.bbc.com/news/world-us-canada-50735371.

6. Leanne Italie, "Merriam-Webster Declares 'They' Its 2019 Word of the Year," AP News, December 10, 2019, https://apnews.com/article/0b88fde3eeb023355fc2be0f8955a0b5.

7. "Merriam-Webster's Words of the Year 2019," *Merriam-Webster*, accessed March 12, 2023, https://www.merriam-webster.com/words-at-play/word-of-the-year-2019-they.

8. "2015 Word of the Year Is Singular 'They,'" *American Dialect Society* (blog), January 8, 2016, https://americandialect.org/2015-word-of-the-year-is-singular-they.

9. Natalie Muller, "Singular 'They' Named Word of the Decade," dw.com, January 4, 2020, https://www.dw.com/en/singular-they-crowned-word-of-the-decade-by-us-linguists/a-51884397.

10. *Oxford English Dictionary*, s.v. "they (*pron., adj., adv., n.*)," accessed March 16, 2023, https://www.oed.com/view/Entry/200700.

11. Ariane de Vogue and Devan Cole, "Supreme Court limits LGBTQ protections with ruling in favor of Christian web designer," CNN Politics, July 1, 2023, https://www.cnn.com/2023/06/30/politics/supreme-court-303-creative-lgbtq-rights-colorado/index.html.

12. Jessica Murphy, "Toronto Professor Jordan Peterson Takes on Gender-Neutral Pronouns," *BBC News*, November 4, 2016, https://www.bbc.com/news/world-us-canada-37875695.

13. Murphy, "Toronto Professor Jordan Peterson."

CHAPTER 7

1. Brandy Schillace, "The Forgotten History of the World's First Trans Clinic," *Scientific American*, May 4, 2021, https://www.scientificamerican.com/article/the-forgotten-history-of-the-worlds-first-trans-clinic/.

2. Joanne Meyerowitz, *How Sex Changed: A History of Transsexuality in the United States* (Cambridge, MA: Harvard University Press, 2004).

3. Schillace, "The Forgotten History."

4. Schillace, "The Forgotten History."

5. Schillace, "The Forgotten History."

6. Meyerowitz, *How Sex Changed*.

7. "David Oliver Cauldwell," Academic Dictionaries and Encyclopedias, accessed March 12, 2023, https://en-academic.com/dic.nsf/enwiki/11600702.

8. Meyerowitz, *How Sex Changed*.

9. Meyerowitz, *How Sex Changed*.

10. Meyerowitz, *How Sex Changed*.

11. "Gender Dysphoria Diagnosis," American Psychiatric Association, https://www.psychiatry.org/psychiatrists/cultural-competency/education/transgender-and-gender-nonconforming-patients/gender-dysphoria-diagnosis.

12. John F. Oliven, *Sexual Hygiene and Pathology: A Manual for the Physician and the Professions*, 2nd ed., fully rev. and enl. (Philadelphia: Lippincott, 1965).

13. "What Does It Mean to Be Transgender?," *Them*, April 25, 2022, https://www.them.us/story/inqueery-transgender.

14. American Psychiatric Association, *Diagnostic and Statistical Manual of Mental Disorders: DSM-5*, 5th ed. (Washington, DC: American Psychiatric Association, 2013).

CHAPTER 8

1. Nick Seip, "Why LGBT Youth Homelessness? Why Not All Youth?," True Colors United, April 26, 2016, https://truecolorsunited.org/2016/04/26/why-lgbt-youth/.

CHAPTER 9

1. KC Clements, "What Does It Mean to Be Cissexist?," Healthline, June 1, 2021, https://www.healthline.com/health/transgender/cissexist.

2. Julia Serano, "Julia's Trans, Gender, Sexuality, and Activism Glossary," juliaserano.com, accessed March 16, 2023, http://www.juliaserano.com/terminology.html.

3. Crissonna Tennison, "Feminism 101: What Is Cissexism?," *FEM*, May 29, 2016, https://femmagazine.com/feminism-101-what-is-cissexism/.

4. Juniper Russo, "Definition of 'Cissexism,'" *The Queer Dictionary*, accessed March 16, 2023, http://queerdictionary.blogspot.com/2014/09/definition-of-cissexism.html.

5. "The Lens of Systemic Oppression," National Equity Project, accessed March 14, 2023, https://www.nationalequityproject.org/frameworks/lens-of-systemic-oppression.

6. "Medical Organization Statements on Transgender Health Care," TLDEF Trans Health Project, accessed March 14, 2023, https://transhealthproject.org/resources/medical-organization-statements/.

7. Barbara Simon, "Medical Association Statements Supporting Trans Youth Healthcare and Against Discriminatory Bills," GLAAD, April 19, 2021, https://www.glaad.org/blog/medical-association-statements-supporting-trans-youth-healthcare-and-against-discriminatory.

8. "Doctors Agree: Gender-Affirming Care Is Life-Saving Care," American Civil Liberties Union, April 1, 2021, https://www.aclu.org/news/lgbtq-rights/doctors-agree-gender-affirming-care-is-life-saving-care.

9. Moira Szilagyi, "Why We Stand Up for Transgender Children and Teens," AAP Voices, American Academy of Pediatrics, August 10, 2022, https://www.aap.org/en /news-room/aap-voices/why-we-stand-up-for-transgender-children-and-teens/.

10. V. Macdonald et al., "The World Health Organization's Work and Recommendations for Improving the Health of Trans and Gender Diverse People," *Journal of the International AIDS Society* 25, no. S5 (October 2022), accessed March 16, 2023, https://onlinelibrary.wiley.com/doi/10.1002/jia2.26004.

11. "Endocrine Society Alarmed at Criminalization of Transgender Medicine," Endocrine Society, February 23, 2022, https://www.endocrine.org/news -and-advocacy/news-room/2022/endocrine-society-alarmed-at-criminalization-of -transgender-medicine.

12. "March 26, 2021: State Advocacy Update," American Medical Association, March 26, 2021, https://www.ama-assn.org/health-care-advocacy/advocacy-update /march-26-2021-state-advocacy-update.

13. "Frontline Physicians Oppose Legislation That Interferes in or Criminalizes Patient Care," American Psychiatric Association, April 2, 2021, https://www .psychiatry.org:443/news-room/news-releases/frontline-physicians-oppose-legislation -that-inter.

14. Lee Savio Beers, "American Academy of Pediatrics Speaks Out Against Bills Harming Transgender Youth," American Academy of Pediatrics, accessed March 16, 2023, https://www.aap.org/en/news-room/news-releases/aap/2021/american-academy -of-pediatrics-speaks-out-against-bills-harming-transgender-youth/.

15. "Discriminatory Policies Threaten Care for Transgender, Gender Diverse Individuals," Endocrine Society, December 16, 2020, https://www.endocrine.org /news-and-advocacy/news-room/2020/discriminatory-policies-threaten-care-for -transgender-gender-diverse-individuals.

16. "AACAP Statement Responding to Efforts to Ban Evidence-Based Care for Transgender and Gender Diverse," American Academy of Child and Adolescent Psychiatry, November 8, 2019, https://www.aacap.org/AACAP/Latest_News/AACAP _Statement_Responding_to_Efforts-to_ban_Evidence-Based_Care_for_Transgender _and_Gender_Diverse.aspx.

17. Jack Resneck Jr., "Everyone Deserves Quality Medical Care Delivered Without Bias," American Medical Association, August 22, 2022, https://www.ama-assn.org /about/leadership/everyone-deserves-quality-medical-care-delivered-without-bias.

18. Kathryn Panek and Gabrielle A. Carlson, "Child Psychiatry Opposes AR HB1570," American Civil Liberties Union, March 31, 2021, https://www.aclu.org /letter/child-psychiatry-opposes-ar-hb1570.

19. Hallie Jackson and Courtney Kube, "Trump's Controversial Transgender Military Policy Goes into Effect," *NBC News*, April 12, 2019, https://www .nbcnews.com/feature/nbc-out/trump-s-controversial-transgender-military-policy -goes-effect-n993826.

20. "Fatal Violence Against the Transgender and Gender Non-Conforming Community in 2021," Human Rights Campaign, accessed March 14, 2023, https://www .hrc.org/resources/fatal-violence-against-the-transgender-and-gender-non-conforming -community-in-2021.

CHAPTER 11

1. Jack Turban, "The Evidence for Trans Youth Gender-Affirming Medical Care," *Psychology Today*, January 24, 2022, https://www.psychologytoday.com/us/blog /political-minds/202201/the-evidence-trans-youth-gender-affirming-medical-care.

2. Jack L. Turban et al., "Psychological Attempts to Change a Person's Gender Identity from Transgender to Cisgender: Estimated Prevalence Across US States, 2015," *American Journal of Public Health* 109, no. 10 (October 2019): 1452–1454, https://doi.org/10.2105/AJPH.2019.305237.

3. James et al., *The Report of the 2015 U.S. Transgender Survey.*

4. Annelou L. C. de Vries et al., "Puberty Suppression in Adolescents with Gender Identity Disorder: A Prospective Follow-Up Study," *The Journal of Sexual Medicine* 8, no. 8 (August 2011): 2276–2283, https://doi.org/10.1111/j.1743-6109.2010.01943.x.

5. Annelou L. C. de Vries et al., "Young Adult Psychological Outcome After Puberty Suppression and Gender Reassignment," *Pediatrics* 134, no. 4 (October 1, 2014): 696–704, https://doi.org/10.1542/peds.2013-2958.

6. Rosalia Costa et al., "Psychological Support, Puberty Suppression, and Psychosocial Functioning in Adolescents with Gender Dysphoria," *The Journal of Sexual Medicine* 12, no. 11 (November 2015): 2206–2214, https://doi.org/10.1111/jsm.13034.

7. Riittakerttu Kaltiala et al., "Adolescent Development and Psychosocial Functioning After Starting Cross-Sex Hormones for Gender Dysphoria," *Nordic Journal of Psychiatry* 74, no. 3 (April 2020): 213–219, https://doi.org/10.1080/08039488.2019.1691260.

8. Diego López de Lara et al., "Psychosocial Assessment in Transgender Adolescents," *Anales de Pediatría (English Edition)* 93, no. 1 (July 2020): 41–48, https://doi .org/10.1016/j.anpede.2020.01.004.

9. Anna I. R. van der Miesen et al., "Psychological Functioning in Transgender Adolescents Before and After Gender-Affirmative Care Compared with Cisgender General Population Peers," *Journal of Adolescent Health* 66, no. 6 (June 2020): 699–704, https://doi.org/10.1016/j.jadohealth.2019.12.018.

10. Christal Achille et al., "Longitudinal Impact of Gender-Affirming Endocrine Intervention on the Mental Health and Well-Being of Transgender Youths: Preliminary Results," *International Journal of Pediatric Endocrinology* 2020, no. 1 (December 2020), https://doi.org/10.1186/s13633-020-00078-2.

11. Laura E. Kuper et al., "Body Dissatisfaction and Mental Health Outcomes of Youth on Gender-Affirming Hormone Therapy," *Pediatrics* 145, no. 4 (April 2020): e20193006, https://doi.org/10.1542/peds.2019-3006.

12. Jack L. Turban et al., "Pubertal Suppression for Transgender Youth and Risk of Suicidal Ideation," *Pediatrics* 145, no. 2 (February 2020): e20191725, https://doi .org/10.1542/peds.2019-1725.

13. Polly Carmichael et al., "Short-Term Outcomes of Pubertal Suppression in a Selected Cohort of 12 to 15 Year Old Young People with Persistent Gender Dysphoria in the UK," ed. Geilson Lima Santana, *PLoS One* 16, no. 2 (February 2, 2021): e0243894, https://doi.org/10.1371/journal.pone.0243894.

14. Connor Grannis et al., "Testosterone Treatment, Internalizing Symptoms, and Body Image Dissatisfaction in Transgender Boys," *Psychoneuroendocrinology* 132 (October 2021): 105358, https://doi.org/10.1016/j.psyneuen.2021.105358.

15. Elizabeth Hisle-Gorman et al., "Mental Healthcare Utilization of Transgender Youth Before and After Affirming Treatment," *The Journal of Sexual Medicine* 18, no. 8 (August 2021): 1444–1454, https://doi.org/10.1016/j.jsxm.2021.05.014.

16. Amy E. Green et al., "Association of Gender-Affirming Hormone Therapy with Depression, Thoughts of Suicide, and Attempted Suicide Among Transgender and Nonbinary Youth," *Journal of Adolescent Health* 70, no. 4 (April 2022): 643–649, https://doi.org/10.1016/j.jadohealth.2021.10.036.

17. Jack L. Turban et al., "Access to Gender-Affirming Hormones During Adolescence and Mental Health Outcomes Among Transgender Adults," *PLoS One* 17, no. 1 (January 2022): e0261039, https://doi.org/10.1371/journal.pone.0261039.

18. Diana M. Tordoff et al., "Mental Health Outcomes in Transgender and Nonbinary Youths Receiving Gender-Affirming Care," *JAMA Network Open* 5, no. 2 (February 2022): e220978, https://doi.org/10.1001/jamanetworkopen.2022.0978.

19. Kristina R. Olson et al., "Gender Identity 5 Years After Social Transition," *Pediatrics* 150, no. 2 (August 2022): e2021056082, https://doi.org/10.1542/peds.2021 -056082.

20. Maria Anna Theodora Catharina van der Loos et al., "Continuation of Gender-Affirming Hormones in Transgender People Starting Puberty Suppression in Adolescence: A Cohort Study in the Netherlands," *The Lancet Child & Adolescent Health* 6, no. 12 (December 2022): 869–875, https://doi.org/10.1016/S2352-4642(22)00254-1.

21. Philip David Zelazo, Clancy B. Blair, and Michael T. Willoughby, "Executive Function: Implications for Education," National Center for Education Research, 2016, https://eric.ed.gov/?id=ED570880.

22. Zelazo, Blair, and Willoughby, "Executive Function."

23. Heather J. Ferguson, Victoria E. A. Brunsdon, and Elisabeth E. F. Bradford, "The Developmental Trajectories of Executive Function from Adolescence to Old Age," *Scientific Reports* 11, no. 1 (January 14, 2021), https://doi.org/10.1038/s41598 -020-80866-1.

24. "What Is Executive Function? And How Does It Relate to Child Development?," Center on the Developing Child, Harvard University, accessed March 16, 2023, https://developingchild.harvard.edu/resources/what-is-executive-function-and -how-does-it-relate-to-child-development/.

25. Adele Diamond, "Executive Functions," *Annual Review of Psychology* 64, no. 1 (January 3, 2013): 135–168, https://doi.org/10.1146/annurev-psych-113011-143750.

26. Marsha M. Linehan, *Cognitive-Behavioral Treatment of Borderline Personality Disorder* (New York: Guilford Press, 1993).

27. John Bowlby, *Attachment and Loss* (New York: Basic Books, 1969).

28. Kara N. Denny et al., "Intuitive Eating in Young Adults. Who Is Doing It, and How Is It Related to Disordered Eating Behaviors?," *Appetite* 60, no. 1 (January 1, 2013): 13–19, https://doi.org/10.1016/j.appet.2012.09.029.

CHAPTER 12

1. "Gender Incongruence and Transgender Health in the ICD," World Health Organizaiton, accessed March 14, 2023, https://www.who.int/standards/classifications /frequently-asked-questions/gender-incongruence-and-transgender-health-in-the-icd.

2. "Pubertal Blockers for Transgender and Gender-Diverse Youth," Mayo Clinic, June 18, 2022, https://www.mayoclinic.org/diseases-conditions/gender-dysphoria/in-depth/pubertal-blockers/art-20459075.

3. Ashley Marcin, "Navigating Puberty: The Tanner Stages," Healthline, February 10, 2023, https://www.healthline.com/health/parenting/stages-of-puberty#tanner-stages.

4. Jordan Weissmann, "So, Let's Talk About Republicans and Sex Crimes," *Slate*, April 9, 2022, https://slate.com/news-and-politics/2022/04/from-hastert-to-gaetz-lets-talk-about-republicans-and-sex-crimes.html.

5. "Perpetrators of Sexual Violence: Statistics," RAINN, accessed March 16, 2023, https://www.rainn.org/statistics/perpetrators-sexual-violence.

6. "Sexualized Violence Statistics," Supporting Survivors, Cal Poly Humboldt, accessed March 16, 2023, https://supportingsurvivors.humboldt.edu/statistics.

7. Jamie Grierson, "Most Child Sexual Abuse Gangs Made Up of White Men, Home Office Report Says," *The Guardian*, December 15, 2020, https://www.theguardian.com/politics/2020/dec/15/child-sexual-abuse-gangs-white-men-home-office-report.

8. "Child Abuse in the U.S.—Perpetrators by Race/Ethnicity 2020," Statista, accessed March 16, 2023, https://www.statista.com/statistics/418475/number-of-perpetrators-in-child-abuse-cases-in-the-us-by-race-ethnicity/.

9. J. West and D. I. Templer, "Child Molestation, Rape, and Ethnicity," *Psychological Reports* 75, no. 3, pt. 1 (December 1994): 1326, https://doi.org/10.2466/pr0.1994.75.3.1326.

10. Weissmann, "So, Let's Talk About Republicans and Sex Crimes."

11. Elizabeth Boskey, Interview, March 10, 2023.

12. "Cosmetic Surgery in Teens: Information for Parents," HealthyChildren.org, accessed March 14, 2023, https://www.healthychildren.org/English/ages-stages/gradeschool/puberty/Pages/Cosmetic-Surgery-in-Teens-Information-for-Parents.aspx.

13. "Sweet 16 Birthday Breast Implants Spark Uproar in Britain," *The Morning Journal*, January 5, 2001, 16, https://www.morningjournal.com/news/sweet-16-birthday-breast-implants-spark-uproar-in-britain/article_1ba78a3c-af99-5660-9058-cc119fa3ef45.html.

14. Zuckerman, Diana, "Teenagers and Cosmetic Surgery," *Virtual Mentor* 7 no. 3 (March 2005): 253–256, https://journalofethics.ama-assn.org/article/teenagers-and-cosmetic-surgery/2005-03.

15. "Cosmetic Surgery in Teens."

16. Turban, "The Evidence for Trans Youth Gender-Affirming Medical Care."

17. Turban et al., "Psychological Attempts."

18. James et al., *The Report of the 2015 U.S. Transgender Survey.*

19. de Vries et al., "Puberty Suppression."

20. de Vries et al., "Young Adult Psychological Outcome."

21. Costa et al., "Psychological Support."

22. Kaltiala et al., "Adolescent Development."

23. López de Lara et al., "Psychosocial Assessment."

24. van der Miesen et al., "Psychological Functioning in Transgender Adolescents."

25. Achille et al., "Longitudinal Impact."

26. Kuper et al., "Body Dissatisfaction."

27. Turban et al., "Pubertal Suppression."

28. Carmichael et al., "Short-Term Outcomes."

29. Grannis et al., "Testosterone Treatment."

30. Hisle-Gorman et al., "Mental Healthcare Utilization."

31. Green et al., "Association of Gender-Affirming Hormone Therapy."

32. Turban et al., "Access to Gender-Affirming."

33. Tordoff et al., "Mental Health Outcomes."

34. Olson et al., "Gender Identity 5 Years After Social Transition."

35. van der Loos et al., "Continuation of Gender-Affirming Hormones."

36. Heather Boerner, "What the Science on Gender-Affirming Care for Transgender Kids Really Shows," *Scientific American*, May 12, 2022, https://www.scientificamerican.com/article/what-the-science-on-gender-affirming-care-for-transgender-kids-really-shows/.

37. Daniel Klink et al., "Bone Mass in Young Adulthood Following Gonadotropin-Releasing Hormone Analog Treatment and Cross-Sex Hormone Treatment in Adolescents with Gender Dysphoria," *The Journal of Clinical Endocrinology & Metabolism* 100, no. 2 (February 2015): E270–275, https://doi.org/10.1210/jc.2014-2439.

38. Janet Y. Lee et al., "Low Bone Mineral Density in Early Pubertal Transgender/Gender Diverse Youth: Findings from the Trans Youth Care Study," *Journal of the Endocrine Society* 4, no. 9 (July 2020): bvaa065, https://doi.org/10.1210/jendso/bvaa065.

39. Julia C. Sorbara et al., "Mental Health and Timing of Gender-Affirming Care," *Pediatrics* 146, no. 4 (October 1, 2020): e20193600, https://doi.org/10.1542/peds.2019-3600.

40. James et al., *The Report of the 2015 U.S. Transgender Survey.*

41. Ashley Austin et al., "Suicidality Among Transgender Youth: Elucidating the Role of Interpersonal Risk Factors," *Journal of Interpersonal Violence* 37, nos. 5–6 (March 2022): NP2696–2718, https://doi.org/10.1177/0886260520915554.

42. Boerner, "What the Science."

43. Jack L. Turban et al., "Sex Assigned at Birth Ratio Among Transgender and Gender Diverse Adolescents in the United States," *Pediatrics* 150, no. 3 (September 1, 2022): e2022056567, https://doi.org/10.1542/peds.2022-056567.

44. Thomas D. Steensma et al., "Desisting and Persisting Gender Dysphoria After Childhood: A Qualitative Follow-Up Study," *Clinical Child Psychology and Psychiatry* 16, no. 4 (October 2011): 499–516, https://doi.org/10.1177/1359104510378303.

45. Devita Singh, "A Follow-Up Study of Boys with Gender Identity Disorder" (PhD thesis, University of Toronto, 2012), 341.

46. Diane Ehrensaft et al., "Prepubertal Social Gender Transitions: What We Know; What We Can Learn—A View from a Gender Affirmative Lens," *International Journal of Transgenderism* 19, no. 2 (April 3, 2018): 251–268, https://doi.org/10.1080/15532739.2017.1414649.

47. Ehrensaft et al., "Prepubertal Social Gender Transitions."

48. Singh, "A Follow-Up Study of Boys."

49. Jack L. Turban et al., "Factors Leading to 'Detransition' Among Transgender and Gender Diverse People in the United States: A Mixed-Methods Analysis," *LGBT Health* 8, no. 4 (June 1, 2021): 273–280, https://doi.org/10.1089/lgbt.2020.0437.

50. Turban et al., "Factors Leading to 'Detransition.'"

51. Turban et al., "Factors Leading to 'Detransition.'"

52. Olson et al., "Gender Identity 5 Years After Social Transition."

53. Olson et al., "Gender Identity 5 Years After Social Transition."

54. Khiara M. Bridges, "Implicit Bias and Racial Disparities in Health Care," *Human Rights Magazine*, accessed March 16, 2023, https://www.americanbar.org/groups /crsj/publications/human_rights_magazine_home/the-state-of-healthcare-in-the -united-states/racial-disparities-in-health-care/.

55. Kelly M. Hoffman et al., "Racial Bias in Pain Assessment and Treatment Recommendations, and False Beliefs About Biological Differences Between Blacks and Whites," *Proceedings of the National Academy of Sciences of the United States of America* 113, no. 16 (April 19, 2016): 4296–4301, https://doi.org/10.1073/pnas.1516047113.

56. "Black Americans Are Systematically Under-Treated for Pain. Why?," Frank Batten School of Leadership and Public Policy, University of Virginia, June 30, 2020, https://batten.virginia.edu/about/news/black-americans-are-systematically-under -treated-pain-why.

57. Samantha Artiga and Latoya Hill, "Health Coverage by Race and Ethnicity, 2010–2021," *KFF*, December 20, 2022, https://www.kff.org/racial-equity -and-health-policy/issue-brief/health-coverage-by-race-and-ethnicity/.

58. Alan Mozes, "Most Transgender Children Stick with Gender Identity 5 Years Later: Study," HealthDay, May 4, 2022, https://consumer.healthday.com/5-4-most -transgender-children-stick-with-gender-identity-5-years-later-study-2657223343.html.

59. Ana Vasuian, "Do You Regret Having Cosmetic Surgery?," Medical Accident Group, May 28, 2014, https://www.medicalaccidentgroup.co.uk/news/do-you-regret -having-cosmetic-surgery/.

CHAPTER 14

1. "The Facts: Bathroom Safety, Nondiscrimination Laws, and Bathroom Ban Laws," Movement Advancement Project, https://www.lgbtmap.org/policy-and-issue-analysis /bathroom-ban-laws.

2. "Local Nondiscrimination Ordinances," Movement Advancement Project, https://www.lgbtmap.org/equality-maps/non_discrimination_ordinances.

3. Amira Hasenbush, Andrew R. Flores, and Jody L. Herman, "Gender Identity Nondiscrimination Laws in Public Accommodations: A Review of Evidence Regarding Safety and Privacy in Public Restrooms, Locker Rooms, and Changing Rooms," *Sexuality Research and Social Policy* 16, no. 1 (March 1, 2019): 70–83, https://doi.org /10.1007/s13178-018-0335-z.

4. "Transgender Teens with Restricted Bathroom Access at Higher Risk of Sexual Assault," Harvard T.H. Chan School of Public Health, May 7, 2019, https://www .hsph.harvard.edu/news/hsph-in-the-news/transgender-teens-restricted-bathroom -access-sexual-assault/.

5. "Transgender Teens with Restricted Bathroom Access."

6. Tim Fitzsimons, "Trans Teens Face Higher Sexual Assault Risk When Schools Restrict Bathrooms, Study Finds," *NBC News*, May 6, 2019, https://www.nbcnews .com/feature/nbc-out/trans-teens-face-higher-sexual-assault-risk-when-schools -restrict-n1002601.

7. "Local Nondiscrimination Ordinances," Movement Advancement Project, https://www.lgbtmap.org/equality-maps/non_discrimination_ordinances.

8. Christopher Zara, "It's 2019, and your boss can still fire you for being gay in these states," *Fast Company*, June 25, 2019, https://www.fastcompany.com/90369004/lgbt-employee-protections-by-state-map-shows-where-gay-workers-can-be-fired.

9. HRC Foundation, "2022 State Equality Index," Human Rights Campaign Foundation, 2023, https://reports.hrc.org/2022-state-equality-index.

10. HRC Foundation, "2022 State Equality Index," Human Rights Campaign Foundation, 2023, https://reports.hrc.org/2022-state-equality-index.

11. German Lopez, "Anti-Transgender Bathroom Hysteria, Explained," *Vox*, February 22, 2017, https://www.vox.com/2016/5/5/11592908/transgender-bathroom-laws-rights.

12. Maya Rhodan, "Why Do We Have Men's and Women's Bathrooms Anyway?," *Time*, May 16, 2016, https://time.com/4337761/history-sex-segregated-bathrooms/.

13. Rhodan, "Why Do We Have."

14. "Victims of Sexual Violence: Statistics," RAINN, accessed March 14, 2023, https://www.rainn.org/statistics/victims-sexual-violence.

15. Ayesha Ahmed, "Quick Facts About Sexual Assault in America," *PlanStreet* (blog), May 25, 2022, https://www.planstreetinc.com/quick-facts-about-sexual-assault-in-america/.

16. James et al., *The Report of the 2015 U.S. Transgender Survey*.

17. "Sexual Assault: The Numbers," Office of Justice Programs, Office for Victims of Crime, accessed March 16, 2023, https://ovc.ojp.gov/sites/g/files/xyckuh226/files/pubs/forge/sexual_numbers.html.

18. "Sexual Assault and the LGBTQ Community," Human Rights Campaign, accessed March 16, 2023, https://www.hrc.org/resources/sexual-assault-and-the-lgbt-community.

19. Ahmed, "Quick Facts About Sexual Assault in America."

20. Chantelle Billson, "Republican Senator Says Gender-Neutral Bathrooms Will Lead to Violence from 'Dads Like Me,'" *PinkNews*, May 24, 2023, https://www.thepinknews.com/2023/05/24/illinois-neil-anderson-gender-neutral-toilets/.

21. "Myths and Facts About Sexual Assault," California Megan's Law Website, accessed March 14, 2023, https://www.meganslaw.ca.gov/mobile/Education_MythsAndFacts.aspx.

22. "Children and Teens: Statistics," RAINN, accessed March 14, 2023, https://www.rainn.org/statistics/children-and-teens.

CHAPTER 15

1. "Super Straight," LGBT+ pride Wiki, accessed March 14, 2023, https://lgbt-pride.fandom.com/wiki/Super_Straight.

2. Steven Asarch, "A Social-Media Trend Has People Identifying as 'Super Straight.' The Transophobic Campaign Was Meant to Divide LGBTQ People," *Insider*, March 8, 2021, https://www.insider.com/super-straight-flag-meaning-tiktok-super-straight-ss-movement-origin-2021-3.

3. "How Common Is Infertility?," NIH Eunice Kennedy Shriver National Institute of Child Health and Human Development, accessed March 14, 2023, https://www.nichd.nih.gov/health/topics/infertility/conditioninfo/common.

4. "1 in 6 People Globally Affected by Infertility," World Health Organization, April 4, 2023, https://www.who.int/news/item/04-04-2023-1-in-6-people-globally -affected-by-infertility#:~:text=Around%2017.5%25%20of%20the%20adult,care %20for%20those%20in%20need.

CHAPTER 16

1. James et al., *The Report of the 2015 U.S. Transgender Survey.*
2. Wikipedia, s.v. "Rape by Deception," accessed March 10, 2023, https://en .wikipedia.org/w/index.php?title=Rape_by_deception&oldid=1143895880.
3. Ashlee Marie Preston, "The Anatomy of Transmisogynoir," *Harper's Bazaar*, September 9, 2020, https://www.harpersbazaar.com/culture/features/a33614214/ashlee -marie-preston-transmisogynoir-essay/.
4. Mila Jam Adderly, Interview, October 27, 2022.

CHAPTER 17

1. "Renée Richards Documentary Debuts at Tribeca Film Festival," *Tennis Panorama*, April 22, 2011, https://web.archive.org/web/20120403155400/http:/www .tennispanorama.com/archives/9472.
2. Jon Wertheim, "She's a Transgender Pioneer, But Renée Richards Prefers to Stay Out of the Spotlight," *Sports Illustrated*, June 28, 2019, https://www.si.com /tennis/2019/06/28/renee-richards-gender-identity-politics-transgender-where-are -they-now.
3. Chris Mosier, "Transgender Athletes in the Olympics," Transathlete.com, accessed March 14, 2023, https://www.transathlete.com/olympics.
4. Mosier, "Transgender Athletes."
5. Mosier, "Transgender Athletes."
6. "IOC Framework on Fairness, Inclusion and Non-Discrimination on the Basis of Gender Identity and Sex Variations," International Olympic Committee, n.d., https://stillmed.olympics.com/media/Documents/Beyond-the-Games/Human-Rights /IOC-Framework-Fairness-Inclusion-Non-discrimination-2021.pdf.
7. Wikipedia, s.v. "Fallon Fox," accessed March 7, 2023, https://en.wikipedia.org /w/index.php?title=Fallon_Fox&oldid=1143444121.
8. Mosier, "Transgender Athletes."
9. Cyd Zeigler, "Read the Olympics' New Transgender Guidelines That Will Not Mandate Surgery," Outsports, January 21, 2016, https://www.outsports.com /2016/1/21/10812404/transgender-ioc-policy-new-olympics.
10. Mosier, "Transgender Athletes."
11. Katie Barnes, "How Two Transgender Athletes Are Fighting to Compete in the Sports They Love," ESPN.com, May 29, 2018, https://www.espn.com/espn/story/_ /id/33460938/how-two-transgender-athletes-fighting-compete-sports-love.
12. Nicholas Rondinone, "Federal Judge Dismisses Lawsuit Seeking to Bar Transgender Athletes from CT Girls Sports," *Connecticut Post*, April 25, 2021, https://www .ctpost.com/news/article/Federal-judge-dismisses-lawsuit-seeking-to-bar-16128048.php.
13. Kevin Baxter, "The First U.S. Boxer to Fight as a Woman, and Then as a Man," *Los Angeles Times*, August 4, 2017, https://www.latimes.com/sports/boxing/la -sp-pat-manuel-20170804-htmlstory.html.

14. Dawn Ennis, "NCAA Champion CeCé Telfer Says 'I Have No Benefit' by Being Trans," Outsports, June 3, 2019, https://www.outsports.com/2019/6/3/18649927 /ncaa-track-champion-cece-telfer-transgender-athlete-fpu-trans-testosterone.

15. Mosier, "Transgender Athletes."

16. Alex Cooper, "Olympic Soccer Player Quinn Becomes First Trans Athlete to Medal," Advocate, August 6, 2021, https://www.advocate.com/sports/2021/8/06 /olympic-soccer-player-quinn-becomes-first-trans-athlete-medal-0.

17. Mosier, "Transgender Athletes."

18. "IOC Framework on Fairness."

19. Joanna Hoffman, "Athlete Ally & Chris Mosier Respond to NCAA New Trans Inclusion Policy," Athlete Ally, January 20, 2022, https://www.athleteally.org /athlete-ally-mosier-respond-ncaa-new-trans-policy/.

20. "Varsity Odds," ScholarshipStats.com, August 31, 2020, https://scholarshipstats .com/varsityodds.

21. Karleigh Webb, "Trans Boxer Patricio Manuel Wins First Match in Four Years, Improves to 2-0," Outsports, March 22, 2023, https://www.outsports.com /trans/2023/3/22/23650980/patricio-manuel-hien-hunyh-boxer-trans-win-long-beach.

22. Colleen De Bellefonds, "Why Michael Phelps Has the Perfect Body for Swimming," Biography, May 14, 2020, https://www.biography.com/athletes/michael -phelp-perfect-body-swimming.

23. Monica Hesse, "We Celebrated Michael Phelps's Genetic Differences. Why Punish Caster Semenya for Hers?," The Washington Post, May 3, 2019, https: //www.washingtonpost.com/lifestyle/style/we-celebrated-michael-phelpss-genetic -differences-why-punish-caster-semenya-for-hers/2019/05/02/93d08c8c-6c2b -11e9-be3a-33217240a539_story.html.

24. De Bellefonds, "Why Michael Phelps Has the Perfect Body for Swimming."

25. Hesse, "We Celebrated Michael Phelps's Genetic Differences."

26. David J. Handelsman, Angelica L. Hirschberg, and Stephane Bermon, "Circulating Testosterone as the Hormonal Basis of Sex Differences in Athletic Performance," Endocrine Reviews 39, no. 5 (October 2018): 803–829, https://doi.org/10.1210 /er.2018-00020.

27. Chris Brummitt, "Serena Williams Says 'Williams Brothers' Comment Was Case of Bullying," The Independent, October 19, 2014, https://www.independent.co.uk /sport/tennis/serena-williams-says-williams-brothers-comment-was-case-of -bullying-sexist-and-racist-9804563.html.

28. IMDb, s.v. Irrefutable Proof That Serena Williams Is a Man (2014), accessed March 16, 2023, https://www.imdb.com/title/tt5282834/.

29. Kylie Cheung, "Simone Biles Should Be Praised, Not Punished for Achieving a Feat That Was Deemed Impossible," Salon, May 26, 2021, https://www.salon .com/2021/05/26/simone-biles-yurchenko-double-pike-gymnastics-scoring/.

30. John Riley, "School Investigated Athlete's Gender After Her Competitors Complained," Metro Weekly, August 19, 2022, https://www.metroweekly.com/2022/08 /school-investigated-athletes-gender-after-her-competitors-complained/.

31. Agence France-Presse, "A Spate of Drownings: Classes Help Black Americans Learn to Swim," VOA, October 22, 2022, https://www.voanews.com/a/a-spate -of-drownings-classes-help-black-americans-learn-to-swim-/6801549.html.

32. Sarah Berman, "2022 NCAA Division I Women's Swimming and Diving Championships Records Roundup," SwimSwam, March 20, 2022, https://swimswam .com/2022-womens-ncaa-division-i-swimming-and-diving-championships -records-roundup/.

33. "Top Times/Event Rank Search," USA Swimming, accessed March 16, 2023, http://www.usaswimming.org/times/popular-resources/event-rank-search.

34. "Nancy Hogshead-Makar Explains Problems with Lia Thomas Situation," *Swimming World News*, December 25, 2021, https://www.swimmingworldmagazine .com/news/nancy-hogshead-makar-explains-problems-with-lia-thomas-situation/.

35. Brooke Migdon, "Sixteen Penn Swimmers Say Transgender Athlete Lia Thomas Holds 'Unfair Advantage,'" *The Hill*, February 4, 2022, https://thehill.com /changing-america/respect/diversity-inclusion/592822-sixteen-penn-swimmers -say-transgender-athlete/.

36. "Top Times/Event Rank Search."

37. Melissa Block, "Idaho's Transgender Sports Ban Faces a Major Legal Hurdle," NPR, May 3, 2021, https://www.npr.org/2021/05/03/991987280/idahos-transgender -sports-ban-faces-a-major-legal-hurdle.

CHAPTER 18

1. Carolina Aragão, "Gender Pay Gap in U.S. Hasn't Changed Much in Two Decades," Pew Research Center, accessed March 16, 2023, https://www.pewresearch .org/fact-tank/2023/03/01/gender-pay-gap-facts/.

2. "Closing Gender Pay Gaps Is More Important than Ever," UN News, September 18, 2022, https://news.un.org/en/story/2022/09/1126901.

3. Maya Salam, "What Is Toxic Masculinity?," *The New York Times*, January 22, 2019, https://www.nytimes.com/2019/01/22/us/toxic-masculinity.html.

4. Emily P. Terlizzi and Benjamin Zablotsky, "Mental Health Treatment Among Adults: United States, 2019," Centers for Disease Control and Prevention, September 2020, https://www.cdc.gov/nchs/products/databriefs/db380.htm.

5. "Gender Affecting Domestic Violence," Counseling Services, Valparaiso University, accessed March 16, 2023, https://www.valpo.edu/counseling-services/gender -affecting-domestic-violence/.

6. "Suicide Statistics," American Foundation for Suicide Prevention, November 15, 2019, https://afsp.org/suicide-statistics/.

7. Markham Heid, "The 7th Most-Common Killer of Men—and How You Can Avoid It," *Men's Health*, June 13, 2016, https://www.menshealth.com/health /a19522651/7th-leading-cause-of-death/.

8. Zack Beauchamp, "Jordan Peterson, the Obscure Canadian Psychologist Turned Right-Wing Celebrity, Explained," *Vox*, May 21, 2018, https://www.vox.com /world/2018/3/26/17144166/jordan-peterson-12-rules-for-life.

CHAPTER 19

1. "Black Trans Women and Black Trans Femmes: Leading & Living Fiercely," Transgender Law Center, accessed March 16, 2023, https://transgenderlawcenter.org /black-trans-women-black-trans-femmes-leading-living-fiercely.

2. Yue Qian, "Asian Guys Stereotyped and Excluded in Online Dating," *The Conversation*, February 9, 2020, http://theconversation.com/asian-guys-stereotyped-and-excluded-in-online-dating-130855.

3. Ravi Mangla, "The Race Dynamics of Online Dating: Why Are Asian Men Less 'Eligible'?," *Pacific Standard*, June 14, 2017, https://psmag.com/social-justice/why-are-asian-men-less-eligible-on-tinder.

4. Mangla, "The Race Dynamics."

5. "Black Trans Women and Black Trans Femmes."

6. Preston, "The Anatomy of Transmisogynoir."

7. Ashlee Marie Preston, Interview, October 25, 2022.

8. Preston, Interview.

9. "Black Trans Liberation," Black Trans Liberation, accessed March 16, 2023, https://www.blacktransliberation.com.

10. Madeline Smith-Johnson, "Transgender Adults Have Higher Rates of Disability than Their Cisgender Counterparts," *Health Affairs* 41, no. 10 (October 2022), https://doi.org/10.1377/hlthaff.2022.00500.

11. Jesper Dammeyer and Madeleine Chapman, "A National Survey on Violence and Discrimination Among People with Disabilities," *BMC Public Health* 18, no. 1 (March 15, 2018): 355, https://doi.org/10.1186/s12889-018-5277-0.

12. Jill Feder, "Why Are Persons with Disabilities 3 Times More Likely to Experience Sexual Assault?," Accessibility.com, June 14, 2022, https://www.accessibility.com/blog/disability-and-sexual-assault.

13. Sarah Parker Harris, Rob Gould, and Courtney Mullin, "Research Brief: Experience of Discrimination and the ADA," ADA National Network, accessed March 16, 2023, https://adata.org/research_brief/experience-discrimination-and-ada.

14. Jaboa Lake, Valerie Novack, and Mia Ives-Rublee, "Recognizing and Addressing Housing Insecurity for Disabled Renters," Center for American Progress, May 27, 2021, https://www.americanprogress.org/article/recognizing-addressing-housing-insecurity-disabled-renters/.

15. Elizabeth W. Diemer et al., "Gender Identity, Sexual Orientation, and Eating-Related Pathology in a National Sample of College Students," *Journal of Adolescent Health* 57, no. 2 (August 2015): 144–149, https://doi.org/10.1016/j.jadohealth.2015.03.003.

16. "Eating Disorders Among LGBTQ Youth," The Trevor Project, February 17, 2022, https://www.thetrevorproject.org/research-briefs/eating-disorders-among-lgbtq-youth-feb-2022/.

17. American Psychiatric Association, *Diagnostic and Statistical Manual of Mental Disorders: DSM-5-TR*, 5th ed., text rev. (Washington, DC: American Psychiatric Association Publishing, 2022), 273.

CHAPTER 21

1. McLean, Interview.

2. McLean, Interview.

3. Kiara Alfonseca, "Why Abortion Restrictions Disproportionately Impact People of Color," *ABC News*, June 24, 2022, https://abcnews.go.com/Health/abortion-restrictions-disproportionately-impact-people-color/story?id=84467809.

4. Christine Dehlendorf, Lisa H. Harris, and Tracy A. Weitz, "Disparities in Abortion Rates: A Public Health Approach," *American Journal of Public Health* 103, no. 10 (October 2013): 1772–1779, https://doi.org/10.2105/AJPH.2013.301339.

5. Megan Diamondstein, "The Disproportionate Harm of Abortion Bans: Spotlight on Dobbs v. Jackson Women's Health," Center for Reproductive Rights, November 29, 2021, https://reproductiverights.org/supreme-court-case-mississippi-abortion-ban-disproportionate-harm/.

6. Nandita Bose, "Roe v Wade Ruling Disproportionately Hurts Black Women, Experts Say," Reuters, June 27, 2022, https://www.reuters.com/world/us/roe-v-wade-ruling-disproportionately-hurts-black-women-experts-say-2022-06-27/.

7. Allison Schrager, "No Abortion Means Poor States Will Get Poorer," *Bloomberg*, May 4, 2022, https://www.bloomberg.com/opinion/articles/2022-05-04/roe-v-wade-outlawing-abortion-will-keep-more-women-poor.

8. Ijeoma Oluo, *So You Want to Talk About Race*, 1st ed. (New York: Seal Press, 2018).

9. Blair Imani (@blairimani), "#SmarterInSeconds: Tone Policing," TikTok, October 10, 2022, https://www.tiktok.com/@blairimani/video/7155978031603944750?lang=en.

10. "Accepting Adults Reduce Suicide Attempts Among LGBTQ Youth," The Trevor Project, June 27, 2019, https://www.thetrevorproject.org/research-briefs/accepting-adults-reduce-suicide-attempts-among-lgbtq-youth/.

INDEX

Addison Rose Vincent (they/them) is a trans feminine non-binary LGBTQ+ inclusion educator and consultant.

Ashlee Marie Preston (she/her) is a self-described fat Black trans woman. She is a writer, speaker, consultant, and media personality.

B. Hawk Snipes (they/she) is a Black, non-binary, trans femme entertainer, style icon, and actor who you may have seen on *Pose*.

Charlie Amáyá Scott (they/she) is a Nádleehí, an Indigenous (Diné) trans femme, non-binary scholar, writer, and content creator.

Devin-Norelle (ze/zim/zis) is a Black and mixed-race trans masculine, non-binary writer, model, and advocate. Ze is a New Yorker, intimately ingrained in Harlem.

Dylan Kapit (they/them) is a queer, trans, non-binary, Jewish, autistic person. A doctoral student in Special Education at the University of Pittsburgh, Dylan's research focuses on creating queer and trans inclusive autistic sexual education materials.

Elle Deran (they/she) is a queer, trans, non-binary actor, singer, and content creator committed to producing educational, entertaining, and queer-affirming content.

Indya Moore (she/they) is a queer, genderqueer, gendervariant, Afro-Taino, mixed-race artist, model, and actress. Known for playing Angel Evangelista in *Pose* and named as one of *TIME* 100's most influential people in the world in 2019, Indya describes herself as "very curious," and "unafraid of people."

Lia Thomas (she/her) is a transgender woman and athlete who swam for the University of Pennsylvania. In 2022, she became the first openly transgender D1 champion in NCAA history.

Meg Lee (they/them) is an Asian American, trans non-binary artist and activist. Meg creates apparel and art that aims to represent and fight for the BIPOC LGBTQIA+ communities.

Mila Jam (she/her) is a pop recording artivist who uses her experience as a Black trans woman to merge her art with her activism.

Pınar Ateş Sinopoulos-Lloyd (they/them) is a Quariwarmi and a non-binary person of Quechua and Turkish ancestry. An award-winning Indigenous multi-species futurist, mentor, consultant, and eco-philosopher, Pınar is cofounder of Queer Nature, a trans-run nature-based and naturalist education project serving mostly the LGBTQ2S+ community.

Dr. shawndeez (they/them) is a trans masculine non-binary Muslim Iranian American scholar who completed their PhD in Gender Studies at the University of California, Los Angeles. Their dissertation explores how queer and trans Iranian Americans engage with the spiritual and mystical dimensions of Islam as a form of resilience and overcoming.

Dr. Shay-Akil McLean (they/he) is a Black non-binary trans masculine evolutionary biologist, geneticist, biological anthropologist, and sociologist whose work as an educator focuses on unpacking systemic oppression disguised as science.

READING DISCUSSION GUIDE FOR *HE/SHE/THEY*

Thank you for engaging with *He/She/They*. My hope in providing this discussion guide is to deepen your learning off the page. *He/She/They* presents vast amounts of information; though useful, I have discovered that new information is better integrated when we apply the concepts and considerations directly to our personal lives. Discussions of gender often alienate trans people, placing us into a category of "other." But everyone has a gender—and everyone can join this fight for gender liberation.

These questions invite you to dig into your own experiences, biases, and growth. Vulnerability is key, but honesty with yourself is paramount.

GROUP DISCUSSIONS: UNDERSTANDING EMOTIONS
AND POWER DYNAMICS

Many of these discussion questions prompt participants to share very personal experiences they've had. Some experiences might elicit feelings of shame or embarrassment. If you feel these, invite them to the conversation too. These are expected emotions and need space to be felt. See if you can release yourself of any obligation to fix or deal with them in these moments. Instead, just let them be true.

Some participants might have reactions to the shares of others, especially those in which someone has made a mistake or behaved in ways that are transphobic, racist, or otherwise not acceptable. Consider sharing the feelings that come up without directly attacking or shaming others in the group.

Crucially, those sharing must always remain mindful of the difference between sharing an experience that is difficult or uncomfortable and causing harm through retraumatizing others.

Harm is often perpetuated when differences in power are present. Consider the following example: George (he/him) is a supervisor who is conducting a discussion group about *He/She/They* with his team. George is a straight white cis man. He is not transgender. Among his team members is one trans person, Ruby (she/her). When George answers Question 9 from "Gender and Me," he reflects on how difficult it is to see his niece, who is trans, as a girl. He describes her appearance and her mannerisms in depth and complains, "He—I mean, she—is just so masculine." When it's Ruby's time to share, she gets very nervous and is unable to say much. After listening to George's perception of his niece, Ruby feels that George will evaluate her in the same way. Ruby quickly internalizes George's judgment and transphobic commentary about his niece and is hurt by what she hears.

In this scenario, George's share could be considered harmful for numerous reasons: (1) George is revealing anti-trans sentiments and transphobia in the presence of another trans person without a facilitator. (2) George has not considered the power dynamic present; he is Ruby's supervisor and is neither trans nor a woman. (3) George has potentially damaged his relationship with Ruby by sharing negative beliefs about trans people's identities from a place of power in the workplace.

This does not mean George cannot share, but caution should be implemented:

1. George—or any other person in a similar position of power, relative to their role at the company/group/institution as well as their relevant identities—should be extremely mindful of how his commentary could affect those in the discussion space, especially those who work for him.

2. The company George works for must take proactive steps to mitigate possible harm during these discussions. Here are a few suggestions:

   a. Create a consent-based atmosphere. No one is required to attend or to share. Information regarding the content of the discussion session is announced prior so that potential attendees can consent to participating from an informed place.

   b. Provide trans people present with extensive support—such as access to a culturally competent counselor or therapist at no cost to the individual, mental health time/days, or a relaxation space for a few minutes alone during the discussion.

   c. Hire a facilitator (must be a trans person) who is capable of managing the dynamics and tension that might arise.

Lastly, in these types of discussions, clearly communicated goals are critical. Discussing many of these questions can cause cis people to reveal—unintentionally or not—transphobic bias and bigotry that can be difficult for trans participants to endure. Ideally, the goal in such conversations is to process these exhibits of bias in conjunction with learnings from *He/She/They* so that individuals may move through bias into a more open, curious, and accepting mindset. The goal is *not* to spew hatred toward trans people under the guise of "being vulnerable."

I strongly encourage beginning a discussion with the following collective agreement:

We are all raised in a transphobic, misogynistic, patriarchal, racist, capitalistic world. Bettering ourselves and society does not begin with a declaration of anti-bigotry but rather the acceptance of the biases we hold—conscious or not. In this discussion, I commit to recognizing bias, accepting its existence, and then fighting to act in radical defiance of it.

Now let's dig in.

PART 1: GENDER AND ME

1. When was the first time you noticed your own gender? Can you remember how you felt?

2. When did you first hear the word *transgender*, and how was the word used? What beliefs or stereotypes have you been able to challenge through reading *He/She/They*?

3. Especially if you are not trans, have you ever felt that (the existence of) trans people takes something away from you and your gender? If you are trans, consider this as well. What messaging have you internalized that transness is somehow detrimental to society? Where did this come from? Does it resonate with your worldview?

4. What is one way in which your gender has limited you? Have you ever felt not man/woman enough or too masculine/feminine? Who first communicated these gender ideals to you? When you've considered violating them, what happens for you? What would liberation from these expectations look like for you?

5. Many of our grade school health classes immersed us in a gender binary and bioessentialism that declares genitals = gender. Can you imagine a world where we are taught differently? How does this imagined reality make you feel?

6. With regard to your gender—or not—who did your eight-year-old self imagine you to be?

7. Without using genitals (or any other facet of your body/biology), anything you use to adorn your body (clothes, jewelry, etc.), or mannerisms, attempt to define *gender*. How about *manhood* and *womanhood*? How about *femininity* and *masculinity*?

8. If you are cisgender: How do you know that you are cisgender?

9. If the world were to erase all gendered labels, who would you be?

10. What fears arise when you consider distancing yourself from or disregarding the gender binary? What excites you about it?

11. Consider a time when you felt that your identity was denied to you—when some part of you (race, gender, sexuality, nationality, citizenship status, ability, religion, etc.) was erased by a person or interaction you had. How did that feel and how did you navigate the situation?

12. Reflect on a time (or times) when you adjusted to "fit in." What motivated you to fit in? What did you feel once you'd adjusted your behavior or expression? How did this facilitate social interactions (or not)?

PART 2: GENDER AND OTHERS

1. Consider a trans person you know well. Do you see them as their gender? If not, what stops you from doing so?

2. For parents or primary caregivers to children: Is gender relevant in how you care for your child? If yes, how so?

3. Consider a time when someone came out to you. How did you feel? Is there something you wish you would have said or done differently?

4. Let's pretend that I am sitting in front of you and I say, "You are transphobic. Yes, you. Regardless of your identity, your actions, your background. You hold transphobic bias." How would you feel? After reading Chapter 9, "So You Think You're Not Transphobic," have your feelings shifted? If so, how?

5. What feelings arise when you consider standing up in the face of transphobia? Trans folks, you're welcome to address this question, but cisgender friends, this is directed at you. What strategies might you use to intervene and protect the trans folks around you?

PART 3: GENDER AND SOCIETY

1. On page 61, I share a photo of my grandfather when he was a toddler. He is dressed in a dress and his hair is curled. When I was a child, I thought he looked like a girl. But his attire was normal for boys of his time! Reflecting on how

gender norms often depend on cultural context and epoch, consider the gender norms of your parents and grandparents. Do they differ from the current social conventions you are used to?

2. Chapter 22, "What Is Gender," discusses the long-documented history of trans and nonbinary people across the world. What did you learn that surprised you? Why isn't content like this frequently taught?

3. From your experience with kids (your own or in life), what strikes you about how they see gender? Does their perspective differ from yours—if so, how?

4. Of the questions elementary school kids ask me (on page 170), which stand out and why?

5. Consider raising children in a gender-neutral manner. This would entail not gendering them as the gender they are assigned at birth until they tell you their gender. What fears and feelings arise? What might you and the child gain? What might you and the child lose? Why?

6. Anti-trans legislation has continued to plague the United States and beyond. What are the smallest ways you can effect change and advocate for equal rights amid this onslaught? What are the biggest?

While the following questions are excellent for people—especially those who are not transgender—to think about and explore as honestly as possible, discussion could also encourage the disclosure of heavy transphobia. As a result, discussion with the following questions could be harmful to trans folks present and this should be considered first and foremost. I strongly encourage exercising restraint, foresight, and compassion as you comb through these and, even better, hiring a facilitator to mitigate potential risks.

7. Consider the truth that you have used/occupied a public restroom alongside a trans person before. How does this make you feel?

8. Would you date a trans person? Why or why not? Did reading Chapter 15, "Trans People and Dating," shift your perspective on dating trans people? How so?

9. Do you feel that a trans person must disclose their transness? Be honest with yourself and the group. Why or why not? Can you reexamine these feelings given what you've read?

10. Did Lia Thomas' story change your perspective on trans athletes? Elaborate.

11. Given evidence that trans women have not and do not dominate women's sports, why do you think the media and sociopolitical atmosphere have placed such a high focus on them?

12. Many people believe that the conjecture "Boys are better than girls at sports" is common sense. How might you approach this sentiment after having read Chapter 17, "Trans Athletes and Sports"?

13. What was your relationship with sports when you were young? Did you play sports? What barriers did you face, if any?

14. Following Chapter 18, "Toxic Masculinity from the Lens of a Transgender Man," what did you learn that surprised you about toxic masculinity?

15. What behaviors or roles do you partake in that perpetuate toxic masculinity? Why do you engage in these? This question is for everyone to consider, not just men.

16. This is an identity exercise that I recommend you practice in groups of two or more people:
    a. Each participant writes down five identities that are most important to themselves.
    b. Pass this list to another person in the group who then arbitrarily crosses one item off and then passes the list back to its writer.
    c. The writer discusses how it feels to have this identity item eliminated.
    d. If desired, repeat the exercise, crossing off another item.

17. Consider your own intersectionality. How does intersectionality impact your life? (Remember that intersectionality is not simply different identities coming together; intersectionality is the various layers of oppression that result from intersecting identities.)

PART 4: BEYOND

1. Especially if you are a white person, reflect on the passage my father wrote about his experiences with me on page 287. What pieces of yourself do you observe in his words? What feelings of resistance do you experience, if any?

2. Taking into consideration your many identities (your gender, race, sexuality, ability, religion, financial background, citizenship status, size, etc.), in what ways has the system been created or set up for you? In what ways have you benefited from the system? In what ways has the system failed you?

3. How can you use your privileges to help others? How can you use power that comes from these privileges to create space for others?

4. Observe / Question / Shift Exercise

    Consider the photos on the following page as you answer the subsequent questions. (*Note: Do NOT use any other photos of anyone else to conduct this exercise. This engages a high level of scrutiny, particularly of one's body, that can be harmful to an individual. I have consented to that scrutiny by sharing these photos with you.*)

    ### Observe

    - How are you gendering the person in these photos?
    - What factors are causing you to gender each photo the way that you are?
    - What assumptions do you have about the person in each photo?

Question

- Consider the factors named in *Observe*. Why do these result in gendering the person the way that you have?
- Where do these factors come from?
- Where do these assumptions come from? Are they your own? Did you learn them somewhere?

Shift

- Can you interrupt this process of automatic gendering?
- What do you observe about the person in these photos that is *not* gendered?
- What information is valuable to you about someone when you view their photo? Why? What do you *hope* would be valuable to you when you view a photo?
- Is it difficult to refer to both photos with he/him pronouns given that both are me, a man who uses he/him pronouns? If so, why?

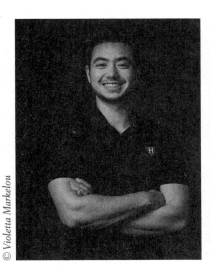 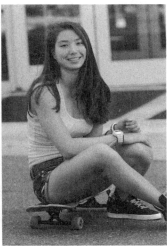

© Violetta Markelou

Photo courtesy of Hong Bailar family

5. What is the smallest thing you can do to show up for a trans person tomorrow? This month? This year? (If you're

trans, consider yourself that person. What is the smallest thing you can do to show up for yourself just a little bit more?)

6. Trans joy is the radical, unbridled freedom I feel in my gender and trans identity. It has taken years of liberation to discover, cultivate, and protect this experience—a process still unfolding and one that I hope never ends. What brings you this internal liberation? What stands in your way of attaining it?